MAGIC FOODS
for better
Blood Sugar

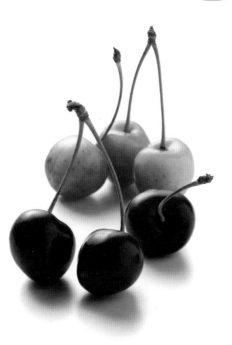

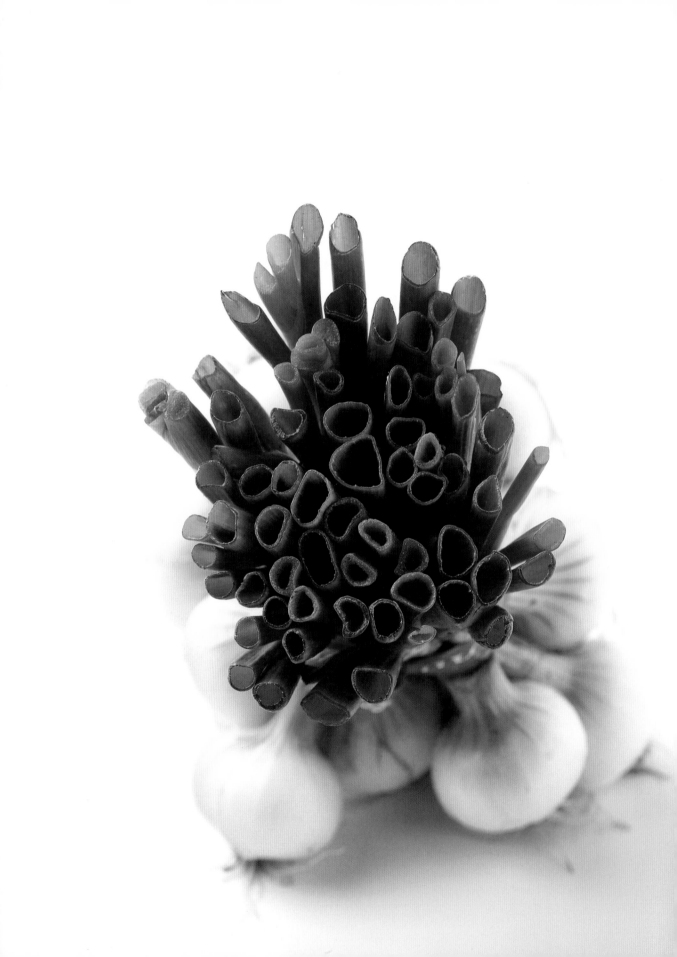

MAGIC FOODS
for better
Blood Sugar

Live longer, supercharge your energy,
lose weight and banish cravings

PUBLISHED BY THE READER'S DIGEST ASSOCIATION LIMITED
London • New York • Sydney • Montreal

CONSULTANTS

UK NUTRITIONIST

Fiona Hunter BSc (Hons) Nutrition
Diploma Dietetics

MEDICAL ADVISER

Dr Penny Preston MB MRCGP

CHIEF NUTRITION ADVISER

Christine L. Pelkman PhD,
Assistant Professor of Nutrition
State University of New York at Buffalo

NUTRITION ADVISER

Brandia Joy Freiman MS RD,
Clinical Nutrition Instructor
State University of New York at Buffalo

RECIPE DEVELOPER

Patsy Jamieson

RECIPE ADAPTATION

Norma Macmillan

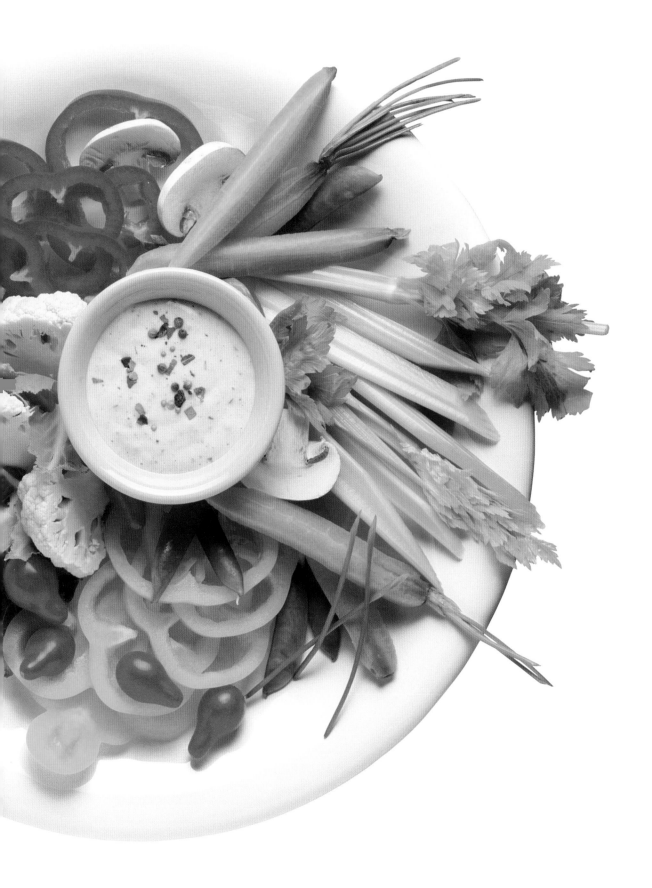

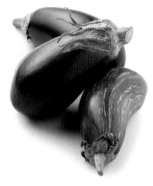
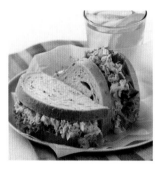
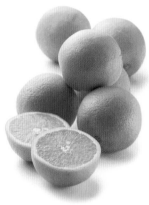
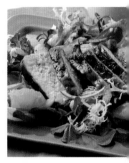

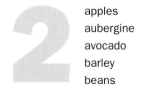

CONTENTS

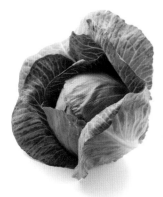
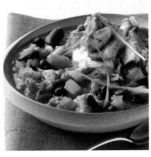
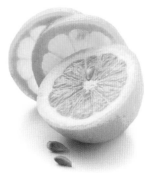
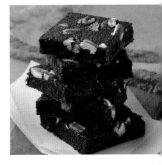

Meal makeovers

Magic recipes and meal plans

Introduction

A major health crisis is emerging – one that most doctors are just beginning to recognise. You may never have heard of it, but it could well be affecting how you feel at this minute. It's not heart disease, diabetes or obesity, although it's linked to all three. It's out-of-control blood sugar, which many people have without even knowing it.

Put it down to modern-day diets, which are often full of foods that send blood sugar levels soaring, then diving back down again. When the drop comes, you may feel listless, irritable, headachy – and ravenously, must-eat-something-sugary-this-minute hungry. Riding the blood sugar rollercoaster is a certain way to send your hunger up, your energy down, and your waistline out.

Our love affair with sugar-raising foods, especially 'white' foods such as white bread, white rice, chips and sugary processed foods, has led to an outbreak of insulin resistance – essentially, what happens when the body's system for handling blood sugar surges becomes worn out from overwork. Insulin resistance is linked to serious problems, ranging from heart disease and memory loss to – you've guessed it – diabetes. A survey, published in the *British Journal of General Practice* in 2008, concluded that more than half a million people in the UK may be at high risk of developing – or already have – diabetes, without knowing it. If you're over 45 and overweight, you could be among them.

Fortunately, insulin resistance is reversible. If eating the wrong foods can cause it, eating the right ones can cure it. And it's not that difficult to do. We have designed this book to help you to avoid blood sugar swings – without turning your diet upside down.

In *Magic Foods for Better Blood Sugar*, you won't find strict dietary rules. What you will find are 57 foods that can help you to nudge your diet into sugar-friendly territory. Add just one to your plate (for instance, eat wholemeal bread instead of white bread), and you could see results straightaway. Add a few more (such as avocados, which contain fats that actually improve insulin sensitivity), and you'll be firmly on the road to feeling better and staving off killer diseases.

Even if you already have diabetes, these strategies can help to make your cells more sensitive to insulin and keep blood sugar swings under control.

You can still eat steak, if you keep it lean, as well as pasta and other carbohydrate foods, if you choose the right ones (whole grains actually reduce your diabetes risk). We'll also show you how adding a few 'secret' ingredients, such as vinegar, to your dishes can yield amazing results.

Magic Foods is based on the latest nutrition science, but it's designed for people like you who just want to know what to eat. For instance, you won't have to look up numbers before you choose a food. Our recipes, meal makeovers, meal plans and Cooks' tips make it incredibly simple to get more of the 57 Magic foods onto your plate. Your meals will still taste delicious – and they'll leave you more satisfied, so you won't be looking around for something else to eat.

At Reader's Digest, we take your health to heart. Here's something you can do to rein in insulin resistance, get rid of dangerous tummy fat, guard against diabetes (or help to reverse it), and feel more fully charged and ready to embrace life every day. Don't wait for your doctor to say you have a problem. Turn the page now and start discovering the good foods and delicious recipes that await you.

The Editors

the new
Blood sugar
solution

1

The nation's secret health crisis

If you're like most people, you've probably never given your blood sugar a second thought unless you have diabetes. But doctors and researchers have recently discovered a shocking truth: if your blood sugar levels regularly soar and crash like a radio-controlled plane, your body may sustain damage, just as the plane does over time. Of course, in your case, the damage will occur on the inside, where you can't see it. The consequences, such as low energy or weight gain, are problematic – and can be life-threatening.

*It's no longer a select group of people who need to worry about their blood sugar. **It's just about everyone.***

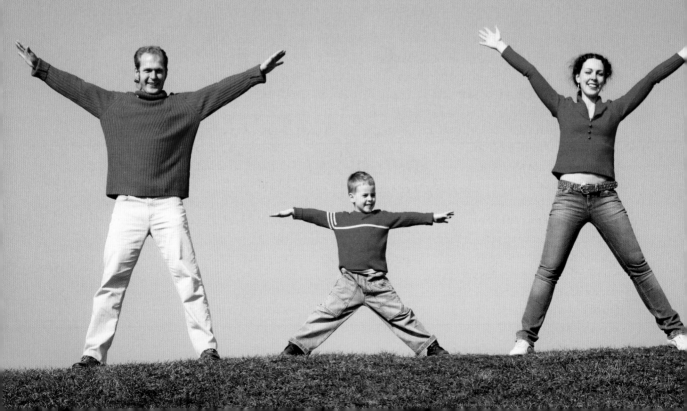

Whether or not you have diabetes, a diet loaded with foods that send blood sugar soaring and plunging can increase your risk of heart disease by damaging your blood vessels and raising your cholesterol. It may even chip away at your memory and increase the risk of certain cancers. You may not notice a problem, but that doesn't mean it's not there. You may be on a path that can shave years off your life.

This new thinking looks set to revolutionise our understanding of diet and health. Luckily, none of the damage happens overnight, and even modest changes in the foods you eat every day can start you on a healthier path and make you feel more alert, alive and energised straightaway.

The lure of 'fast-acting' foods

When you need a quick pick-me-up, what do you reach for? Perhaps a bar of chocolate, a biscuit or a packet of crisps. It makes sense. These 'fast-acting' foods take no time at all to dissolve in your stomach. Like lightning, they race into your bloodstream, flooding your body with blood sugar (glucose), and you're raring to go! The trouble is, the surge doesn't last long. In fact, it's over just as quickly as it started, leaving you feeling worse off than before – and hungry again well before your next mealtime.

Without knowing it, you may be starting your day with foods that fizzle out in a hurry, leaving you in a slump. Think back to the last time you ate slices of white toast with jam for breakfast, a bowl of cornflakes, or a hot, buttery croissant. You probably felt fine at first, but later in the morning you may have noticed your energy levels beginning to sink. Perhaps you started to become irritable. Once your energy hit rock bottom, you may have found yourself hungry again – or more likely starving. So naturally, you ate a large lunch and probably a fast-acting one to boot: maybe a sandwich or a giant white roll, with a few handfuls of crisps, a large fizzy or fruity drink to wash them down, and a biscuit (or two) for dessert. And the cycle started all over again.

Unfortunately, our diets are packed full of foods that send us for a white-knuckle ride on the blood-sugar rollercoaster. It's no wonder most of us have less energy than we'd like and feel listless so often. It's also no wonder most of us weigh more than we want to. Yes, eating too much and exercising too little get the lion's share of the blame, but the erratic blood sugar rollercoaster contributes too, by setting in motion a chain of events that eventually sends you shopping for outsize jeans.

If you think that sounds bad, read on. Low energy and weight gain are just the tip of the iceberg in terms of what happens when your blood sugar swings high and low.

Why blood sugar matters

For most of us, even when blood sugar skyrockets after a big meal, our bodies have little difficulty restoring it to normal within a few hours. Only people with untreated diabetes have blood sugar levels that stay quite high most of the time. Thus, for many years, doctors thought that only those people needed to be concerned about the effect of food on blood sugar.

Now we know that even in healthy people, high blood sugar after meals can, over time, damage the body, even if it never causes diabetes.

In short, it's no longer just one group of people who need to worry about their blood sugar; it's just about everyone. It should concern you even

High blood sugar after meals can, over time, damage the body, even if it never causes diabetes.

HEALTH EFFECTS
of fast-acting foods

Diets full of fast-acting carbohydrates such as these send blood sugar on a wild ride, which can wreak havoc on our bodies, contributing to:

- diabetes
- fatigue
- heart attacks
- hunger

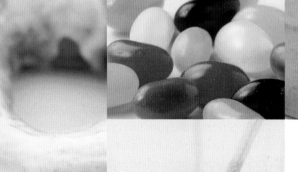

- low energy
- memory loss
- mood swings
- weight gain

if you're thin and healthy, and especially if you don't get much exercise or you carry extra weight around your middle. Does that describe you? It describes most people.

By now you're wondering, 'How can I get off the rollercoaster?' It's not that difficult – and the book you're holding will show you how. Later, we'll get into much more detail about how our diets contribute to unstable blood sugar (hint: foods such as white bread, white rice, potatoes and sugary drinks are major culprits) and which foods can help solve the problem and keep our blood sugar steady. But for now, let's take a deeper look at why you should care and how you stand to benefit from this book.

Energy and weight gain

Eating makes you feel full, doesn't it? Well, actually, that depends. When you eat a big meal, especially one with a lot of starchy or sugary foods, the food makes its way through your stomach and intestines and is then converted into glucose, the main fuel for your muscles and even your brain. Voilà, instant energy.

But a big starchy meal can give the body more glucose than it needs. In fact, it can raise blood sugar levels twice as much as another, healthier meal would. Most people's bodies can bring blood sugar down quite quickly, within an hour or two of eating. The body does this by releasing insulin, a hormone produced by beta cells in the pancreas. Insulin tells the body to allow blood sugar into cells to use as fuel and to store the rest in the muscles.

But if you eat a huge pile of chips or a large slice of white bread, your body has to deal with a serious flood of blood sugar, so it overreacts, pumping out too much insulin. If you're overweight, it may pump out even more. All that extra insulin brings blood sugar crashing down too far. And the insulin hangs around in the bloodstream for a long time, keeping your blood sugar low for hours.

As a result, you can fall into a semi-starved state. Ironically, your blood sugar may be even lower than it was before you ate the starchy meal. At this point you're really struggling and you may feel quite uncomfortable. Your energy is low and you may get a headache.

Your body recognises that your blood sugar is too low, so it reverses course, spewing out hormones that raise blood levels of sugars and fats (the kind that could trigger a heart attack). Your brain also produces signals that tell you that you're hungry. Even though you consumed more calories at lunch than you really needed, your blood sugar is so low that your body thinks it needs more food. The biscuit tin in the kitchen looks increasingly attractive.

MEALS THAT MAKE YOU HUNGRY

It's not just low blood sugar but also rapidly falling blood sugar that triggers a powerful hunger signal. In 16 studies, 15 of them found that meals that raise blood sugar quickly resulted in people feeling hungrier before the next meal. For example, in a study of 65 women, those whose meals were designed to keep blood sugar stable felt less intense hunger and less desire to eat, especially in the afternoon.

These kinds of meals increase levels of leptin, a hormone that decreases hunger, helps to burn fat and lowers levels of ghrelin, a hormone that increases hunger. The women who ate blood sugar-boosting meals reported that they felt hungrier sooner.

In many studies, people who ate such meals also ate more at the next meal. In a study of overweight teenage boys, the boys ate 500 more calories within 5 hours after eating blood sugar-boosting breakfasts and lunches than they did when they ate meals that were kinder to their blood sugar. In other studies, the differences were more modest, about 150kcal (what we loosely call 'calories' are strictly 'kilocalories', as you'll see on food labels). Still, eating even 100kcal a day may mean the difference between losing weight and gaining it.

We all know that it is possible to lose weight on any diet that cuts calories. But losing weight is only half the battle – and often it's the easiest part. Sticking to a healthy eating plan that enables you to keep the weight off is the hard part. But help is at hand. Making sure that your diet if full of Magic foods is a key solution.

A MOMENT ON THE LIPS ...

When you eat a meal that makes your blood sugar soar, your body pumps out lots of insulin to bring it down, as you've just learned. But it also stops burning fat for fuel so it can use up the blood sugar instead. Your stomach (or hips or thighs) pays the price. People whose diets boost blood sugar the most tend to have more body fat, especially around the abdomen, the most dangerous place for it to accumulate.

Getting off the blood sugar rollercoaster can make losing that spare tyre a lot easier. In studies involving everyone from obese men to pregnant women to children, a diet that stabilised blood sugar levels led to more body fat loss (or, in the case of the pregnant women, less body fat gain during the pregnancy).

In a cruel twist of fate, a diet that causes your blood sugar to surge and plunge may even slow your metabolism. Compared to a diet that keeps blood sugar levels stable, it reduces the rate at which you burn calories when you're sitting still.

In a study of 39 overweight men and women, the difference worked out to about 80 extra calories burned each day. That's an extra 1lb (0.5kg) lost about every six weeks, or more than 8lb (3.5kg) a year. The more overweight you are, the greater the difference may be.

A threat to your heart

It's fairly easy to imagine how a diet that's rough on your blood sugar can contribute to weight gain. It's a little harder to understand how it can also contribute to a heart attack – yet it can. It can lead to clogged arteries and higher blood pressure, and it can raise the level of inflammation in the body, which doctors now know is intimately connected with an increased risk of heart attack.

High blood sugar produces unstable forms of oxygen called free radicals. These nasty molecules damage the arteries, so it is harder for blood vessels to do their job of keeping blood pressure normal, while cholesterol is more likely to stick like glue to artery walls.

The high levels of insulin that your body needs to tame all this blood sugar are pretty nasty, too. They can set in motion changes that

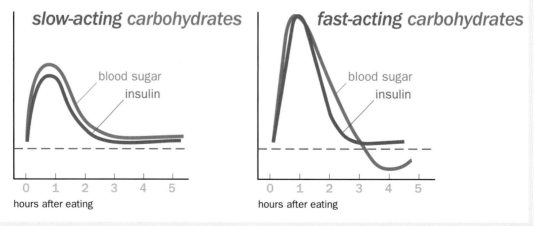

BLOOD SUGAR ups and downs All carbohydrates raise blood sugar. But some carb foods, such as white potatoes and white bread, raise it higher and faster than others, such as sweet potatoes and barley. Higher peaks mean steeper drops – your blood sugar may sink lower than before you ate (below the dotted line) – and that's when energy stalls and hunger strikes anew.

slow-acting carbohydrates
blood sugar
insulin

0 1 2 3 4 5
hours after eating

fast-acting carbohydrates
blood sugar
insulin

0 1 2 3 4 5
hours after eating

raise blood pressure, make blood more likely to form heart-threatening clots, and increase inflammation – all of which are known to raise your risk of heart disease.

Over time, meals that cause blood sugar to surge also tend to lower 'good' HDL cholesterol and raise triglycerides, fats that are toxic to cells, increasing the risk of heart disease – and of sudden cardiac arrest.

Large, prestigious studies have shown how powerful these damaging effects can be to the heart. In a study of more than 43,000 men aged 40 and older, those whose diets boosted blood sugar the most were 37 per cent more likely to develop heart disease in the following six years. In the Nurses' Health Study of more than 75,000 middle-aged American women, those whose diets boosted blood sugar the most were twice as likely to develop heart disease over 10 years. For overweight women, such a diet was even more threatening. For instance, their triglycerides were 144 per cent higher than those of women who ate a healthier diet, compared to 40 per cent higher for women who weren't overweight.

Fortunately, the phenomenon works in reverse, too. The kinder your meals are to your blood sugar, the kinder they'll be to your heart. Several studies have found that people who ate the fewest blood sugar-boosting foods had higher levels of HDL cholesterol, lower triglycerides, and fewer heart attacks.

The cancer connection

It's even harder to imagine how seesawing blood sugar levels could possibly lead to cancer, but high insulin levels seem to promote an environment that makes it easier for certain tumours to grow. Research is still continuing, although it's too early to make definitive statements about the connection between blood sugar levels and cancer. But there may be cause for concern with the following cancers.

■ **Colon and rectal cancer** In the Health Professionals Follow-up Study, conducted by the Harvard School of Public Health and involving more than 50,000 middle-aged men, those whose diets were most likely to raise blood sugar fast and high were 32 per cent more likely to develop colon or rectal cancer over 20 years. The heavier the men, the stronger the effect. The Women's Health Study, funded in part by the US National Cancer Institute, and involving more than 38,000 women, also suggested an increased risk.

■ **Breast cancer** In the US Women's Health Study, sedentary women who followed a blood sugar-boosting diet were 135 per cent more likely to develop breast cancer over seven years than women whose diets were more blood sugar friendly. These women had not yet entered menopause. On the other hand, a Canadian study of nearly 50,000 women found no link to breast cancer before the menopause, but among postmenopausal women, there was an 87 per cent increase in breast cancer risk – and it was even higher if the women did little or no vigorous exercise. A Mexican study comparing women who got breast cancer with those who didn't found the risk was 62 per cent greater with blood sugar-boosting diets. A similar Italian study found an 18 per cent increase.

■ **Endometrial cancer** In the Iowa Women's Health Study in the USA, which involved more than 23,000 postmenopausal women, those who didn't have diabetes and followed blood sugar-spiking diets were 46 per cent more likely to get this cancer over 15 years. An Italian study that compared women who developed endometrial cancer with a similar group of women who didn't found a 110 per cent increase in risk linked to this type of blood sugar-boosting diet.

■ **Prostate cancer** An Italian study looked at men aged 46 to 74 who developed prostate cancer and compared their diets with those of a similar group of men who didn't get the cancer.

Those whose diets were most likely to raise blood sugar were 57 per cent more likely to have prostate cancer. A similar Canadian study found a 57 per cent increase in risk.

The mood and memory connection

We began this chapter by showing how a meal that raises blood sugar fast and furiously can seriously deplete your energy levels. Not surprisingly, it doesn't do much for mood, either.

Our moods are intimately affected by the levels of hormones in our systems, including the hormone insulin. These hormones in turn affect neurotransmitters, chemical messengers in the brain. The different types of nutrients we eat, including carbohydrate and protein, affect these transmitters differently, triggering drowsiness or alertness. But the brain may be most sensitive to one simple compound: blood sugar.

Unlike muscles, the brain can't store sugar. It needs just the right amount of it at all times to function best, so it's not surprising that it's sensitive to even small differences in the amount of blood sugar available. A steady supply, which the foods in this book will help you to achieve, is by far the best.

Both low and high levels of blood sugar can cause trouble when it comes to mood and memory. People report feeling more symptoms of depression when their blood sugar is low. Memory is affected, too. In one study, people with diabetes had more trouble processing information, remembering things and paying attention – besides being in a bad mood – when their blood sugar was low. In people with Type 2 diabetes, blood sugar swings are linked not only with poor memory but also, over time, with cognitive decline and dementia.

High blood sugar levels spell trouble, too. Long before they cause diabetes, they can impair the brain, affecting the storage of memories and increasing the risk of Alzheimer's disease. In one study at New York University, researchers found that in people who tended to have high blood sugar levels after meals, a part of the brain called the hippocampus, which is associated with memory, was smaller than in people whose post-meal blood sugar levels were lower.

On the positive side, keeping your blood sugar on an even keel can help you to feel better and stay mentally sharp. People with diabetes who control their blood sugar well report better moods, less depression and less fatigue than those who don't. Careful studies have found that the better they control their blood sugar, the better they are able to recall a paragraph after reading it and to remember words from a list.

Eating a good breakfast is the best way to improve mental functioning later in the day. Studies show that eating breakfast of any sort improves mood, mental alertness, concentration and memory. Eating the right breakfast, one that keeps blood sugar on an even keel until lunchtime, is likely to work even better.

The road to diabetes

Perhaps the worst thing about eating meals full of fast-acting foods is that, over time, they can greatly increase your risk of Type 2 diabetes, the kind that's related to lifestyle. In Type 2 diabetes, which we'll just call diabetes from now on, the body cannot make enough insulin or the body cells are resistant to the effects of the insulin that is produced. Often, both problems are present. In all cases, blood sugar levels are not controlled effectively.

In major long-term studies, eating fast-acting meals increased the risk of diabetes by 40 per cent in middle-aged men and by 50 per cent in middle-aged women. Fortunately, it doesn't happen overnight. It's not as if you eat a Danish pastry on Tuesday and wake up with diabetes on Wednesday. It takes years, even decades, for your body to get to the point where it can't keep blood sugar under control on its own. It is fair to say, though, that many of us are certainly heading in the wrong direction.

The good news is that the slow journey towards diabetes may be redirected *at any point along the path*. The earlier you start, of course,

FIGHTING
insulin resistance

Eating foods that keep blood sugar levels stable is key to preventing or reversing insulin resistance. Try these steps, too.

■ **Exercise** Even if you don't lose weight, exercising reduces insulin resistance. In one study, spending 30 minutes on an exercise bike three or four times a week cut insulin levels by 20 per cent and lowered blood sugar levels by 13 per cent – enough to take someone from 'pre-diabetes' to 'normal'.

■ **Get enough sleep** Having less than a full night's sleep increases insulin resistance, possibly by disturbing hormone balance. Studies suggest that doing so for years increases the risk of diabetes.

■ **Cut calories** Eating less, even before you lose any weight, can improve insulin sensitivity and reduce levels of circulating insulin. In one study of sedentary men and women, consuming 25 per cent fewer calories than they were used to over six months resulted in significantly lower fasting insulin levels. Other studies have found that cutting calories improves insulin sensitivity – sensible advice for anyone who spends most of the day sitting down.

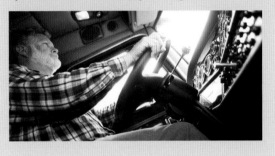

the easier and more effectively you can change direction. Eating meals that are gentler to your blood sugar is an important step.

Insulin resistance: a growing epidemic

Have you ever damaged the head of a screw in the middle of a DIY project? Suddenly, you need to use real elbow grease to turn it very slightly. The more you damage it, the harder it is to turn.

Your body can be a bit like that. The more foods you eat that send your blood sugar soaring, the more insulin your body has to pump out to handle the load. Over time, repeated surges of insulin can affect your cells' insulin receptors so that they don't work as well, and the insulin can't be used as efficiently – a condition called insulin resistance. When you have this, your body has to pump out more insulin to do the same job.

In the West, where the super-sized meal and the sedentary lifestyle are all too pervasive, insulin resistance is increasingly common. An estimated 25 per cent of adults have it. And if

you're overweight and over 45, the chances that you have it may be as great as one in two. You're much more likely to develop insulin resistance if you're overweight and sedentary.

If you have insulin resistance, your blood sugar levels may still be normal, although they may be on the high side after meals. You don't have diabetes – yet. But you are going in a direction that's putting a lot of stress on your blood-sugar control system, and you're doing some damage along the way.

The extra insulin your body has to churn out can raise blood pressure, cause cholesterol problems and even make it easier for certain cancers to grow. It also paves the way for weight gain. And here's a real scare: there's growing evidence that the brain itself can become insulin resistant, which impairs the function of nerves and increases the risk of dementia, including Alzheimer's disease. And, of course, insulin resistance increases the risk of diabetes. High blood sugar and extra insulin can damage the beta cells in the pancreas – the ones that make

Do you have METABOLIC SYNDROME?

Metabolic syndrome is a cluster of risk factors that often occur together and increase susceptibility to diabetes and heart disease. Many medical experts – including the World Health Organisation – define the syndrome by looking at five measurements. The first you can measure, the others should be tested by your GP or at your local hospital.

Once you know your numbers, take this test.

☐ **Waist size** Check this box if yours is more than 102cm (40in) for men or more than 88cm (35in) for women.

☐ **Triglycerides** A normal level is below 1.70mmol/l* (150mg/dl) Check this box if yours is 1.70mmol/l (150mg/dl) or higher.

☐ **HDL cholesterol** This is the 'good' cholesterol, so a higher number is better. Check this box if yours is lower than 1.00mmol/l (40mg/dl) for men or 1.30mmol/l (50mg/dl) for women.

☐ **Blood pressure** A normal level is less than 120/80mm/Hg. Check this box if yours is 130/85mm/Hg or higher.

☐ **Fasting blood glucose** This is the level of blood sugar after you haven't eaten for 8 hours. A normal level is 4.0 to 5.5mmol/l (70 to 100mg/dl). Check this box if yours is 6.0mmol/l (110mg/dl) or higher.

*The UK measures blood glucose, blood cholesterol and triglycerides by millimole per litre (mmol/l). The milligram per decilitre (mg/dl) method is the US standard. The measurements used may vary a little: those above come from the US National Institute of Health's National Cholesterol Education Program.

Your SCORE Add up all the boxes you ticked, then find your results here.

0 Congratulations; you have no signs of metabolic syndrome. Keep up the good work.

1 You don't have metabolic syndrome, but each of these is an independent risk factor for heart disease, so you should still take action.

2 You don't have metabolic syndrome, but you do have two of the risk factors, so ask your doctor to help you to remedy them.

3 You have metabolic syndrome. You are at increased risk of developing diabetes and heart disease in the years ahead, but you can reverse the trend by losing weight, taking more exercise and eating better. Talk with your doctor about ways to reduce your risk factors. The dietary approach outlined in this book is particularly important for you.

4 You have metabolic syndrome and then some – the more risk factors you have, the greater your overall risk. Get medical help and follow the dietary approach in this book.

5 You have all the risk factors of metabolic syndrome and are at very high risk of developing diabetes and heart disease. Talk to your doctor and follow the guidance provided in this book.

insulin – so they become fatigued or die off. When that happens, you have diabetes.

Insulin resistance starts slowly. It has no symptoms. But once you develop it, it's easier to become even more insulin resistant. In a vicious cycle, the more insulin your body has to produce to keep blood sugar down, the more insulin resistant you become – unless you do something to reverse the trend. Changing your eating style to include more of the slow-acting foods in this book is one of the key ways to prevent or reverse the condition. (For other ways, see 'Fighting insulin resistance' on page 17.)

Metabolic syndrome: a collection of problems

Insulin resistance on its own can be dangerous, but there's worse news: if you have it, you may also have a host of related problems that tend to cluster together. Each of them on its own raises your risk of heart disease, but if you have three or more of them, your risk is double what it would be if you had only one. You are at a greatly increased risk of having a heart attack, even if your levels of 'bad' LDL cholesterol are normal.

This cluster of problems has been given the term 'metabolic syndrome'. If you have this condition, which is becoming increasingly prevalent worldwide, you're also susceptible to diabetes, even if your blood sugar levels aren't yet high. About 85 per cent of people with Type 2 diabetes are thought to have metabolic syndrome.

Metabolic syndrome may affect as many as one in four adults. Anyone can develop it, but you're much more likely to get it as you get older. In one large study of men and women aged 50 and older, 44 per cent had it. If you're carrying extra pounds, you're even more likely to have it. Getting older and being sedentary contribute to the syndrome but, in many ways, it is a condition that you eat your way into.

Diets low in fibre, high in calories, full of saturated fat and packed with foods that boost blood sugar quickly can all contribute. In the

If you have metabolic syndrome, you're an excellent candidate for diabetes, even if your blood sugar levels aren't high yet.

Framingham Heart Study, one of the longest and largest studies of diet and disease, those who ate foods which raised their blood sugar the highest after meals were 40 per cent more likely to have metabolic syndrome than those who usually ate foods. such as those recommended in this book.

According to the World Health Organisation, you have the syndrome if you have three or more of these problems.

■ **Abdominal fat** From your body's standpoint, fat around the middle is very different from the kind of fat on your thighs or around your hips. It's easier for abdominal fat to get into the bloodstream, where it can wreak havoc and increase the risk of heart disease. Indeed, researchers now suspect a large waist may be a stronger marker for heart disease risk than being overweight or obese in general.

■ **High triglyceride levels** These fats are stored in fat tissue and carried in the blood. They are broken down for energy. Even a mild elevation can increase your risk of heart disease.

■ **Low HDL cholesterol levels** You've probably heard a lot of talk about 'good' HDL cholesterol. It's the kind your body uses to pull excess LDL cholesterol out of the blood and transport it back to the liver, where it's broken down. High levels of LDL cholesterol can cause fatty deposits to develop on the lining of the arteries (atherosclerosis). Levels of HDL are often low in people with metabolic syndrome.

■ **High blood pressure** Blood pressure is also often elevated in metabolic syndrome. It may not be high enough for your doctor to diagnose you as having high blood pressure but, together with the other factors, it's bad for your heart.

■ **High fasting glucose levels** Your blood sugar may not be high enough to qualify you as having diabetes, but it still increases your risk of developing both diabetes and heart disease. The cause is insulin resistance.

Do you have
PRE-DIABETES?

Only a blood glucose test can tell for sure. If your fasting blood glucose level (after 8 hours of not eating anything) is between 5.5 and 7.0mmol/l (100 and 126mg/dl), you have pre-diabetes. (Some doctors prefer a different test, measuring your blood glucose levels after you've had a sugar-rich drink.)

Should you ask your doctor to test you? Here's how to decide.

■ **If you're 45 or older**, consider being tested. Testing is strongly recommended if you are overweight or have any of the following risk factors:

☐ **You have a parent**, brother or sister with diabetes, or with a history of diabetes during pregnancy (gestational diabetes).

☐ **Your ancestry** is African, Caribbean, South Asian or Arabic.

☐ **You're a mum** who has had a baby weighing 9lb (4 kg) or more at birth, or you had gestational diabetes.

☐ **Your blood pressure** is 140/90mm/Hg or higher, or you've been told you have high blood pressure.

☐ **Your cholesterol levels** aren't normal: your HDL cholesterol is 0.90mmol/l (35mg/dl) or lower, or your triglycerides are 2.80mmol/l(250mg/dl) or higher.

☐ **You are fairly inactive**, or you exercise less than three times a week.

Even if you are younger than 45, you should consider being tested if you are overweight or have one or more of the other risk factors listed above.

Some of these numbers, such as those for blood pressure and HDL, are different from those in the quiz for metabolic syndrome. One reason is that borderline risk factors become more significant when they're combined, as they are in metabolic syndrome.

Do you have DIABETES?

If your blood sugar level after not eating for 8 hours (fasting blood glucose level) is 7.0mmol/l (126mg/dl) or higher, you may have diabetes. Ideally, you would have been tested when you showed any of the risk factors for pre-diabetes (*see* 'Do you have pre-diabetes?' on the opposite page), but many people don't find out they have diabetes until they start to have symptoms. That's unfortunate, because even though diabetes may cause no symptoms for years, it's increasing your risk of heart disease, blindness and nerve problems. The sooner you get your blood sugar levels under control, the better your chances of avoiding these complications.

See your doctor at once if you have any of these symptoms:

☐ **Increased urination, often at night** This is the result of the body trying to remove the excess glucose from the bloodstream.

☐ **Increased thirst** When blood glucose is not being controlled adequately the body increases the throughput of urine to try to remove it from the body – resulting in a constant thirst.

☐ **Increased appetite** The body is not absorbing the glucose from foods properly, so the individual feels hungry.

☐ **Fatigue** With the body's cells starved of glucose, even the simplest of tasks can feel exhausting.

☐ **Weight loss without dieting** Since glucose is not being absorbed, the body resorts to mobilising fat stores and so the diabetic loses weight.

☐ **Blurred vision** The shape of the lens in the eye may alter, affecting vision.

☐ **Cuts and sores that heal very slowly** The high levels of sugar constantly in the blood and urine impair the body's ability to repair and heal itself.

QUIZ

Pre-diabetes

Even if you have insulin resistance and metabolic syndrome, a test of your blood sugar in a doctor's surgery may show perfectly normal levels. For a while – for years, really – your body may be able to cope with too much blood sugar after meals by pumping out extra insulin.

In some people, though, the insulin-producing beta cells in the pancreas just can't keep up. They become less effective and some of them die. Then your body can't make enough insulin to keep blood sugar levels under control.

Your blood sugar may be a little high when you wake up in the morning. A normal level after a fast (that is, after 8 hours of not eating anything) is between 4.0 and 5.5 millimoles (mmol) of glucose for every litre (l) of blood/70 to 100 milligrams (mg) of glucose for every 10th of a litre (dl) of blood. If yours is between 5.5 and 7.0mmol/l (100 and 126mg/dl), you have pre-diabetes. You don't have full-blown diabetes yet, but you're on the route that takes you there.

Your chances of developing diabetes are high over the next few years, but you may still be able to avoid it. That was shown in a major piece of US research, called the Diabetes Prevention Program, which studied men and women with pre-diabetes. Some of these people made lifestyle changes, such as eating healthier meals, losing weight and taking regular exercise. Such measures were associated with a 58 per cent reduction in the incidence of the disease.

Diabetes

If insulin resistance has damaged your pancreas so much that you have pre-diabetes, and you do nothing to change your lifestyle, it's almost inevitable that you will develop diabetes. Your beta cells are exhausted and just can't produce nearly enough insulin to do their job. Your blood sugar levels are above 7.0mmol/l (125mg/dl) even when you wake up in the morning.

At this stage, your diet will now be an essential part of your treatment plan. You'll need to work with your doctor to take the right medication to improve your insulin sensitivity and insulin production. Losing weight, exercising, and choosing foods that are gentle to your blood sugar levels are key to the effectiveness of those medications.

Take this book to your doctor or dietician and discuss how to work our recommendations into your lifestyle plan. Working with your doctor, you may be able to reduce the medications you take. In some cases, under medical supervision, you may even be able to stop stop taking your medications altogether.

The *Magic Foods* solution

The nation's hidden health crisis – insulin resistance and the closely related threats of diabetes, heart disease, and other health problems – is a secret no longer. The way we eat affects our moods, appetite, weight and, in the end, our longevity. But once you know what to do, you can make simple changes that will help you to feel better and be healthier within days and for the next 20 years.

Magic Foods for Better Blood Sugar isn't a radical diet. It doesn't turn basic nutrition upside down. You'll find many of the same building blocks of a healthy diet here that you've heard about for decades: whole grains, fruits and vegetables, nuts, seeds, beans, eggs, lean meats and poultry, seafood and low-fat dairy products. But we've improved this to help you to keep your blood sugar in balance before, during, and after each meal. You'll do it with the Magic foods in Part 2, the meal makeovers in Part 3, and the recipes and meal plans in Part 4.

The differences between the *Magic Foods* approach and a basic healthy diet are subtle but powerful. Whether you're young or not so young, thin or not so thin, with normal blood sugar levels or high ones; whether you are insulin resistant or not; and indeed, whether you have diabetes or not, this way of eating can make all the difference in the world to your health. Read on to learn more.

The hidden effects of food

2

Now you know the situation: most of us are damaging our health by eating too many foods that send our blood sugar soaring. Besides contributing to diabetes and other serious illnesses in the long term, meals full of these foods also leave you tired, grumpy and hungry again in next to no time after you've eaten them. But there are other foods that barely move the blood sugar needle or at least move it very gradually, keeping you feeling full and energised for much longer.

Your body's glycaemic load is a more powerful factor in keeping you healthy than the amount of carbohydrate – or fat – you eat.

Carbohydrates are the foods that raise blood sugar. Plain and simple, right? But not all carbs are created equal.

Unfortunately, foods don't

come with labels explaining which ones make your blood sugar rise sharply and which ones don't. After reading this chapter, though, you'll know how to tell the difference.

In the end, it's as simple as choosing wholemeal pasta over white rice, baked beans instead of mashed potatoes, oil-and-vinegar dressing instead of Thousand Island, and other easy fixes. Read on to discover what makes these particular foods Magic.

First, we'll talk about the three so-called macronutrients in food – carbohydrate, fat and protein – from which we get almost all of our calories, and we'll tell you how they affect your blood sugar. Then we'll talk about two 'magic' food components you can use for amazingly effective blood sugar control: soluble fibre and acetic acid (found in sour foods).

Carbohydrate

We'll reveal the main plot twist immediately: carbohydrates are the foods that raise blood sugar. That's plain and simple, isn't it? The trouble is, not all carb foods are the same.

In fact, carbohydrates are found in most foods except fats and oils, meats, poultry and fish. But some foods contain more carbs than others. Beans are about 25 per cent protein and 75 per cent carbohydrate. Rice, on the other hand, is more than 90 per cent carbohydrate.

It's the quantity of carbohydrate in foods (and of course, how much of the food you eat) that primarily affects blood sugar, but the type of carbohydrate also has an effect.

Introducing the glycaemic index

To find out which carbs are best and worst for blood sugar, scientists had to do some serious detective work. First, they needed to come up with a way to measure a particular food's effect on blood sugar. In 1981 nutrition scientist Dr David Jenkins PhD developed a system that could indicate the extent to which certain foods affect blood sugar levels. He called it the glycaemic index (GI) – the prefix 'glyc' means 'sugar'. He asked volunteers to eat different foods, all containing 50g of carbohydrate. Then he measured the volunteers' blood sugar over the following 2 hours to see how high it went. As a control he used pure glucose, the form of sugar that's identical to blood sugar – your body converts glucose very quickly to blood sugar – and assigned it the number 100 on his new index.

The glycaemic index opened a lot of eyes. Almost everyone had assumed that table sugar would be the worst offender, much worse than the complex carbohydrates found in starchy staples such as rice and bread. But this didn't always prove true. Some starchy foods, such as potatoes and cornflakes, ranked very high on the index, raising blood sugar nearly as much as pure glucose. That's why you won't see these foods in our list of Magic foods.

WHERE THE GLYCAEMIC INDEX FELL SHORT

Something was wrong, however. Some of the results pointed the finger at healthy foods, such as carrots and strawberries. Watermelon was just about off the top of the GI chart. But no one ever gained weight from eating carrots, nor do carrots, in the real world, raise blood sugar. What was the GI missing?

The GI measured the effects of a standard amount of carbohydrate: 50g, or about 1½oz. But you'd be awfully hard-pressed to eat enough carrots – seven or eight large ones – to get 50g of carbohydrate. The same holds true for most other vegetables and fruits. They're full of water, so there's not much room in them for carbohydrate. Bread, on the other hand, is crammed with carbohydrate. You get 50g by eating just one slice.

To solve the problem, scientists came up with a different measurement: the glycaemic load (GL). This takes into account not only the type of carbohydrate in the food but also the amount of carbohydrate you would eat in a standard serving. To get a bit technical, a food's GL is the GI multiplied by the amount of carbohydrate in one serving.

This made more sense. By this criterion, carrots, strawberries and other low-calorie foods are clearly good to eat – they all have low GL values, since the amount of carbohydrate they contain is low.

The GL has turned out to be a powerful way to think not just about individual foods but also whole meals and even entire diets. When scientists looked at the GL of typical diets in different populations, they found that the higher the GL, the greater the incidence of obesity, diabetes, heart disease and cancer. You may remember a study we mentioned in Chapter 1 in which men who ate the most sugar-boosting foods were 40 per cent more likely to get diabetes. That's GL we were talking about. We also talked about the Nurses' Health Study finding that women were twice as likely to develop heart disease over 10 years if they ate more sugar-boosting foods. Again, the GL. The converse is also true: the lower the GL of your diet, the more likely you are to keep your weight under control and stay free of chronic disease.

When it comes to eating properly, controlling weight and preventing disease, the GL is a key player. It's a more powerful factor in keeping you healthy than the amount of carbohydrate – or even fat – you eat.

What makes some carbohydrates better than others?

Why would one high-carb food have a different GL from another? Why does white rice, for instance, have a higher GL than, say, honey? It has to do with the way Nature constructed them.

Carbohydrates consist of starches and sugars. Starch – think of starchy foods such as beans and potatoes – is made up of sugar molecules bound together in long chains. When you eat a carbohydrate-rich food, your body converts those starches and sugars into glucose, or blood sugar. Some starches, such as those in white rice, are extremely easy for the body to convert, and therefore blood sugar levels rise like a hot

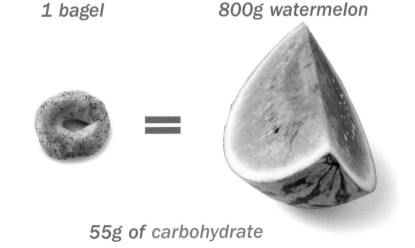

CARB DENSITY counts The glycaemic load takes into account how much carbohydrate a serving of food contains. The amount in one bagel equals the amount in four or five helpings of watermelon.

1 bagel *800g watermelon*

55g of carbohydrate

temper after you eat them. Others, like those in beans, take a lot more work to break down, so blood sugar levels simmer rather than explode. Four factors determine how fast the body breaks down carbohydrate.

THE TYPE OF STARCH – OR WHY YOU SHOULD AVOID STICKY RICE

Remember, starches are made of sugar molecules chained together. Some chains are straight, while others are branched. The straight-edged type, called amylose, is harder for your body to break down and turn into blood sugar. The branched type, called amylopectin, is much easier to break down because there are so many places for the enzymes to get at it. Think of a tree with lots of branches – there are a lot more spots for birds to land on compared to a simple post.

White potatoes are very high in amylopectin, the branched kind of sugar chain, which is why they raise your blood sugar in the blink of an eye. Peas and lentils are high in amylose, the straight-edged kind of starch, so they're converted to blood sugar at a snail's pace.

Basically, the more amylose a food contains, the slower it will be digested and converted into blood sugar. Take rice, for instance. Some types contain more amylose than others. In general, the softer and stickier the rice is after cooking, the lower its amylose content; this is why 'sticky rice' is dastardly to your blood sugar. The firmer the rice, the higher the amylose and the harder it is for your body to turn into blood sugar quickly – making brown rice a better choice. Some genetic variants of rice – such as some sold in Australia, for example – are particularly high in amylose (as much as 25 per cent), but unfortunately, most of the rice we eat is low in amylose and therefore has a high GL.

THE TYPE OF SUGAR – OR WHY FRUIT IS ALWAYS GOOD

Sugar is the molecule that makes up carbohydrates, but there is more than one kind of sugar. There's table sugar (sucrose) as well as the kind found in fruits and grains (fructose), the kind in milk (lactose) and the kind in malted barley (maltose). The sugar in milk and fruit tends to be absorbed more slowly than other sugars because it needs to be converted into glucose by the liver first, which is why these foods are gentle to your blood sugar.

Ironically, table sugar, which is half fructose and half glucose, is turned into blood sugar more slowly than some starches, like bread or potatoes. That doesn't make sugar good for you, of course. One reason is that fructose, especially in the amounts contained in packaged foods loaded with high-fructose corn syrup, raise triglycerides, blood fats that increase the risk of heart attack.

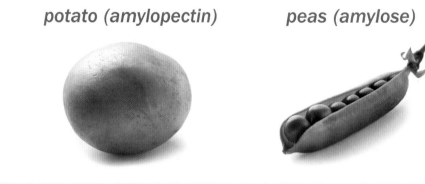

NOT ALL STARCHES are equal **Potatoes raise blood sugar fast because the type of starch they contain is easily broken down. Peas contain a type of starch that's broken down much more slowly.**

potato (amylopectin)   *peas (amylose)*

(Fruit, by contrast, contains a little fructose plus plenty of water, fibre and nutrients.) Sugar also packs a lot of carbohydrate calories in a small amount. A large cola (525ml), for instance, contains 55g sugar and 225kcal – and it will send your blood sugar sky high.

HEAT – OR WHY YOU SHOULD NOT OVERCOOK RICE OR PASTA

All starch, whether it's made of straight or branched chains, is composed of crystals, which don't dissolve in cold water. Think of a grain of rice or a piece of raw potato – put it in water and it stays the same. But heat breaks down those crystals so the starch can dissolve in water. When you cook a starchy food, it absorbs water and becomes easier to digest.

The more overcooked rice or pasta is, the faster it makes your blood sugar rise. When starch is heated and then cooled, it can return, in part, to its crystal form; that's why hot potatoes have a high GL, while the GL of potato salad is slightly lower. Just make it with olive oil instead of mayonnaise to keep it healthier.

PROCESSING – OR WHY YOU SHOULD AVOID WHITE FLOUR

Have you ever noticed that some brown breads are as smooth as white bread, while others have crunchy kernels in them? Those kernels take a long time for your body to break down, as do any whole, intact grains.

Modern commercial flour, on the other hand – especially white flour – is extremely easy for the body to turn into blood sugar. This is why we suggest throughout this book that you choose whole grains that are still intact and foods such as beans and lentils instead of those made from white flour. (Unfortunately, we're surrounded by white-flour foods. You'll need to make a conscious effort to cut back.)

Until the 19th century, the main way to turn grain into flour was to grind it between stones, sometimes powered by a waterwheel. Making very fine flour took a lot of work, and it was available only in small amounts to the wealthy.

PASTA
gets the green light

Bread, even some wholemeal breads, can raise your blood sugar pretty quickly. Yet pasta, even if it's made from white flour, has a much lower GL. How can that be?

Imagine putting cooked pasta and a piece of bread in a bowl of water. The bread will fall apart, but the pasta won't. That's because in pasta dough, the starch granules get trapped in a network of protein molecules, so it takes more work – and more time – to get at them. That's why pasta releases its carbs much more slowly than potatoes or most breads do, especially if it's served *al dente* (slightly undercooked). Similarly, gnocchi, a pasta-like product made from durum wheat and potato flour, has a lower GL than potatoes. You'll find pastas, especially wholemeal pastas, on our list of Magic foods in Part 2.

Pasta is particularly good for you if you eat it as the southern Italians do: cooked *al dente*, prepared with olive oil and beans or vegetables, served in modest portions, and followed by a piece of fish or lean meat and side vegetables, with fruit for dessert.

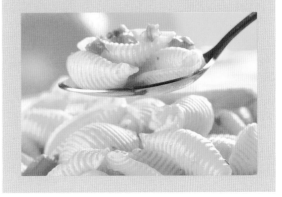

In a study, people who ate a high-protein diet consumed 25 per cent fewer calories than those in the high-carbohydrate group.

Then high-speed, high-heat steel rollers, which make very fine flour quickly and inexpensively, were invented, almost instantly transforming our diets into blood sugar nightmares.

Modern manufacturing also allows grains to be turned into highly processed forms such as cornflakes or puffed corn snacks, which tend to have higher GIs than grains left intact, like popcorn, or those milled in an old-fashioned manner, such as coarse, stoneground wholemeal flour used in stoneground bread.

Protein

Unlike carbohydrate, protein doesn't raise blood sugar. Your body breaks it down into amino acids, which it uses as building blocks for muscles as well as many compounds such as neurotransmitters, the brain's chemical messengers. Unless you're on a diet that has no carbs, your body won't even try to convert protein into blood sugar.

That's why you'll find protein foods such as fish, chicken, lean meat, soy, milk, eggs and cheese on our list of Magic foods. If you substitute calories from one of these foods for some of your carbohydrate calories, you'll be helping to keep your blood sugar steady. For instance, if you add prawns or chicken to a rice dish, you'll eat less rice, and the meal will have less impact on your blood sugar.

While we're fans of protein, we're not suggesting a diet of fatty bacon, greasy burgers and the like. These are packed with saturated fat, and as you'll read a bit later, saturated fat increases insulin resistance, which is bad for your blood sugar. Lean protein foods, such as skimmed milk and chicken breast without the skin, are far better choices because they contain fewer calories and less saturated fat. Fish and shellfish are definitely on the menu because

they're not only low in saturated fat but also high in heart-healthy omega-3 fatty acids. Beans, peas and lentils, all high in protein, have the added plus of being rich in fibre.

Though we are promoting protein, we're not suggesting an extremely high protein, low carb diet. You'll find out why in the next chapter.

More pluses for protein

There are also other benefits to protein. Some of the compounds our bodies make from protein's amino acids help to regulate blood sugar, so including protein in a meal means your body will handle the carbohydrates in that meal more efficiently.

Another reason to increase the protein is that your body takes a while to break down protein in the foods you eat. This has the effect of slowing the digestion of the whole meal, including the carbohydrates it contains, making for a slower rise in blood sugar.

In one recent study, healthy volunteers ate a starchy breakfast (white bread) followed by a starchy lunch (mashed potatoes and meatballs). On some days, however, they got extra protein in the form of whey (dairy protein). On days when they ate more protein, their blood sugar levels were more than 50 per cent lower in the following 2 hours than on days when they ate mostly carbs. Another study, of people with diabetes, found that adding whey reduced their blood sugar response by 21 per cent over the following 2 hours.

Protein, especially the kind found in milk, also stimulates the pancreas to produce insulin. That may not sound like a good idea as having high levels of insulin over long periods of time is unhealthy. But the earlier your body makes insulin in response to a rise in blood sugar, the less insulin it may need to make – and the less likely you are to become insulin resistant.

Protein and weight loss

Eating more protein-rich foods should even help you to lose weight. Protein makes you less hungry, expanding the time between when you eat and when your stomach starts rumbling again. Research proves it. In a six-day study, one group of volunteers went on a low-GI, high-protein diet. The other group followed a low-protein, high-carb diet. Both groups were allowed to eat as much as they wanted. The people who ate the high-protein diet consumed 25 per cent fewer calories than those in the high-carb group. In a study lasting six months, high-protein dieters lost more weight than high-carb dieters. They ate less because they felt fuller.

Getting enough protein can also help to keep your metabolism running at full speed. Usually, when you really cut back on calories – especially if you go on a very low carb diet – your body resorts to breaking down muscle tissue for energy. But muscle tissue burns up a lot of calories even when you're not flexing a thing, so breaking it down ultimately slows your metabolism. Eating plenty of protein helps your body keep its muscle tissue.

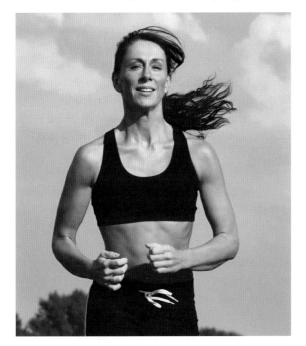

In diet studies, people following moderately high protein diets lost more body fat and less muscle than those on low protein diets. A moderately high protein diet might obtain as much as 30 per cent of its calories from protein, rather than the 15 to 20 per cent most people get. We recommend an intake of 20 to 30 per cent.

Fat

For a long time fat has had a bad reputation, to the point where most people think the less fat you eat, the better. But research is now proving that this just isn't true.

THE POWER of protein Adding protein to a carbohydrate dish lowers the glycaemic load of the dish – assuming you eat the same amount – because you end up eating less carbohydrate. Protein itself also helps to steady blood sugar.

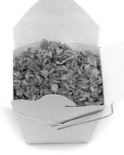

fried rice

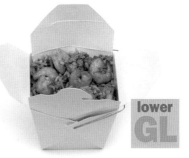

lower
GL

fried rice with prawns

A moderate-fat diet can be every bit as effective as a low-fat diet in helping you lose weight.

During the height of the low-fat craze, people filled up on carbohydrates such as fat-free crisps and low-fat biscuits – foods laden with fast-acting carbohydrates – thinking they were doing themselves good. In fact, they were wreaking havoc on their blood sugar and consuming just as many calories into the bargain.

The fact is, fat is no demon. In fact some fats are positively good for you and your blood sugar, and they absolutely belong in your diet. Like protein, fat doesn't raise blood sugar, so swapping carb-rich foods such as crisps for fat-rich foods such as nuts can be an excellent trade.

Also, like protein, fat takes a while to digest. Because it slows the rate at which food leaves your stomach, it can blunt the blood sugar effect of a whole meal, even if that meal includes carbs. Tossing your salad with olive oil or drizzling some on your pasta, adding some nuts to your rice, grilling some fatty fish for dinner, or using slices of ripe avocado in your sandwich won't magically lower your blood sugar, but it will help.

Good fat, bad fat

Notice that we've talked about nuts, oils and fish instead of other fat sources such as burgers or butter. It's true that adding fat lowers the GL of a starchy food, but adding butter or sour cream to a heap of mashed potatoes doesn't make it healthy. Quite the contrary.

Butter is an animal food and, as with many animal foods, most of the fat it contains is saturated. That's the kind that clogs arteries. It's also bad for blood sugar. In both animal and human studies, a diet high in saturated fat has been shown to trigger insulin resistance, which it does in many ways. Saturated fat increases inflammation, which is toxic to cells, including those that handle glucose. It also makes cell membranes less fluid, so the insulin receptors there are less responsive to insulin.

It's clear that people who eat the most saturated fat are at the highest risk of developing insulin resistance and metabolic syndrome. And, as you read in Chapter 1, these conditions increase your risk of heart disease and diabetes. The trick, then, is to avoid the worst of the 'bad' fat foods, such as fatty meats, butter, whole milk, full-fat cheeses and ice cream, and choose instead lean cuts of meat and poultry, skimmed or semi-skimmed milk, low-fat cheese, and lean cold meats such as turkey, chicken and ham.

Even better, stick to unsaturated fats, which can actually improve insulin sensitivity, thus benefiting your blood sugar. These fats come mainly from plants – think avocados, nuts and seeds, olives and olive and rapeseed oil – and fish and seafood. The Mediterranean diet, one of the healthiest diets in the world, gets a moderately high 30 to 35 per cent of its calories from fat, mostly the unsaturated kind. This is the fat ceiling we recommend.

Protecting your heart

'Good' fats are also good for your heart. Swapping that cheeseburger for seafood or butter for peanut butter (a good source of unsaturated fat) lowers your 'bad' LDL cholesterol while leaving 'good' HDL cholesterol alone. In fact, eating just a handful of nuts a few times a week can slash your risk of getting heart disease by 25 per cent.

So can eating fish a few times a week. Seafood contains omega-3 fatty acids, which do a world of good for your heart by lowering triglycerides, helping to prevent blood clots, reducing inflammation and promoting normal heart rhythm. Eating just two servings of fish a week – especially oil-rich fish such as salmon or mackerel – can reduce your risk of heart disease by a third or more.

Losing weight

You'd think that if you want to lose weight, you should cut way back on fat, which is high in calories. Pretty obvious, right? Surprisingly, recent research has shown it's not necessarily true. A moderate-fat diet can be every bit as effective as a low-fat diet in helping you to lose weight – but you must choose mostly 'good' fats.

A bit of fat also makes meals more satisfying, which can make it easier to stick to a healthy eating plan in the long term. If you try to adopt a diet that is too low in fat, you're likely to give up at some point, probably sooner rather than later. In one study of overweight men and women, those on a moderate-fat diet lost about 9lb (4kg) over 18 months, while those on a low-fat diet actually ended up gaining more than 6lb (3kg). One key reason was dieting fatigue: only 20 per cent of those on the low-fat diet were still actively participating by the end of the study, while 54 per cent of those on the moderate-fat diet stayed with it.

Lower blood sugar with soluble fibre

Carbs, protein and fat are all macronutrients – nutrients that provide the vast majority of our calories. Fibre doesn't count because it isn't digested by the body, so it provides not a single calorie. Nevertheless, it's an extremely important element in a Magic diet.

There are two types of fibre: soluble and insoluble. Soluble fibre is found in oats, barley, beans and some fruits and vegetables. Insoluble fibre is found mostly in whole grains and some fruits and vegetables. Both types are very good for you, but only soluble fibre will help to lower your blood sugar. But it does so in a big way.

How big? Researchers at a US Department of Agriculture nutrition laboratory tested porridge oats and barley (which is even richer in soluble fibre than porridge) on overweight middle-aged women. On days when the women ate porridge for breakfast, their blood sugar levels over the following 3 hours were about 30 per cent lower than when they ate a sugar-laden pudding. On days when they ate barley cereal, it was about 60 per cent lower.

BEST FOODS FOR
soluble fibre
Here you'll find the amount of soluble fibre per serving of various foods. Remember, you're aiming for about 10g a day.

GRAINS (80g COOKED)	
Barley	1g
Oats	1g

BEANS AND PEAS (125g COOKED)	
Black beans	2g
Cannellini beans	1g
Kidney beans	3g
Lima beans	3.5g
Haricot beans	2g
Pinto beans	2g
Black-eyed peas	1g
Chickpeas	1g

VEGETABLES (80g COOKED)	
Broccoli	1g
Brussels sprouts	3g
Carrots	1g

FRUIT (1 MEDIUM FRUIT, EXCEPT WHERE NOTED)	
Apple	1g
Blackberries (80g)	1g
Grapefruit	2g
Orange	2g
Pear	2g
Prunes (40g)	1.5g

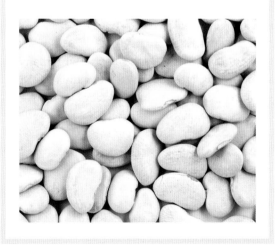

***Eating more foods rich in soluble fibre** is a key strategy for lowering your blood sugar after meals.*

How does soluble fibre work its magic? When it mixes with water, it forms a gum. Think of porridge; you can pick out the flakes when it's dry, but once you add water and cook it, it' becomes mushy. This mush forms a barrier between the digestive enzymes in your stomach and the starch molecules in food. It not only locks up the starch in the porridge but also in the toast you ate with it. This means that it takes longer for your body to convert the whole meal into blood sugar.

Eating more foods rich in soluble fibre is a key strategy for lowering blood sugar after meals. It will also improve your health in other ways. Studies have shown that oats can help to lower cholesterol – porridge manufacturers can claim this in their advertising – and oats may lower high levels of triglycerides and reduce blood pressure as well. Lots of other foods are also rich in soluble fibre (*see* 'Best foods for soluble fibre' on page 31).

Nutrition experts tell us to aim for at least 18–24g of total fibre a day, both insoluble and soluble. A good target for soluble fibre is 9–12g. Does that sound like a hard goal to reach? Here are some foods you might eat in a typical day that would add up to 10g:

Breakfast: A big bowl of porridge with a chopped medium apple (soluble fibre: 3g).

Lunch: Add a side dish of black beans (soluble fibre: 2g) and a pear or orange (soluble fibre: 2g).

Dinner: Add a side dish of Brussels sprouts (soluble fibre: 3g).

Not surprisingly, many of these fibre-rich foods also have low GLs, so they can help lower the GL of a meal if you use them to replace other carbs. For instance, if you ate a combination of 90g rice and 125g beans instead of 180g rice, you'd reduce the GL by almost half.

Sour power

Wouldn't it be terrific if there were a simple ingredient you could add to your meals that would act like an anchor, keeping blood sugar from rising too high? As it turns out, there is. It's acetic acid, the sour-tasting compound that gives that characteristic tang to vinegar, pickles and sourdough bread.

The effect can be quite dramatic. In one small study, people who ate a buttered 85g bagel and orange juice (a high-GL breakfast) saw their blood sugar shoot up in the next hour. But when they also drank about a tablespoon of apple cider vinegar (with artificial sweetener added to improve the taste), their blood sugar levels after the meal were 50 per cent lower. A similar 50 per cent reduction in blood sugar occurred when the participants had the vinegar along with a chicken-and-rice meal.

How does acetic acid make it happen? Scientists aren't sure, but they do know that it interferes with the enzymes that break apart the chemical bonds in starches and the kinds of sugars found in table sugar and milk. This means it takes your body longer to break down those foods into blood sugar. Other researchers believe acetic acid keeps foods in the stomach longer so they aren't digested as quickly. Acetic acid may also speed up the rate at which glucose is moved out of the blood and into muscle cells for storage.

No matter how it works, it does, and taking advantage of it is as easy as adding vinegar to salads and other foods and having a pickle with your sandwich at lunchtime. You'll read more about this in Part 2.

The secrets of a Magic diet

Now you understand why rice raises blood sugar fast while porridge raises it more slowly and chicken doesn't raise it at all. And why the soluble fibre in beans and the acetic acid in vinegar help to keep your blood sugar steady. If

WHAT ABOUT wine?

Alcohol, in the right amounts, can benefit blood sugar. Moderate drinking – from one drink a few times a week up to one a day for women or two a day for men – is associated with lower fasting insulin levels, higher levels of 'good' HDL cholesterol, smaller waist circumference, and lower triglycerides. in other words, a lower risk of metabolic syndrome (see page 19).

Alcohol also lowers the risk of developing diabetes by between 33 and 56 per cent,

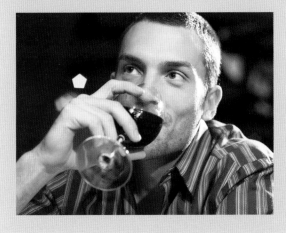

according to a comprehensive review of more than 30 studies. And if you have diabetes, it reduces your risk of developing heart disease by 34 to 55 per cent.

Wine, especially red wine, may have extra benefits. It contains antioxidants that, in animal studies, help to prevent insulin resistance. Wine is also acidic, so in theory, it should reduce the blood sugar effect of foods you eat. But beer is fine, too; despite what you may have heard, even regular beer is fairly low in carbohydrates.

The main benefits come from the alcohol itself, but moderation is important. People who have three or more drinks a day have a much higher risk of diabetes and heart disease. One drink is defined as 340ml of beer, 150ml of wine or a 45ml shot of spirits, such as vodka.

If you have diabetes, ask your doctor about drinking. Because alcohol lowers blood sugar, it could cause hypoglycaemia.

you don't feel like remembering the details, then don't. You don't need to. In Chapter 4 we'll reveal to you the seven secrets of Magic eating, and if you follow these simple rules, you'll be eating for better blood sugar.

You don't even need to bother with the exact GL numbers of the foods you eat (although we do supply them for some common foods on pages 55–58). In this book, we've simply classified foods according to very low, low, medium, high and very high GL. The foods you'll read about in Part 2 have very low, low, or medium GLs – part of what makes them Magic.

It's important to note that you don't always have to choose foods in the 'low' category. Eating just one low-GL food in a meal in place of a high-GL food is enough to tame your blood sugar

response to the whole meal. But you should also remember that a food's GL is based on a moderate portion; if you eat twice as much, the effect on your blood sugar will be twice as great. Of course, the converse is also true: if you eat 50 per cent less of a starchy food, your blood sugar response will be 50 per cent lower.

In each Magic food entry in Part 2, you'll find out the size of an appropriate serving of that food. Keeping your portions under control is, of course, the best way to lose weight, whether or not you choose low-GL foods.

You'll learn much more about how to focus on Magic foods later in the book. First, in case you're tempted after reading this chapter to switch to a very low carb diet, let us explain why that's a bad idea.

Why low-carb diets aren't the answer

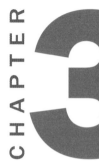

CHAPTER 3

What raises blood sugar? The simple answer is carbohydrates. So why not just remove them from your diet like weeds from your garden? Why not reduce blood sugar by cutting out bread, pasta, rice and cereal? But we've been there, done that. The low-carb craze is on the downswing and that's a good thing because, in the long run, very low carb diets simply aren't good for you, as you'll discover in this chapter. That doesn't mean it's not sensible to cut back on carbohydrates – but don't go overboard.

Many low-carb diets have turned out to be less effective and less healthy than originally claimed.

When low-carb diets first

became popular, they seemed to be a breath of fresh air after the low-fat (and high-carb) diets that preceded them. Remember low-fat biscuits, low-fat cakes and low-fat everything else? With low-carb diets, suddenly people could fill up on bacon and still lose weight, as long as they were willing to eat hamburgers without buns and pretty much give up sandwiches and spaghetti. People were amazed at how effective these diets could be. Weight loss could happen very quickly, sometimes within days. And amazingly, it often seemed to come with added health benefits, including lower cholesterol, blood pressure and triglycerides (blood fats linked to heart attacks).

The most extreme kind of low-carb diet was pioneered by the late Dr Robert Atkins, whose first book, *Dr Atkins' Diet Revolution*, came out in 1972. It promised quick and long-lasting weight loss and prevention of chronic disease, all while allowing you to eat fatty meat and ice cream. Since then other, more moderate low-carb diets have permitted small amounts of carbohydrate-rich foods, but they still cut out most grains as well as starchy vegetables and even fruit.

The drawbacks of low-carb diets

The Atkins diet and the many other low-carb diets that followed in its footsteps have turned out to be less effective, and less healthy than originally claimed. Often, the weight that was initially lost soon returned, and as it did, problems such as high cholesterol and high blood pressure came back, too. Also, many people decided they didn't want to go through life without ever eating pasta again.

Let's look at what would happen if you followed an extreme low-carb diet.

You'll feel terrible

Low-carb diets usually begin with an 'induction' phase that eliminates nearly every source of carbohydrate. Often, you'll consume as few as 20g of carbohydrate a day. That's less than 100kcal – about as much as a small bread roll contains. On a 1,200kcal diet it accounts for 8 per cent of your daily calories. By contrast, health experts recommend that we get between 45 and 65 per cent of our calories from carbs.

When carbohydrate consumption falls below 100g, the body responds by burning muscle tissue for the glycogen (stored glucose) it contains. When those glycogen stores start to run out, the body resorts to burning body fat. But that's an inefficient, complicated way to produce blood sugar. The body tries to do it only when it absolutely has to (such as when it's starving) – and for good reason. Turning fat into blood sugar comes at a price in the form of by-products called ketones. They make your breath smell funny. They can also make you tired, lightheaded, headachy and nauseated. Feeling lousy is certainly one way to dampen the appetite, but not one that most people would choose.

With virtually no carbs in your system, you may even have trouble concentrating. According to the Institute of Medicine of the National Academy of Sciences in the USA, the human brain requires the equivalent of 130g of carbohydrate a day to function optimally – and that's a minimum. It's no wonder that people on very low carb diets, who are trying to exist on an input of 20g a day, find themselves feeling flat and exhausted.

Your health may suffer

If you're overweight or obese, and you have insulin resistance – especially if you have pre-diabetes or diabetes – cutting way back on carbohydrates can have immediate health benefits. Your blood sugar and insulin levels will go down, your triglycerides and blood pressure may fall, and your levels of

> *Burning fat for blood sugar produces ketones, which can make you tired, lightheaded, headachy and nauseated.*

'good' HDL cholesterol may rise. But the low-carb diet will also wreak some havoc. When your body breaks down lean body mass – muscle – for energy, your metabolism slows because muscle tissue burns up a lot of calories. This may be one reason that the weight often comes back after you've been shunning carbs for a while.

The effects on your heart are also questionable. If you switch to a high-saturated-fat diet, as people do when they start eating their fill of steak and bacon, your 'bad' LDL cholesterol will go up. Levels of homocysteine, an amino acid that increases the risk of heart disease, may also rise if you eat a lot of meat and too few vegetables. And to get rid of the ketones produced when your body burns fat for energy, your kidneys need to work overtime, which raises your risk of kidney stones.

Ironically, low-carb diets may even interfere with insulin sensitivity; a certain amount of carbs in your diet may be needed in order for the pancreas, which produces the insulin that keeps blood sugar in check, to work well.

You'll miss out

It's not just that you'll feel deprived because you've had to give up bread, fruit and all the rest. Your body will actually be deprived of foods and nutrients that are known to be essential for good health, including the following:

■ **Whole grains** These are packed with nutrients and are thought to protect against metabolic syndrome, diabetes, heart disease, stroke and some types of cancer.

■ **Fruits and vegetables** Fresh produce helps to prevent heart disease, stroke and some cancers. Most fruits and vegetables are very filling while providing few calories, so they can help you to cut calories without feeling deprived. Indeed, the more fruits and vegetables people eat, studies show, the thinner they tend to be.

■ **Beans** Rich in protein, complex carbohydrates and B vitamins, beans contain no saturated fat and lots of soluble fibre. They also contain plant chemicals that are thought to protect against heart disease and cancer.

■ **Low-fat dairy foods** Of course, you *can* have butter and cream on a carb-restricted diet, but you won't get much calcium or protein from them. Fat-free and low-fat versions of milk and yoghurt are excellent sources of those nutrients.

■ **Fibre** You'll get fibre from these foods (except dairy foods), which helps to reduce the risk of heart disease and diabetes. Beans and many fruits and vegetables are particularly rich in soluble fibre, which helps to lower blood sugar, curbs hunger and lowers LDL cholesterol.

■ **Vitamins, minerals and health-protective plant chemicals** Whole grains, for example, are rich in components such as lignans, which may protect against diabetes independently of their effects on blood sugar. And without fruits and vegetables, you'd be awfully hard-pressed to get enough vitamin C or other disease-fighting antioxidants.

You'll eat too much 'bad' fat

The original Atkins diet became popular largely because it allowed people to eat foods that are traditionally forbidden on most other diets, such as cheese and cream. More recently, the diet has been revised to include sources of healthier fats, such as fish and olive oil, and other low-carb diets have shied away from saturated fats as well. But in practice, once you cut out bread, fruit and beans, it's all too easy to eat too many fatty animal foods. After all, how many foods is it possible for you to take out of your diet?

If you fill up on saturated fats – the original Atkins diet got as much as 26 per cent of its calories from saturated fat versus the 10 per cent or less most experts recommend – it's bad for your health. Saturated fats are still the major culprits behind elevated LDL cholesterol. The latest revisions to the diet, to be fair, do emphasise lean poultry and seafood, but in practice many people are attracted to this diet for the bacon and butter.

What's more, saturated fats also directly impair the body's ability to react to insulin, so following a low-carb, high-saturated-fat diet may help you to lose weight in the short term, but it may also speed the development of insulin resistance. Eventually, that can lead to metabolic syndrome, diabetes and heart disease.

The weight will come back

Two major studies of low-carb diets, published in the *New England Journal of Medicine*, looked at obese men and women who kept to either a low-carb, high-fat diet or a low-fat, high-carb diet. Both diets were low in calories.

In one study, which lasted six months, the low-carb diet seemed to win hands down. The people on it lost nearly 13lb (6kg); the low-fat dieters shed just 4lb (2kg). But the second study lasted six months longer, revealing a truth about low-carb diets: the results don't last. This study too found that the low-carb dieters lost more weight in the first six months, but in the second half of the year the weight came roaring back. By the end of a year there was no significant difference in weight loss between the two groups. This weight regain may be one reason that extreme low-carb diets have fallen out of favour.

Take the good, leave the bad

The good news? Many of the weight-loss advantages of low-carb diets may have nothing at all to do with restricting carbohydrates. The main benefit may be due to the extra protein – and you can add protein to your diet even if you don't drastically cut carbs. As you discovered in Chapter 2, protein-rich foods can really help with weight control. One reason may be that protein stimulates the body to burn slightly more calories than carbohydrates or fats do.

The main reason, though, is that protein foods curb hunger better. When people eat protein-rich foods, they feel fuller longer, and when they diet, they consume fewer calories and lose more weight when they eat

The main benefit of low-carb diets may be due to the extra protein in them.

a lot of protein. One recent study puts it in perspective. Researchers at the University of Washington School of Medicine in Seattle gave volunteers a diet that got 50 per cent of its calories from carbohydrates. That's certainly not a low-carb diet, though it's not a high-carb diet either. It's actually a good goal, on par with what we suggest in this book.

To start with, the volunteers got only 15 per cent of their calories from protein and 35 per cent from fat. That's about what most people get. Then they switched: carbohydrate consumption stayed the same, but their fat intake was decreased to 20 per cent of calories, and protein was doubled to 30 per cent. Throughout the experiment the participants were allowed to eat as much as they wanted – but they actually ate less. Over 14 weeks, they lost an average of 11lb (5kg), including 8lb (3.5kg) of body fat, thanks to the extra protein.

More protein and carbohydrates in moderation

No matter how you calculate it, we eat too many carbohydrates. We consume many more calories than we need to, and most of those extra calories come from extra carbs (so many chips, cakes and and biscuits). Therefore, it makes sense to cut back a little on carbs. It also makes sense to choose lower-GL carbohydrate foods instead of 'fast-acting' carbs that send your blood sugar soaring. These strategies are a big part of the *Magic Foods* approach to eating.

That approach, which we spell out in the next chapter, provides the benefits of a drastically low carb diet with none of the hazards. You'll get the blood-sugar advantages, including lower insulin levels. By eating plenty of lean protein, you'll feel satisfied and less hungry. And by choosing 'good' fats and limiting 'bad' ones, you'll keep LDL cholesterol from rising and protect your heart in the process. You'll also discover a way of eating that you can enjoy – rather than endure – for the rest of your life.

A breakthrough eating approach

4

Now that you know how important it is to eat foods that help to keep your blood sugar steady, you're probably wondering, 'So what's for dinner?' We've given you some strong hints already, but it's time to spell it all out so you know exactly how to eat the *Magic Foods* way. Get ready for an easy-to-follow, sugar-beating, health-enhancing diet. You'll feel so good on it, you'll never want to go back to your old way of eating again.

This is not a 'diet' in the usual sense. It's a delicious, practical, long-term strategy for healthy eating.

In this chapter, you'll discover the 'seven secrets of Magic eating' and how to put them to practical use. The great news is that it's easier than you may think. In fact, changing just a few of the foods you eat every day can help you to feel more energised and prevent the chronic diseases that slow us all down as we age.

This is not a 'diet' in the usual sense. It's a delicious, practical, long-term strategy for healthy eating. It will not only help to stabilise your blood sugar but it will also make it easier to leave that extra weight behind. The best part is that you can start by making as many or as few changes to your current diet as you like. You can decide to do only one or two new things – for instance, switching from white rice to brown rice and snacking on carrots instead of crisps – until you're ready for another change. Or you can be a bit more ambitious right from the start. Our aim is to give you the tools you need to eat for better blood sugar, to use as you wish.

With the *Magic Foods* approach to eating, you don't have to give up bread, although you will want to navigate the bread aisle carefully and eat a little less. You don't have to give up potatoes and white rice, although you'll definitely eat them more sparingly than you do now. You can also have pasta, in moderation (we'll explain which types are best for better blood sugar). And we encourage you to have cereal for breakfast – assuming it's one of the kinds we describe in this chapter.

You'll enjoy eating more protein-rich foods to keep you full and help keep your blood sugar low and steady. And while you'll say goodbye to unhealthy fats, your diet will actually contain plenty of fat in the form of 'good' fats to add appeal to meals and blunt the blood sugar effects of the carbs you eat.

Along the way, you'll learn a few clever tricks of the trade, such as how to finish your salad with a dressing that can lower the blood sugar impact of your entire meal, how to use a little-known Middle Eastern spice to pull the plug on blood sugar, which sour fruit has a sweet benefit and which little seeds pack a powerful health kick. We're not asking you to throw your current diet out of the window – just to tweak it a bit. Magic eating is really a series of very small, simple steps, such as adding a chopped apple to your porridge, choosing sourdough bread instead of regular white bread and making sweet potato fries your fries of choice (try them; you'll love them). Whether you make one change per meal, one change a day, or only one change in all, your blood sugar will benefit.

Although the changes are easy to make, the rewards are substantial. The benefits include more energy, less weight, a healthier heart, lower risk of diabetes, protection against certain cancers and a greatly improved quality of life.

The seven secrets of Magic eating

If you remember only one strategy from this book, remember the seven secrets of Magic eating. Some of them may sound unusual, while others seem like the tried and tested rules of healthy eating you already know about. But each one was chosen for a specific reason: to keep your blood sugar levels steady throughout the day. Here's a quick summary. You may even want to jot down the seven secrets and post them on your fridge as a daily reminder to keep you on the *Magic Foods* course. You'll read more about each of these secrets shortly.

1 **Choose low-GL carbs and limit carb portions** Carbohydrate-rich foods, especially grains and starchy vegetables, are the main contributors to high blood sugar. By choosing 'slow-acting' (low-GL) carbs instead of 'fast-acting' (higher-GL) carbs, you can help to keep blood sugar low and steady. You'll also want to limit your portions no matter what kind of carbs you choose.

2 **Make three of your carb servings whole grains** You're not eating as many carbs, so make sure that those you do eat count by always choosing whole grains. These nutritious foods

contain vitamins and fibre and are known to help prevent heart disease and diabetes independently of their effects on blood sugar.

3 **Eat more fruits and vegetables** Aim for at least seven to nine small servings a day. Most fruits and vegetables contain little carbohydrate and are packed with vitamins, fibre and health-protective compounds, with few calories. Eating fruits or adding vegetables to carbohydrate-rich dishes helps make your diet blood-sugar friendly.

4 **Eat protein at every meal** Protein lowers the GL of meals and helps curb hunger, making weight loss easier.

5 **Favour good fats** The 'bad' saturated fats can interfere with your ability to control blood sugar, but 'good' unsaturated fats help your body to control it better. Good fats also help to lower the GL of meals.

6 **Add acidic foods to your meals** It's an amazingly simple way to blunt the blood sugar effect of a meal.

7 **Eat smaller portions** We're not just talking about carb-rich foods here but about all foods. Even when you eat a low-GL diet, calories count. Cutting calories can help you to fight insulin resistance – and of course, along with exercise, it's still the way to lose weight.

secret 1 Choose low-GL carbs and limit carb portions

Most of the carbs we eat are the kind that send blood sugar soaring. We eat lots of potatoes, often fried as chips. We consume enormous quantities of bread in all forms, but most of it is bread that's made with refined white flour and has little fibre. We eat a lot of rice, most of it white. We treat ourselves to muffins, cakes and pastries made with white flour. We snack on bags of crisps and pretzels (pretzels are low in fat, but they're more or less just empty carbs). And we wash it all down with sugar-sweetened fizzy drinks and fruit drinks. If you're going to tackle your dietary weak points, this is the place to start. The good news is that it's relatively easy to make improvements. Because we eat so many of these foods to begin with, any change is a change for the better.

'Just say less'

One approach is to simply eat fewer of these high-GL foods. In the past decade or two, we've started to eat more calories, nearly all of them from carbohydrates – and nearly all of those carbohydrates are high GL. So it's time to rein in the carbohydrate mania: eat fewer salty snacks out of bags, fewer chips, less bread, fewer pastries, and cut right down on fizzy pop and other sweetened drinks. Ask yourself, 'Do I really need that sugar-coated cereal, that whole takeaway container of white rice, those chips on the 'side' (which take up half the plate), or that giant slice of leftover birthday cake?'

We're not talking about a 'just say no' policy but a much easier 'just say less' approach.

Let's say you start your day with a great big bowl of cornflakes or Rice Krispies or Cocoa Pops. If you measured how much you poured into the bowl, it would probably be at least twice the serving size suggested on the box. So the 'just say less' approach is to pour out less cereal. Fill the rest of the bowl with berries – low-GL fruits that will bring down the overall GL of your breakfast. And like many fruits, berries are rich in fibre that can help to fill you up and has other health benefits, too.

Go low GL

Even better, why not choose a lower-GL breakfast cereal? If you fill your bowl with a single serving of a medium-GL cereal – such as Grape-Nuts, Cheerios or Special K – instead of a high-GL one, your blood sugar will be lower after breakfast. And it'll be even lower if you choose a low-GL cereal, such as All-Bran, Bran Buds or muesli; or, if you like hot cereal, porridge. Keep watching portion size and slicing berries or an apple into your bowl, and you'll really lower your blood sugar response to breakfast. Plus, you'll give yourself a seriously healthy start to last until lunchtime, without that mid-morning slump.

If you like numbers, consider this: a 60g bowlful of Kellogg's Cornflakes has a GL of 48; a 30g bowlful of All-Bran cereal plus a whole medium apple has a GL of 15. That's more than two-thirds less. It means your blood sugar will rise two-thirds less as well.

Here's another example. For your evening meal, instead of a jacket potato, you might decide to make pasta as it has a lower GL. That's a good substitution. A 140g baked potato has a GL of 26; the same size serving of pasta has a GL of 17. So the switch itself lowers the GL of that side dish by 9 points, changing it from a 'high' to a 'medium' GL choice. You could serve the pasta with a little olive oil, freshly ground black pepper and a tablespoon of Parmesan cheese and never miss the potato at all.

Now, to lower the GL of your pasta side dish even further, you could cut some red peppers into strips, microwave them for a minute and toss them with the pasta, oil, pepper and cheese. Because the vegetables add volume to the dish, if you serve yourself the same 140g portion, you'll eat half as much pasta, so the GL of the dish has been cut in half – to 4.5. This means the GL of your side dish is only 20 per cent of what it would have been if you'd had the baked potato. When you put all this together, you reduce the rise in blood sugar by as much as 80 per cent!

Take a look at 'The glycaemic load of common foods' on page 55 and 'The magic carb pyramid' on page 43. Pick out a high-GL food that you eat frequently and figure out ways to eat less of it – such as substituting a low-GL or a medium-GL food for it and eating small portions. Now you're cooking.

A final note: even if you're choosing lower-GL foods, it's still important to watch your portion sizes. If you eat twice the recommended portion of the food, the GL will double. It's a simple concept, but one that many people miss. Even if you choose beans – a low-GL food – doubling the serving size will double the GL.

WHAT'S BOOSTING your blood sugar the most?

The best way to lower the GL of your diet is to figure out which high-GL foods you eat the most and then eat less of them, either by cutting back on portions or choosing different foods in their place.

In a study of middle-aged women, these five foods were the biggest contributors to GL in the diet. Together, they made up about 30 per cent of the GL of the women's diets. Try the healthier substitutions instead. Each of them has a GL that's at least 50 per cent lower than the food it replaces.

FOOD	PER CENT OF GL IN THE DIET	SMART SUBSTITUTION
Cooked potatoes	7.7	Pasta
Highly refined cereal	6.5	Porridge
White bread	5.2	Sourdough bread
Muffin	5.0	Apple
White rice	4.6	Lentils

For children, studies show that the biggest contributors to a high-GL diet are sweets, soft drinks, cakes, biscuits and salty snacks. So this age group require a different strategy. For them, encouraging fruits as snacks and low-fat milk as a beverage may be the best thing you can do.

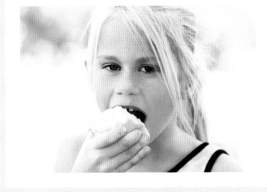

secret 2 Make three of your carb servings whole grains

If we are gorging ourselves on refined carbs, we're doing it largely at the expense of whole grains. And that's a shame because whole grains have many health benefits. There's clear, strong evidence that if you eat at least three servings of these foods a day, you'll substantially lower your risk of developing metabolic syndrome, diabetes, heart disease and cancer. Most of us, though, have less than one serving a day. Eating more whole grains has been shown to cut the risk of heart disease by 25 per cent in women and 18 per cent in men, while reducing the risk of diabetes by 35 per cent in both. One key way whole grains may protect against these diseases is by helping to prevent a root cause: metabolic syndrome (described on page 19).

In one study of more than 750 men and women over age 60, those who ate about three servings of whole grains a day were 54 per cent less likely to have metabolic syndrome than people who ate less than one serving a day. Their fasting blood sugar levels were lower, and they tended to have less body fat. They also had 52 per cent fewer fatal heart attacks. In fact, just six weeks on a whole grain diet can markedly improve insulin sensitivity, according to one study of overweight men and women.

Whole grains are good for us because they contain all the parts of the grain, not just the starchy low-fibre centre (endosperm) but also the nutrient-rich germ layer and the outer fibre-rich bran layer. Whole grains are packed with fibre, antioxidants, vitamins, minerals and a wide range of plant compounds that protect against chronic disease in many different ways.

Most whole grains have lower GLs than most refined grains, but there are exceptions. Finely milled 100 per cent wholemeal bread, for instance, actually has a fairly high GL, while some refined foods, such as pastas made from white semolina flour, have medium GLs. In general, though, you're better off with whole grains, which offer benefits to blood sugar that are totally unrelated to their GLs.

When it comes to the grain-based carbohydrates you eat, don't be a perfectionist. As long as you get three servings of whole grains a day, there's room for some refined grain foods, especially if they're low GL. Just watch portion sizes no matter what kind you're eating.

How many carbs should you eat in total? In the *Magic Foods* approach, your goal is to get 45 to 55 per cent of your calories from carbs every day. Turn to the 'Magic meal plans' in Part 4 to see what this looks like in an actual menu.

WHAT COUNTS AS whole grain?

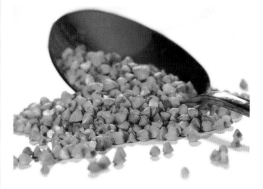

■ **Bread** with the word whole in the first ingredient (such as whole-grain wheat)

■ **Brown rice**

■ **Whole-grain barley** (pearl barley isn't technically a whole grain, but it is good for you)

■ **Oats**

■ **Wholemeal pasta**

■ **Popcorn**

■ **Oatcakes**

■ **Exotic grains**, including amaranth, buckwheat, and quinoa

THE NEW BLOOD SUGAR SOLUTION

42

THE MAGIC
carb pyramid

CHOOSE least often

- potatoes
- chips
- white bread
- overcooked pasta
- Japanese udon noodles
- white rice
- sticky rice
- rice-based cereal
- cornflakes
- millet
- bagel
- most baked goods
- non-diet fizzy drinks
- sweetened fruit drinks
- dried dates
- raisins

CHOOSE more often

- basmati rice
- wild rice
- brown rice
- bulghur wheat
- pasta cooked *al dente*
- wholemeal pasta
- rye crispbread
- chocolate milk
- apple juice
- pineapple juice
- dried figs
- bananas
- sweet potatoes
- black-eyed peas
- whole-grain cereals
- low-sugar cereals
- whole-grain and sourdough bread

CHOOSE most often

- coarse barley bread
- whole-grain pumpernickel
- pearl barley
- porridge
- bran cereal
- muesli
- rye bread
- split peas
- low-fat milk
- oatcakes
- tomato juice
- prunes
- dried apricots
- popcorn
- yoghurt
- most vegetables (except potatoes)
- lentils
- beans (except black-eyed peas)
- most fresh fruits (and 100% fruit juice if limited to 180ml)

secret 3 Eat more fresh fruits and vegetables

It's no secret that fruits and vegetables are good for you. You probably already know some of their health benefits, such as lower blood pressure and lower risk of heart disease, diabetes, stroke and certain cancers. You may even know that eating fresh produce can reduce your risk of losing your vision as you age. Yes, fruits and vegetables are rich in vitamins, thousands of health-protective compounds and fibre.

But did you know that eating more of them is a key strategy in losing weight and keeping it off? With the exception of a few starchy vegetables, the vast majority are very low in calories. That's largely because they're mostly made up of water and fibre (both of which have no calories). Studies consistently show that the more fruits and vegetables people eat, the less they tend to weigh.

It can be as simple as eating a salad. In one study at Pennsylvania State University, women who started a meal with a low-calorie salad and then ate a pasta dish consumed about 12 per cent fewer calories in total than women who skipped the salad and started with the pasta. In another study, adding about 170g of vegetables (in this case, carrots and spinach) to dinner helped people feel fuller on fewer calories.

With a few exceptions, there is no need to avoid this fruit or that vegetable because it contains sugar or will raise your blood sugar. Most fruits and vegetables are actually quite low in total carbohydrates and contain fibre – often the soluble fibre that slows blood sugar's rise – so their GLs are quite low. So feel free to snack on apples and pile your plate with vegetables.

Foiling high-GL carbs

You'll lower the GL of a typical portion of any carb dish by mixing in almost any vegetable or fruit (again, potatoes don't count). If you add tomatoes, carrots and spinach to a pasta salad, for example, you'll eat less pasta. If you add chopped broccoli to a rice side dish, you'll eat less rice; the same goes for adding strawberries to hot or cold cereal. And fewer carbs equals lower blood sugar.

Let's consider a rice side dish. A portion of 180g of cooked long-grain white rice has a GL of 23, making it a high-GL food. But the same weight of boiled dried peas has a GL of only 3, so if you mix an equal amount of peas with the rice, a 150g portion of the side dish would have a GL of only 13, changing it from a high- to a medium-GL food. Really, mixing any vegetable into your rice – chopped cooked onions or carrots or asparagus – similarly lowers its GL.

Snack perfection

Whole fruit is almost always a good snack choice. For example, a 50g pack of potato crisps has a GL of 14 – making it a medium-GL food (but only if you eat this much and no more). But a medium peach or plum has a GL of only 5, and the GL of a similar sized apple is 6. Plus, you're eating twice as much food, so which do you think is likely to satisfy your hunger best? Even if you ate a plum, a peach and an apple, the GL would be only 16. On the other hand, if you munched your way through 100g of crisps, the GL for your snack would be a much bigger 28.

Raw veggies are also Magic snacks, dipped in low-fat sour cream, low-fat dressing, or one of the bean dips on pages 206–209. Pack some carrot sticks or cherry tomatoes in a sandwich bag and you'll have no reason to hit the vending machine – very likely devoid of Magic foods – in the afternoon. Fill up on veggies of different colours, since different hues indicate different health-protective compounds. You don't want to miss out on any!

You'll find plenty of tips for adding specific fruits and vegetables to your meals in Part 2, where the book

Studies show that the more fruits and vegetables people eat, the less they tend to weigh.

introduces you to all the Magic foods. And it's important to have plenty of them, particularly the non-starchy fruits and vegetables.

A few exceptions

Just about all fresh garden produce is good for us, but certain types aren't as good for our blood sugar. When we tell you to eat more fruits and veggies, we're talking about colourful veggies (not starchy vegetables or potatoes) and fresh, whole fruit. Here's the low-down.

■ **Potatoes** These are the big exception: they're dense in easily absorbed carbohydrates, so their GL is quite high. In fact, the more potatoes, including chips, that people eat, the higher their risk of diabetes. Many nutritionists think potatoes should be classified with grains rather than with vegetables, and even then they're at the top of the carbohydrate pyramid.

■ **Other starchy vegetables** Sweet potatoes and winter squash are rich in carotenoids and other important nutrients as well as fibre, which is also beneficial. But they're also high in carbohydrates, although their carbs aren't as easily absorbed as those in white potatoes. That makes them a better choice than white potatoes, and we include some delicious recipes for them in Part 4. But, as with other carbohydrate-rich foods, watch your portion size.

■ **Dried fruits** Drying concentrates the sugars in fruit and can make for intensely calorific treats. It's fine to have some raisins, dried plums, dates, figs and apricots, but don't overindulge in them. Consider what happens when grapes (GL 8) turn into raisins (GL 28) or plums (GL 5) turn into dried prunes (GL 10). A handful, or 60g, of dried dates has a whopping GL of 25.

■ **Juices** By drinking just the juice, you'll miss out on most of the fibre and some of the vitamins in the whole fruit, and you'll get a lot more calories and a higher GL. If you eat 125g of fresh pineapple, for example, the GL is 6. But if you drink a small glass (180ml) of pineapple juice, the GL is 12. The same is true for an orange (GL 5) versus a small glass of juice (GL 10), and for grapefruit (GL 3) versus a small glass of

WHAT ABOUT
tropical fruits?

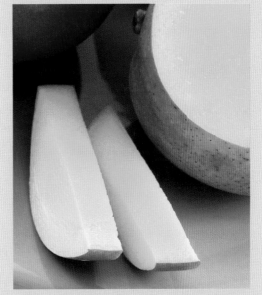

Some nutritionists warn against tropical fruits, which can be starchy, but on the whole these foods are good for you. It's true that bananas are starchy and are a medium-GL fruit, while nearly all others are low GL, so you shouldn't overeat them, but don't exclude them either. And mangoes, which are extraordinarily nutritious (and oh, so good), have been given a bad reputation, but they are low GL, so keep them on the menu. Papayas are fine, too, as are pineapple and watermelon. Coconut isn't the best choice, but this has nothing to do with GL; it's high in saturated fat, which is bad for the heart and insulin sensitivity.

grapefruit juice (GL 7). And if you go for a large sweetened fruit drink, the GL soars: a 375ml glass of cranberry juice cocktail has a GL of 36. So when you drink juices, be careful to keep portions small, and make sure they're unsweetened (read the labels carefully).

THE MAGIC
protein pyramid

CHOOSE least often

- marbled beef
- mince
- pork ribs
- sausage
- bacon

- corned beef
- salami
- hot dogs
- chicken with skin
- whole milk

- butter
- cream
- full-fat cheese

CHOOSE more often

- lean beef
- extra-lean mince
- lean pork

- lean ham
- lean lamb
- rabbit

CHOOSE most often

- poultry without skin
- fish and shellfish
- soya foods (tofu)
- nuts
- seeds

- low-fat cheese
- skimmed or semi-skimmed milk
- fat-free or low-fat yoghurt
- eggs

- split peas
- lentils
- green peas
- all dried beans (except black-eyed peas)

secret 4 Eat protein at every meal

If you want to control your blood sugar and your weight, be sure to get enough protein. A moderately high protein diet may get as much as 30 per cent of its calories from protein, rather than the 15 to 20 per cent most people get. In the *Magic Foods* approach, 20 to 30 per cent of the calories you eat should come from protein.

Protein has little or no effect on your blood sugar, so whenever you mix protein-rich foods with carbohydrate-rich foods, you automatically lower the GL of each portion. But protein has other benefits, as you saw in Chapters 2 and 3. It helps to keep hunger at bay between meals. And if you're trying to lose weight, taking in more protein will help your body to hold on to its calorie-burning muscle tissue so the weight comes off more easily.

There's no need to go overboard, though. A serving of a protein-rich food such as chicken breast or sirloin steak should be a mere 60 to 85g, although a more typical portion is 170g. The main thing to focus on is having at least a small portion of a protein-rich food at every meal (and as part of as many snacks as you can). It can be a side dish of beans, a glass of skimmed milk, a slice or two of lean turkey, a small amount of sirloin steak in a stir-fry, a snack of unsweetened yoghurt, or a handful of nuts. Among the list of Magic foods in Part 2, you'll find these excellent protein sources.

■ **Beans, lentils and peas** These 'vegetarian' sources of protein are excellent. They have essentially no saturated fat and they're very low GL, largely because they contain so much soluble fibre. And they also contain a lot of minerals. Try to eat meals based on these foods at least once or twice a week.

■ **Soya foods** Like beans, these are low saturated-fat, low-GL, high-protein foods. Try a stir-fry with tofu; experiment with soya milk on your cereal

SNEAKING IN protein
It's easy to add protein to your meals and snacks. A little here and there soon adds up.

■ Starting the day with whole-grain toast? Instead of buttering it, spread it with a tablespoon of peanut butter.

■ Making a salad? Toss in some chickpeas or leftover chicken.

■ Centre your lunch around bean soup, either vegetarian or flavoured with a little pork.

■ Buy single-serving packs of nuts to take to work for a quick snack.

■ Keep some hard-boiled eggs in your fridge as snacks or easy protein-rich additions to salads and sandwiches.

■ Keep soya-based veggie burgers in your freezer for quick dinners or high-protein, meaty boosts to pasta sauce (just crumble them into the sauce).

■ When summer berries are in season (or frozen berries are on sale), make a quick smoothie with fat-free yoghurt, a good protein source.

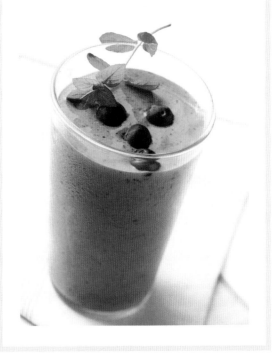

(it tastes better than it once did, so give it a chance); and grill some tempeh, a textured soya-bean product with a nutty flavour. Or stock up on frozen soya-based vegetarian burgers.

■ **Nuts and seeds** It's hard to find a protein-rich snack, but nuts are one of the few. These little nuggets serve up not only protein but also healthy fats. Just stick to a handful as they're high in calories.

■ **Fish and shellfish** All fish and shellfish are low in saturated fat, so they're excellent protein choices. Oil-rich fish are also rich in omega-3 fatty acids, which help to prevent heart disease and may improve insulin sensitivity. You'll make a good choice either way: low-fat fish such as cod and haddock are sources of low saturated-fat protein, while fattier fish such as wild salmon and rainbow trout provide both protein and omega-3s. For a healthy heart, aim for two or three servings of fish or shellfish a week.

■ **Chicken and turkey** These are also low in saturated fat and quite low in calories if you choose white meat without the skin.

■ **Eggs** Eggs are nutritious and versatile. A large egg has only 1.5g of saturated fat, and even though it's high in cholesterol, an egg a day won't raise most adults' cholesterol levels. Have eggs for breakfast or enjoy an egg salad sandwich on whole-grain bread with low-fat mayonnaise. A hard-boiled egg is a good high-protein snack.

■ **Red meat** Beef, pork, lamb and other red meats are major contributors to saturated fat in our diets, but that doesn't mean you can't eat them. The key is to choose the leanest cuts, which have more protein – and less saturated fat. And don't eat red meat every day; leave room for meals centred on fish, beans and so on.

■ **Dairy foods** Skimmed or semi-skimmed milk, low-fat or fat-free yoghurt and low-fat cheeses contribute high-quality protein with very little saturated fat. Like all dairy foods, they're high in calcium, a key mineral. But full-fat cheeses, along with butter and high-fat dairy desserts such as ice cream, are major contributors to saturated fat in our diets. Have milk and other dairy products every day, but stick to low-fat products.

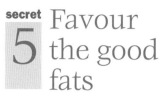

secret 5 Favour the good fats

With all the emphasis on low-fat foods in recent years, you might think we'd be advocating a low-fat diet. But we're not. Instead of following a low-fat diet, which is almost by necessity a high-carbohydrate diet, you can get as much as 35 per cent of your calories from fat in the *Magic Foods* approach. Look at the Magic meal plans in Part 4 to see what this amount looks like.

Fat, as you found out in Chapter 2, isn't all bad, especially where your blood sugar is concerned. Fat doesn't raise blood sugar, and it doesn't require insulin in order to be metabolised, so it doesn't raise insulin levels either. Its GL is zero. Because it slows the rate at which food leaves your stomach, it can blunt the blood sugar effect of a whole meal, even if that meal includes carbs.

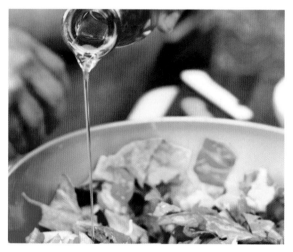

Including fat-rich foods in your meals can also help your body to metabolise carbohydrates better – provided they're the right fats. That means monounsaturated fat (the kind in olive oil, nuts and avocados) and omega-3 fatty acids (found in oil-rich fish) instead of saturated fat (the kind in red meat and dairy foods). Good fats are remarkable because they can actually help to reverse insulin resistance (*see* page 30). Saturated fat, on the other hand, not only raises 'bad' LDL cholesterol and increases heart disease risk, but we now know that it increases insulin resistance, too. Opting for good fats means eating fish at least once a week; adding avocado instead of full-fat cheese to your salads; mixing your pasta salad with, say, olive oil and toasted walnuts instead of salad cream. Adding good fats to foods means each portion will have a lower GL.

Making the switch

If you're used to steaks and butter, how do you make the switch to better fats? With these steps.

■ **Cut back on the major sources of saturated fat in your diet** Start by identifying them: look at the top tier of 'The Magic fats pyramid' below and 'The top 10 sources of saturated fat' on page 51. How often do you eat these foods? What single change do you think you could make in

THE MAGIC
fats pyramid

CHOOSE least often

- marbled beef
- fatty red meats
- butter
- cream
- full-fat cheese

- whole milk
- ice cream
- solid shortening
- solid margarine
- lard

- hydrogenated vegetable oils
- coconut oil
- crème fraîche

CHOOSE more often

- corn oil
- soybean oil
- safflower oil

CHOOSE most often

- sunflower oil
- olive oil
- rapeseed oil
- nuts

- nut oils
- seeds
- flaxseeds (linseeds)
- oil-rich fish

- avocados

FATS at a glance

THE GOOD FATS

Monounsaturated fats: in olive oil, rapeseed oil, avocados, peanuts, almonds, cashews and most other nuts. When they replace saturated fats, they have a beneficial effect on cholesterol and help to reverse insulin resistance.

Omega-3 fats: oil-rich fish. Related fats, which the body can convert – to a degree – into the more active form found in fish, are found in flaxseed and canola oil. Omega-3 fats, especially from fish, help to prevent heart disease and may improve insulin sensitivity.

Polyunsaturated fats: corn, soya bean and safflower oils can be beneficial, but most of us already get plenty of polyunsaturated fats. You're much more likely to need more monounsaturated fat in your diet.

THE BAD FATS

Saturated fats: red meats; full-fat dairy foods; and a few vegetable oils, such as coconut oil. These increase levels of 'bad' LDL cholesterol in the blood, promote heart disease and reduce insulin sensitivity.

Trans fats: solid margarine, vegetable shortening, partially hydrogenated vegetable oils and many deep-fried snacks, fast foods, and refined baked goods. They raise 'bad' LDL cholesterol, lower 'good' HDL cholesterol, increase heart disease risk, and may increase insulin resistance.

the next week – using a leaner sandwich meat at lunch, having steak instead of ribs, choosing low-fat frozen yogurt instead of ice cream? Make that one change, and when you have, start thinking about your next one. Work toward eating more foods from the bases (and middle tiers) of the fat and protein pyramids – and much fewer from the top tiers. Just cutting back on cheese, full-fat yogurt and regular sour cream – or choosing low-fat substitutes – can substantially reduce the amount of saturated fat you eat with very little effort. So can switching from whole milk to semi-skimmed milk.

■ **Avoid trans fats** Over half the products on supermarket shelves may contain trans fats. All packaged foods in the USA must list the levels of trans fats on the label but this is not necessary in Europe. Hydrogenated and partially hydrogenated fats are usually listed, however. If an item contains these you can assume it contains trans fats and is best avoided.

■ **Eat more non-meat protein** We're talking beans, lentils, peas and soya foods. By swapping a few meat-based meals a week for vegetarian options, you can go a long way toward building a healthier diet. Aim for one new vegetarian meal each week for a month. Ultimately, turn it into a lifetime habit.

■ **Eat fish or shellfish twice a week** It can be fresh, canned or frozen. Experiment with different cooking methods but avoid fried and battered fish. As a start, try our recipe suggestions in Part 4.

■ **When you eat red meat, choose lean cuts** It can make a big difference in how much saturated fat you get and you won't need to sacrifice taste. For example, 85g of cooked regular minced beef has 6g of saturated fat, while the same amount of extra-lean minced beef has only 2.5g.

■ **Cook and season with olive oil** Use it for sautéing, grilling and roasting; as an ingredient in salad dressings; or drizzled over vegetables, grains and fish. Reach for the olive oil instead of butter whenever you cook. You'll hardly notice the difference in most foods and making this change can dramatically decrease the amount of

Certain acidic foods, though, such as vinegar (acetic acid), seem to work in additional ways, making them more effective. So dispense with those creamy salad dressings and buy or make dressings that combine vinegar with olive oil, such as vinaigrette. It takes just a tablespoon of vinegar per serving to substantially lower the GL of a meal.

Eat a small green salad drizzled with vinaigrette before lunch or dinner several times a week. You'll get some acetic acid in your meals and squeeze more vegetables into your diet. But don't stop there. Soak fish in vinegar and water before cooking; it'll be sweeter and more tender and hold its shape better. When poaching fish, toss a tablespoon of vinegar into the simmering water. Make a vinegar-based marinade for meat destined for the grill. Mix in a little vinegar when cooking canned soup to perk it up and add some to the water in which you simmer vegetables. See the Vinegar entry in Part 2 for more suggestions.

If you like Japanese food and you're having sushi, you can feel a little better about the rice, as sushi rice is made with rice wine vinegar.

saturated fat you add to your diet. If you crave the taste of butter in a dish, add a teaspoon or two to olive oil to impart that buttery flavour.

■ **Make rapeseed oil your second choice** Use it for a more neutral taste when frying and in baking. It's very versatile yet low in saturated fat.

■ **Add more nuts, seeds and avocado to your menus** You can add nuts to practically any main dish or baked item, while avocado is an easy addition to salads and sandwiches. Or simply carve up a few slices of avocado, drizzle with lemon juice and enjoy as a snack. See the Nuts and Avocado entries in Part 2.

secret 6 Add some acidic foods to your meals

As you discovered in Chapter 2, even a few acidic ingredients can lower your blood sugar response to a carbohydrate-rich meal. Making foods more acidic slows the breakdown of starches into blood sugar, so your blood sugar rises more slowly.

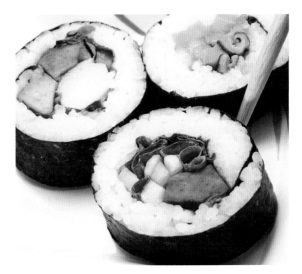

More ways to add acids

These tips will also add bite to your meals.

■ **Use mustard,** which is made with vinegar, instead of mayonnaise on sandwiches, as a base to coat chicken and meats, and in bean dishes.

■ **Eat that pickle** with your sandwich. It gets its sour taste from vinegar.

■ **Go beyond pickled cucumbers** and try pickled tomatoes, carrots, celery, broccoli, cauliflower florets and red and green peppers. If you're at a Japanese restaurant, ask for a side helping of oshinko (pickled vegetables).

■ **Don't throw out the pickle liquid** It makes an excellent marinade, especially when mixed with a little olive oil and chopped fresh herbs.

■ **Eat sauerkraut,** which is pickled cabbage. Look for low-salt varieties.

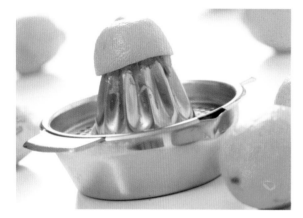

■ **Squeeze lemon juice,** which is also acidic, over fish and seafood. Fresh lemon juice can add zest to a soup or stew, green vegetables, rice and chicken.

■ **Try lime juice** on fish, turkey, avocados, melon, sweet potatoes and black beans.

■ **Eat more citrus fruit** such as fresh grapefruit, which, as your tongue has already told you, is somewhat acidic.

■ **Ask for sourdough bread** As the dough ferments, it releases lactic acid, which, like vinegar, has a beneficial effect on the food's GL.

■ **Cook with wine** It's acidic, too, and gives a tasty tang to sauces, stews, soups and roasts. Try cooking fish in wine: sauté garlic (and onions if you like) in olive oil, add seasoning, then pour in some wine and reduce the heat. Add the fish and cook in the simmering liquid. Squeeze in a little lemon juice at the end.

■ **Drink wine with your dinner** It's another way to include an acidic liquid with your meal. Drinking wine (as well as other alcoholic beverages) in moderation – a glass a day for women, up to two for men – can help to keep blood insulin levels low and is linked with a lower risk of developing diabetes. Moderate alcohol consumption also raises 'good' HDL cholesterol levels and helps protect against heart disease. (If you have diabetes, check with your doctor first.)

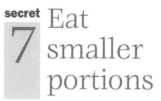

secret 7 Eat smaller portions

We've already stressed the importance of dishing out smaller portions of fast-acting carb foods, such as mashed potatoes and rice, and even slower-acting foods such as whole-grain cereal. But portion sizes count for practically everything you eat – because calories are significant.

Eating fewer calories is one of the best ways to improve your insulin sensitivity. You'll do better if you go ahead and lower the GL of your overall diet, with the help of the Magic foods in this book, but simply eating less also helps by improving your insulin sensitivity (which ultimately lowers your blood sugar). It does this even if you don't lose weight. But of course, eating less does help you to shed pounds – another key element in preventing insulin resistance, diabetes and heart disease.

So where should you cut back on calories? Everywhere. Carbohydrates are, of course, a main target, especially high-GL carbs such as rice, fizzy drinks and white bread. So is anything you tend to eat to excess. Yes, we want you to make protein a part of every meal, but that doesn't mean that gorging on a doorstep-sized steak is okay. Just 170g of a lean sirloin is plenty. We also recommend eating nuts, but again, not too many. About 25 almonds (weighing 30g) has about 165kcal. That's fine. But be vigilant with your portions as it can be tempting to go on picking at nuts and, before you know it, you've eaten three times as much, taking in 500kcal – more than you should get from an entire meal.

WHAT DOES A
serving look like?

Here are some images to keep in mind. Each is one serving.

An 85g serving of cooked meat is the size of a deck of cards.

An 85 g serving of fish is the size of a cheque book.

A 30g portion of cheese is the size of a small matchbox.

A 30g serving of sliced cheese is the diameter of a CD.

A 50g portion of pasta or rice is a pile the size of a computer mouse.

A medium baked potato is the size of a regular bar of soap.

Two tablespoons of peanut butter are the size of a ping-pong ball.

Two tablespoons of salad dressing are the size of a shot glass.

A 180ml serving of juice is the size of a small yoghurt container.

A medium piece of fruit, such as an apple, is the size of a tennis ball.

Few of us have the room in our diets to eat that many extra calories without gaining weight, which increases insulin resistance. Olive oil is great for your heart and your blood sugar, but don't soak your bread in it. At 119kcal per tablespoon, you won't want to consume more than 1 or 2 tablespoons a day.

Fortunately, there's one category of food that doesn't require much portion control: non-starchy fruits and vegetables. It's quite difficult to eat too many apples, carrots, tomatoes, salad greens or raspberries. They'll fill you up, with few calories and a low GL, and take the place of more caloric foods.

How much should you eat?

Of course, the answer to this depends on how much you currently weigh and how active you are. If you know approximately how many calories you want to aim for each day, see our Magic meal plans in Part 4 to get a good sense of how much food this means.

Not sure how many calories you need each day? Nutritionists have calculated that to lose 1lb (500g) of fat in a week you must create a deficit of 3500kcal (about 500kcal a day). So most women should be able to lose weight by restricting their energy intake to 1400kcal/day and most men by restricting their energy intake to 2000kcal/day.

It's worth keeping a food diary for a few days to see how many calories you're really eating; the number may well be more than you think (and aren't you a little curious?). Use the nutrition labels on packaged foods to find out the calories per serving (be careful; some packages contain two servings, so you'll have to double that number if you eat the whole thing). For fresh foods, use a website such as: www.calorie-count.com, www.thecaloriecounter.com, www.nal.usda.gov/fnic/foodcomp/search or www.calorieking.com to get the calorie counts of common foods.

Another way to understand and control portion sizes is to train your eye to identify what a reasonable serving looks like (*see* 'What does a serving look like?', above). Bring these images to mind when you're serving food, ordering food, and of course, eating food. The serving sizes are quite small, so don't feel bad if your portion is twice as large. A serving of pasta or rice should be about 50g, but most people eat twice that. It takes a little time to retrain our eyes. Most of us need no more than six servings of grains a day –

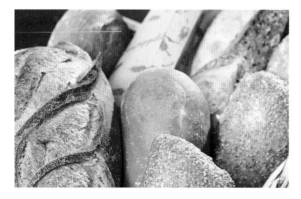

preferably low or medium-GL grains – so if you're eating three or four servings at a sitting, that's too much. A single dense roll or bagel can equal six servings of grains – a day's worth.

A serving of meat or chicken is about 85g, but most people can eat two servings a day – the size of two decks of cards.

Cutting back

Unfortunately, in this age of super-size servings, we've been trained to eat a lot. If you want to be healthier, it's up to you to fight back.

Start by putting less food on your plate or in your bowl. Studies show that when large portions are put in front of us, most of us eat more – often 50 per cent more at a single meal. Put your meals on plates in the kitchen rather than putting a big plate or bowl on the table for everyone to dig into at will. Buy small single-portion bags of snacks rather than eating out of a big bag (which always disappears). If you do buy a big bag, dole out a reasonable portion onto a small plate or a napkin, then close the bag and put it away out of sight before you sit down to munch.

When you're eating out, order smaller dishes (don't be afraid to order from the children's menu at fast-food restaurants) or ask the waiter to put half the dish in a doggie bag before you start to eat. It's also a good idea to share one main dish and a separate dish of vegetables or share one main dish and fill up with a salad or soup.

In general, though, try to eat most of your meals at home. It's much easier to control your calorie intake as well as the amount of fat and number of high-GL foods that go into your meal.

Putting it all together

Are you ready to eat the *Magic Foods* way? In the first chapter, you learned how important it is to your health and well-being to eat in ways that keep your blood sugar levels stable throughout the day. In the second chapter, you found out what makes certain foods send your blood sugar, soaring, while others keep it humming steadily. In the third chapter, you learned the pitfalls of a quick-fix low-carb approach. And now you've learned the seven secrets of magic eating. In the next chapter, you'll quiz yourself to see where your diet stands now, discover some fixes for your dietary downfalls, and find out some sensible strategies for eating out.

Then it's on to the real meat of the book (lean meat, of course). In Part 2, you'll find profiles of the 57 Magic foods, from apples to yoghurt. Each profile tells you the GL of the food (either very low, low, or medium; you won't find Magic foods with a high or very high GL) plus other important health benefits it offers. You'll also learn the proper portion size – because remember, portions count – as well as menu suggestions and cooking tips.

In Part 3, the 'Magic meal makeovers' show you how to make simple changes to your breakfasts, lunches, snacks, dinners and desserts to help you to make your meals more blood-sugar friendly without a lot of fuss.

To help you to put Magic eating into action, in Part 4 we've supplied more than 100 Magic recipes. These make low-GL cooking come alive, incorporating the Magic foods in clever, simple and delicious ways. Each recipe includes full nutritional information, but you don't have to worry about that if you don't want to; we've made sure the dishes are good for your blood sugar.

You'll even find meal plans that fit these recipes into a week's worth of eating based on three different calorie goals to help you to manage your weight. All the tools you need are at your fingertips. So what are you waiting for?

THE GLYCAEMIC LOAD
of common foods

The GL is the best measure of a food's effect on blood sugar. Here, we've listed some common foods and grouped them into three categories: low GL (10 and under), medium GL (11 to 19) and high GL (20 and up). You should aim for as many low-GL foods as possible and eat high-GL foods more sparingly.

Because carbohydrate foods are the ones that contribute most to the GL of your diet, we've focused on those foods here. Foods that are mostly protein or fat – such as meats, fish and cheeses – have little or no GL, so you won't find many of them in this list, although you will find them in the Magic foods entries in Part 2. Including protein-rich foods and 'good' fats in your meals and snacks will help keep your GL score for the day moderate. Remember that portion size makes a big difference: if you eat two servings of a medium-GL breakfast cereal, it suddenly qualifies as a high-GL food. On the other hand, if you just love a food in the high-GL category, go ahead and eat a small portion, preferably along with a small portion of a low or medium-GL food.

 LOW (GL = 10 or less)

Breads, tortillas, grains	Serving size	GL
Soya and flaxseed (linseed) bread	2 slices	10
Whole-grain pumpernickel bread	2 slices	10
Pearl barley	160g	8
Popcorn	15g	8
Wheat tortillas	15cm	6
Breakfast cereals	Serving size	GL
Muesli	30g	10
Porridge	30g (dry weight)	10
All Bran	30g	9
Bran Buds	30g	7
Porridge made from rolled oats	30g (dry weight)	7
Beans and peas	Serving size	GL
Lima beans	250g (cooked)	10
Pinto beans	250g (cooked)	10
Chickpeas	250g (cooked)	8
Baked beans	250g (cooked)	7
Haricot beans	250g (cooked)	7
Kidney beans	250g (cooked)	7
Butter beans	250g (cooked)	6
Green peas	145g (cooked)	6

GL **LOW (GL = 10 OR LESS)**

Beans and peas	Serving size	GL
Split peas, yellow	200g (cooked)	6
Lentils, green or red	200g (cooked)	5

Dairy and soya drinks	Serving size	GL
Low-fat yoghurt with fruit and sugar	200ml	9
Soya milk	250ml	7
Low-fat chocolate milk, sweetened with aspartame	250ml	3
Low-fat yoghurt with fruit, sweetened with aspartame	200ml	2

Fruits and Vegetables	Serving size	GL
Prunes, pitted, chopped	60g	10
Apricots, dried, chopped	60g	9
Peaches, canned in light syrup	125g	9
Grapes, medium bunch (about 50)	125g	8
Mango, sliced	125g	8
Pineapple, diced	125g	7
Apple	1 small	6
Kiwi fruit, sliced	125g	6
Beets, sliced	85g	5
Orange	1 small	5
Peach	1 small	5
Plums	2 small	5
Pear	1 small	4
Strawberries	about 6 medium	4
Watermelon, chopped	125g	4
Carrot, raw	1 large	3
Cherries	125g	3
Grapefruit	½	3

Beverages	Serving size	GL
Orange juice, unsweetened	180ml	10
Grapefruit juice, unsweetened	180ml	7
Tomato juice	180ml	4

Sweets	Serving size	GL
M&Ms with peanuts	30g	6
Nutella (chocolate hazelnut spread)	4 tbsp	4

Nuts	Serving size	GL
Mixed nuts, roasted	45g	4
Cashew nuts	about 13 (45g)	3
Peanuts	45g	1

MEDIUM (GL = 11–19)

Bread, tortillas, crackers, crisps	Serving size	GL
High-fibre white bread	2 slices	18
Crisps	50g	14
100% whole-grain bread	2 slices	14
Sourdough rye bread	2 slices	12
Stone-ground wheat thins	4	12
Corn tortillas	15cm	11
Rye crispbreads	2½	11
Grains	Serving size	GL
Brown rice	130g (cooked)	18
Quinoa	120g (cooked)	16
Wild rice	110g (cooked)	18
Basmati rice	100g (cooked)	24
Bulghur	120g (cooked)	12
Pasta	Serving size	GL
Spaghetti (cooked 15 minutes)	140g (cooked)	17
Wholemeal spaghetti	140g (cooked)	13
High-protein spaghetti	140g (cooked)	12
Beverages	Serving size	GL
Low-fat chocolate milk	250ml	12
Pineapple juice, unsweetened	180ml	12
Apple juice	250ml	8
Fruits, vegetables, beans	Serving size	GL
Sweetcorn	160g	18
Sweet potato	1 medium (140g)	17
Figs, dried, chopped	60g	16
Banana	1 small (125g)	11
Black beans	250g (cooked)	11
Breakfast cereals	Serving size	GL
Grape-Nuts	30g	16
Cheerios	30g	15
Fruit and Fibre	30g	14
Special K	30g	14

GL high | HIGH (GL = 20 or higher)

Potatoes	Serving size	GL
Baked potato	1 medium	26
French fries	140g	22
Grains	**Serving size**	**GL**
Sticky white rice	125g (cooked)	31
Millet	116g (cooked)	25
Couscous	105g (cooked)	23
Long-grain white rice	100g (cooked)	23
Pasta	**Serving size**	**GL**
Japanese Udon noodles	115g cooked	25
Spaghetti (cooked 20 minutes)	140g	22
Breads	**Serving size**	**GL**
French baguette	2 slices	30
Middle Eastern flatbread	1 large	30
Italian white bread	2 slices	22
Hamburger roll	1	21
Light rye bread	2 slices	20
Mini-bagel	1	20
White bread	2 slices	20
Breakfast Cereals	**Serving size**	**GL**
Cornflakes	30g	24
Coco Pops	30g	20
Rice Krispies	30g	22
Dried Fruit	**Serving size**	**GL**
Raisins	50g	28
Dates, dried, chopped	50g	25
Sultanas	50g	20
Beverages	**Serving size**	**GL**
Ocean Spray Cranberry Juice Cocktail	375ml	36
Coca-Cola	375ml	24
Sweets	**Serving size**	**GL**
Mars Bar	60g	26
Jelly beans	20	22
Betty Crocker chocolate cake with chocolate icing	125g	20

Sources: "International Table of Glycemic Index and Glycemic Load Values 2002," Kaye Foster-Powell, Susanna H. A. Holt, and Janette C. Brand-Miller, American Journal of Clinical Nutrition vol. 76, no. 1 (2002), 5–56. Additional data from www.glycemicindex.com, www.mypyramid.gov, www.ars.usda.gov.

The *Magic Foods* approach in action

5

Now that you're armed with the seven secrets of Magic eating – described in full in the last chapter – where do you go from here? Trying to modify your diet may appear to be a difficult task – particularly if you've tried numerous diets before – but this book will show you that it doesn't have to be, especially if you make one tiny change at a time. A good first step is to take stock of your eating habits and find out what you're doing right – and where you could possibly make some small adjustments.

You'll be amazed *how the simple act of acknowledging your eating habits can make you more open to changing them.*

How Magic is YOUR DIET?

Circle the **number** next to your answer for each question, then add up your **score**. Turn to page 62 to see how you did.

1 If you were in my kitchen in the morning, you'd see me drinking:

a Coffee or tea, plain or with low-fat milk and/or a little sugar or sugar substitute — 1

b Coffee or tea with full-fat cream and/or loads of sugar — 2

c A soft drink — 3

2 When I eat cereal for breakfast, I'm most likely to pick one like:

a Cornflakes, Rice Krispies or Coco Pops — 3

b Grape-Nuts or Cheerios — 2

c All Bran, Bran Buds or muesli — 1

3 When I drink juice, it's:

a A small glass of unsweetened juice such as orange or grapefruit — 1

b A large glass of unsweetened juice such as orange or grapefruit — 2

c A large glass of juice drink (5 to 30% juice) — 3

4 When I drink milk (or pour it over my cereal), it's:

a Whole — 3

b Semi-skimmed — 2

c Skimmed — 1

5 The bread on my counter right now is:

a 100% whole grain (wheat, rye, pumpernickel or sourdough) — 1

b Made with white flour and some wholemeal flour (brown bread as opposed to 'wholemeal' bread) — 2

c White — 3

6 Potatoes (including mashed, chips, roast and fried potatoes, etc) are:

a On my plate every day — 3

b On my plate two or three times a week — 2

c On my plate once a week or less — 1

7 Spinach, broccoli and other dark green vegetables are:

a Strangers in my house — 3

b Welcome as occasional visitors, if they keep quiet — 2

c Practically family — 1

8 When I make or buy a sandwich, I:

a Pile on the corned beef, salami or other full-fat meats — 3

b Use roast beef — 2

c Have low-fat meats such as sliced turkey breast or lean ham — 1

9 When I'm hungry in the afternoon, I grab:

a Some fruit, nuts or low-fat yoghurt — 1

b Crackers and cheese or a cereal bar — 2

c Crisps or a chocolate bar — 3

10 I eat nuts:

a Rarely — 3

b By the bagful; can't get enough — 2

c By the small handful every day or two — 1

11 **I eat at** fast-food places:

a At least twice a week — **3**

b Once a week or so — **2**

c Less than once a week — **1**

12 **In my refrigerator** you're most likely to find:

a Soft drinks or sports/energy drinks **3**

b Diet soft drinks — **2**

c Water or sparkling water — **1**

13 **When I get pizza** I usually eat:

a One or two slices with a side salad **1** and a low-calorie drink

b One or two slices, no salad and **2** a soft drink

c Two or more slices plus a big **3** soft drink and some garlic bread

14 **My favourite** salad dressing is:

a Something creamy or cheesy — **2**

b Olive oil and vinegar — **1**

c Who eats salad? — **3**

15 **When I eat** pasta, I:

a Pile it high and top it with cheese **3** sauce or meat sauce

b Have a moderate amount paired **1** with chicken, fish or shellfish

c Enjoy it as a side dish with some **1** olive oil and grated cheese

16 **When I'm offered** vegetarian bean chilli for dinner, I think:

a Looks good! — **1**

b Okay, I guess, but I hope I'm **2** not hungry later

c Where's the beef? — **3**

17 **When I eat beef** for dinner it's likely to be:

a A large juicy steak, **3** like T-bone or prime rib, or a big serving of pot roast swimming in gravy

b A moderate serving **2** of lean grilled beef, such as sirloin, with rice or potatoes

c A small serving of **1** lean beef that's grilled or mixed into a stir-fry

18 **Fish?** I'll eat it:

a Only if it's battered **3** and deep-fried, if ever

b Baked or grilled, a **1** couple of times a week

c Baked or grilled, **2** every couple of weeks or so

19 **When I eat** Chinese food, I eat this much rice:

a About 50g — **1**

b About 100g — **2**

c Lots – as much as it takes **3** to soak up all the sauce

20 **When it comes to** dessert, I:

a Live for them – usually a big slice of pie or cake or a bowl **3** of full-fat ice cream

b Eat it once in a while when I feel **1** like indulging

c Have fruit or a small bowl of **1** reduced-fat ice cream or sorbet

Your **SCORE**

30 or under
You're generally eating the *Magic Foods* way – choosing low-GL carbs most of the time, keeping portions under control, limiting saturated fats, and getting some fruits and vegetables. Use the *Magic Foods* profiles, recipes and meal plans in the rest of the book to help you further fine-tune your eating.

31 to 40
You could improve your diet. Pay particular attention to answers that were 3 points – these are your dietary downfalls. You do have some good things going for you in your diet, though, so build on them. Use the rest of this book to strengthen healthy habits and change less healthy ones.

41 or over
No medal for you – which means that there are plenty of small improvements you can make. Look back carefully over your answers and pick out some '3s' that you can edge into '2s' or '1s'. You'll find lots of tips, tools, suggestions and recipes in this book to help you to improve your diet.

Understanding the **QUIZ QUESTIONS**

1 Having a little sugar in your coffee isn't a big deal, but add 3 teaspoons and you add nearly 50kcal and 12g of carbohydrate. Starting the day with a soft drink – an increasingly common habit – is a dietary downfall. One 473ml bottle of cola has the equivalent of 11 or 12 teaspoons of sugar and will push up your day's GL before you even get out the door.

2 The (a) cereal choices have the highest GLs, the (b) choices are medium GL and the (c) cereals have the lowest GLs and are kindest to your blood sugar. If you like a higher-GL cereal, try mixing it with a lower-GL kind and/or pouring it into a smaller bowl.

3 Orange juice is a healthy beverage, but it has a fair amount of sugar and calories, so don't drink it like water. Use small juice glasses for juice and save large glasses for water and low-calorie drinks only. Juice 'drinks' are mostly sugar and water, so we suggest you avoid them altogether.

4 Whole milk is a major source of saturated fat in our diets, and that's bad for your heart and insulin sensitivity. Drinking semi-skimmed milk is better, but this type still gets about a third of its calories from fat, much of it saturated. Fat-free and skimmed milk are the best choices.

5 When choosing bread, 100 per cent whole-meal varieties are best. If they're made from coarsely ground flours with kernels and seeds, so much the better. Brown breads made with some white flour are second choices and white bread comes in last in terms of its effect on blood sugar.

6 Potatoes are a high-GL food; there's no getting around it. You don't need to exclude them, but don't rely on them as a staple. Sweet potatoes, on the other hand, are a much better choice.

7 You're not surprised, are you? These dark green veggies are incredibly nutritious and have very little carbohydrate. Adding them to any dish or meal – a side dish of sautéed spinach, lightly steamed broccoli florets in a pasta salad – lowers the meal's overall GL per portion. So does adding nearly any other vegetable.

8 Processed meats can be a major source of saturated fat in our diets. Lean meats, on the other hand, provide protein without all the fat. Roast beef is in-between – better than salami and corned beef but fattier than turkey breast. Ask for your roast beef on rye or sourdough and the sandwich is a step better already. Add mustard instead of mayo for the best blood sugar–lowering effect (it contains vinegar, a Magic food).

9   You can't go wrong with low-cal, high-fibre fruit. Low-fat yoghurt, with its sugar-stabilizing protein, is another good choice if it's not overly sweetened. Crackers and cheese are okay, too, especially if the biscuits are whole grain (with no trans fats) and you keep your portions in check. Crisps, though, have easily digested starches, and chocolate bars offer nothing much but fat and sugar.

10 Nuts are a Magic food thanks to their 'good' fats and blood sugar-stabilising protein. People who eat just a handful each day tend to have healthier hearts and may even have an easier time losing weight (nuts are very filling). But eat too many, and the benefits will vanish.

11 If you often eat at fast-food restaurants, the chances are you're eating lots of fried foods, with too much saturated fat, as well as high-GL carbs in the bread and fries. Have fast-food meals a few times a month (or less), not a few times a week.

12 The GL of soft drinks isn't as sky-high as you might expect, but it's easy to down huge amounts. Remember, GL is related to portion size; double the amount you drink, and the GL doubles as well. Switching to water or sparkling water can have a dramatic effect on your calorie and sugar intake – and your waistline.

13 Pizza is another food that's okay in moderation, but more than one slice can really pile on the blood sugar-raising carbs and cheesy fat. When ordering, favour a thinner crust and lots of veggies on top. Don't tip the scales by adding a big soft drink; have a small one or, better still, water or unsweetened iced tea.

14 A green salad topped with a vinegar-based dressing is perhaps the ideal Magic side dish. The vinegar even helps to lower the GL of whatever you eat with your salad. Creamy dressings don't have the same effect and they add a lot more calories, but even a salad with a little creamy dressing is better than no salad at all; try to limit dressing to a tablespoon or less.

15 Pasta's not bad for you; in fact, it's a Magic food. For a carbohydrate food, its GL is not very high, but it's still best to eat it in moderation, as a base for lean protein or vegetables. Most cheese and meat sauces, though, are anything but low fat.

16 Beans are a high-protein, low-GL food, making them ideal for anyone concerned about heart health, weight and blood sugar. Try to have a meatless main meal a few times a week.

17 Beef is a Magic food, but only when it's lean (and eaten in moderation). Even a 'lean' hamburger has more saturated fat than the same amount of sirloin or chuck steak.

18 All fish is low in saturated fat, and the oil-rich varieties have omega-3 fatty acids, which are good for your heart and even your blood sugar. Try to eat a couple of fish meals a week. Eating fish or seafood deep-fried erases all the benefits.

19 Rice has a surprising number of calories (about 200kcal in a serving of 150g), and if you're eating white rice, a high GL. Stick with brown rice and keep portions small.

20 Everyone should indulge in dessert once in a while, because eating well is not about depriving yourself. If you eat it every day, though, you're probably getting too many calories (unless your dessert is virtuous fruit, of course).

Find – and fix your dietary downfalls

All of us have dietary strengths and weaknesses, just as we have strengths and weaknesses in other areas of our lives. No one is perfect – and that's fine! But if you're like most people, there are a few things you're doing out of habit that are sabotaging your efforts to control your blood sugar and lose weight. If you change just one or two of them by setting your mind to it, you'll reap rewards in spades. First, though, you have to recognise them.

Problem I like a big bowl of cereal in the morning.

solution Your first course of action is to make sure you're eating a low-GL cereal, such as porridge, All-Bran, or Bran Flakes, or at least a medium-GL type such as Kellogg's Special K (*see* 'How cereals rate' on page 85). If you're not used to these cereals, mix them with a bit of your usual cereal at first to make the transition easier. Second, pour less into the bowl and add something else to fill it up. You can top your cereal with fresh fruit, such as chopped apples, pears, strawberries or blueberries. Sprinkling on a tablespoon of chopped nuts such as hazelnuts or toasted sliced almonds is an excellent strategy because nuts add protein and 'good' fat, both of which help to stabilise your blood sugar and keep you feeling full. There is nothing to stop you adding both nuts and fruit and even a little natural yoghurt – another low-fat source of protein. Experiment until you find a breakfast that fills you up.

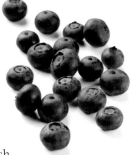

Problem I don't eat breakfast until I get to work, and then I'm tempted by toast and Danish pastries.

solution Pack your breakfast in an insulated cool bag the night before so you can grab it on the way out of the house. An example of a good breakfast is a piece of fruit, a small handful of nuts and 250ml of low-fat yoghurt. Or make a batch of healthy bran muffins (*see* our recipe on page 198) over the weekend and grab one along with an orange. Another option: keep a box of high-fibre, low-GL breakfast cereal (along with plastic spoons and bowls) at your desk and bring the milk, fruit and nuts with you.

Problem I like sweet drinks, not water.

solution That's okay. But think of these drinks, whether they're soft drinks, sweetened iced tea, or sugary fruit drinks, as a treat, like dessert. You wouldn't eat dessert more than once a day, so don't indulge in these drinks more often than that either. Wait until the afternoon and then get the smallest size you can find. In the meantime, cultivate another habit – sipping sparkling water. Some flavoured varieties have few or no calories, and a good squeeze of lemon or lime juice makes plain sparkling water much more interesting and palatable. Buy mineral water in bulk and make sure there's plenty at home and at the office. Changing this one habit can be a really effective way of improving your diet and even losing weight.

Problem There's nowhere to get a healthy lunch close to where I work.

solution One strategy is to think through what changes would make it easier for you to bring lunch from home. If you're lucky, your workplace has a refrigerator, a microwave, or even a toaster oven. If so, get into the habit of making more of whatever you're having for dinner, then pack up the leftovers for lunch the next day. If there's no fridge, pack your lunch in a small insulated cool bag with an ice pack. It will stay cold through lunchtime. On days when you don't pack your lunch, look at page 71 for our tips on eating better at fast-food restaurants.

Problem I like pizza. Is that so bad?

solution It depends. The thicker the crust, the higher the GL of the meal. If you add pepperoni, you really sabotage yourself with extra calories and saturated fat, which contributes to insulin resistance. For a healthier pizza think thin crust with veggies on top. Go for a wholewheat crust if it's available. Stick to one or two slices. Add a salad with vinaigrette dressing so you get enough food to feel full; the vinegar in the dressing will also help to lower the GL of the meal. And make the soft drink a small one or, better still, have sparkling water.

Problem When I get salad from the salad bar, I tend to pile on cheese, croutons and creamy dressing. Is it still good for me?

solution You might as well eat a hamburger with a side of lettuce. Full-fat cheeses and creamy dressings are high in saturated fat, which is bad for insulin sensitivity. They and the croutons (which are fried) are also loaded with calories. Don't abandon salads, just look for ways to keep them interesting and healthy. Add toasted sunflower seeds for crunch (and healthy fat) or a few black olives for richness (and again, 'good' fat). Add hot peppers, if you like them, for kick. Throw on some chickpeas for additional

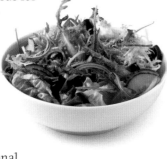

texture and low-fat protein. Top it all off with a vinegar-based dressing; experiment to find a tasty one you like, such as mustard vinaigrette for extra flavour.

Problem I am starving by about 3pm and I eat whatever junk food is in sight.

solution If you eat Magic foods at breakfast and lunchtime, this won't happen. And that's good, because research shows that when they're really hungry, people may eat 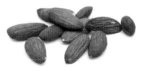 twice as much food as they normally would. Snacking itself isn't bad at all, though, as long as the snack is a healthy one as it can help to keep blood sugar levels steady. So keep healthy snacks to hand (think carrot sticks, apples, low-fat yoghurt, a few whole-grain biscuits , or a handful of peanuts or almonds) to bridge the gap between lunch and dinner.

Problem I eat carbohydrate foods when I'm stressed or anxious.

solution A lot of people reach for carbs when they're stressed. (The scientific jury is out as to whether carbs actually help to calm you down or not. The soothing effect may simply be due to a sense of comfort from a familiar food.) There's no quick solution here. The key is to try to find ways to cope with the stress other than eating. Practise deep breathing or distract yourself by taking a 10-minute stroll, after which the craving should have passed.

One of the best ways to deal with anxiety in general is regular exercise; even a brisk 20-minute walk can lift your mood and calm you down. Try to introduce more activity into your daily routine. Studies show that people who exercise regularly have lower responses to stress than people who don't. You can also help yourself out when you are at the supermarket: avoid buying high-GL carbohydrates so they aren't within temptation's reach.

Problem I know portion sizes are important, but it's difficult not to finish what's on my plate.

solution Why not try using a smaller plate? Manufacturers are actually making many plates and bowls larger because we eat so much bigger portions than we used to. Fight the trend by eating all your meals off smaller plates instead. Serve juice in wine glasses or small tumblers. Instead of using a big bowl for cereal, try a smaller dessert bowl. And always spoon out your dinner onto individual plates rather than leaving serving bowls or platters on the table within easy reach for second helpings.

Problem I'd like to eat more beans, but I don't know how to cook them.

solution You don't have to make bean dishes from scratch. Canned beans can be no-fuss additions to something you're already making. Making a salad? Rinse some canned chickpeas and toss them on top. Add canned kidney beans to nearly any vegetable soup. For a quick bean side dish, drain a can of white beans, put them into a microwaveable bowl, then add some olive oil, grated Parmesan and fresh pepper. Microwave for a minute or two, then mash for a delicious, high-protein, low-GL dish.

Problem When I eat small portions at dinner, I'm still hungry.

solution First, make sure your dinner contains protein and 'good fat', not just carbs. That way, it will keep you full for longer (plus, you're less likely to overeat grilled chicken breast than buttery mashed potatoes). Second, try to eat a little slower so that your stomach has more time to send the message back to your brain that you're full. Take plenty of time between bites for conversation or sips of water. If these don't do the trick, start the meal with clear soup or a large green salad (watch the dressing though). Both of these starters will occupy a lot of space in your stomach and help you to put down your fork sooner. And remember: it's okay to leave the dinner table a tiny bit hungry. You'll feel fuller as your food digests.

Problem I'd like to snack on fruit, but I just don't think of it.

solution Put it in front of your face, literally. Studies show that people eat more fruit when it's in a bowl on the table rather than tucked away in the refrigerator. Lots of fruits will stay perfectly fresh out of the fridge, such as apples, pears, plums, nectarines and bananas. (But don't place oranges next to bananas as this can speed up the ripening process and the bananas can turn black.) When you buy fruit, wash it as soon as you come home, then put it in a bowl – for easy access. If you keep fruit in the fridge – such as grapes, which taste great cold – make sure it's on the top shelf where it's easy to see and grab. Like melon? Cut it into slices or cubes and refrigerate it in an airtight container so it's ready to eat come snack time.

Problem My pitfall is late-night desserts.

solution Try to have your dessert earlier. If you normally eat it at 10pm, aim for 8:30pm, and then brush your teeth so you're not tempted to eat again. Another strategy is to keep those devilish desserts out of the house. Avoid bringing home the kinds of desserts that you most tend to overeat – most people won't leave the house at night just to get dessert.

Finally, train yourself to enjoy healthier desserts, such as a bowl of berries with a dollop of low-fat ice cream or low-fat Greek yoghurt; or a single portion of a light pudding. Then you won't have to worry as much.

The art of eating out healthily

If most restaurants offered menus full of Magic fare such as lean grilled meats, whole-grain side dishes, and fruit-based desserts, it would be easy to eat out the Magic way. But they don't. Nearly all of the most common carbohydrate-rich foods on menus reflect those in the typical Western diet. In other words, they are high-GL foods. And at most restaurants, from fast-food joints to the fanciest white-tablecloth establishments, the food is floating in butter and stuffed with extra calories. Add to that the large portions that we have grown to expect for our money, and eating out seems impossible to do well.

But it can be done and learning how is a survival skill because we eat out – or have takeaway meals – so often now. Fifty years ago, eating out was largely a luxury; today, according to the Food Standards Agency, men consume a quarter of their daily calories outside the home and women a fifth.

The first step is to accept how commonly you eat meals you haven't made yourself, then plan to order better.

Be careful where you eat

Make the challenge of eating out easier by choosing carefully where you eat out. Avoid the temptation of all-you-can-eat places, or buffet-style restaurants, where portions are hard to control. Avoid places that are known for their large portions, such as many pubs.

And it is probably safe to say that you won't find a lot of Magic foods on the menu at eateries that specialise in deep-frying an entire breaded onion. Enjoy a meal at one of these on your birthday, for sure, but don't do it on a regular basis. Not if you want to do your blood sugar and health a favour.

Make friends with the waiter

Once you're in the right kind of restaurant, get ready to befriend the waiters or waitresses. Ask them to hold back the bread basket so you're not tempted to fill up on usually high-GL carbs while waiting for your meal to arrive. If it doesn't come automatically, ask for water as soon as you sit down. Drinking water can help to fill you up. Before you order, take a look around the restaurant to see what other people are ordering. If the portions are huge then go for two starters or share a main course with a friend.

Order creatively

When you order, be bold: order soup or salad to start with, rather than an entrée; or split an entrée and share a side order of vegetables to get more veggies into your meal – and fewer calories. If a main dish comes with a potato, ask if you can have an extra vegetable instead. If you plan to order dessert, plan to share it, too. The best policy is to get to know a restaurant, what they serve and the size of their portions and to use that knowledge to make sensible choices from the menu.

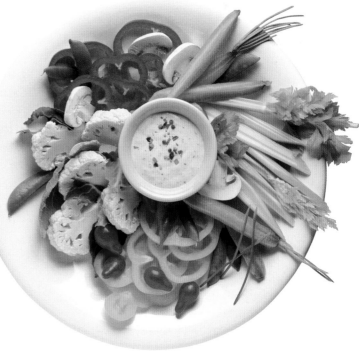

EATING OUT
CHINESE

The traditional Chinese diet is a healthy one, with lots of vegetables, stir-fries with small chunks of meat or fish and soy foods. But that's not evident in the typical fare on offer in a Chinese restaurant here, where the meal is likely to be heavy on greasy meats and swimming in sauces with lots and lots of calories. Even the vegetables are usually served in a fat-laden sauce.

Do you have to give up Chinese takeaways? Of course not; that would be almost unthinkable. But to get a Magic meal, you do have to order carefully.

JUST SAY NO!

Prawn crackers
Crispy noodles
Egg rolls
Fried wontons
Fried rice
Pan-fried noodles
Chow mein
Crispy beef or chicken
Sweet-and-sour pork, chicken and other meat dishes
Szechuan spicy fish
Spicy eggplant
Banana or pineapple fritter

YOUR GAME PLAN

1 **Ask for a half portion of rice**
Most restaurants will allow this. Remember, white rice is a blood sugar disaster waiting to happen. And make sure that you order boiled rice, not fried. Do as a Chinese native would: put a small amount in a small bowl and hold the bowl up, using your chopsticks (or fork) to eat a little rice in between bites of your main dish. Or be bold and don't have any rice at all.

2 **Start your meal with** wonton, chicken noodle, or hot-and-sour soup. This will take the edge off your hunger without a lot of calories (avoid soups with coconut milk). If you want a ravioli-type starter, order steamed vegetable dumplings, but nothing fried.

3 **For the main dish**, order from the 'health' menu. Here is where you'll find steamed chicken and vegetables with sauce on the side and similar low-fat choices. Another good choice is *moo goo gai pan* (chicken with mushrooms).

If you like stir-fries, ask the waiter or waitress to have yours prepared with less oil and more veggies and get the sauce on the side.

4 **Make sure you order** plenty of vegetables. If you really want to make the meal healthier, order a plate of steamed vegetables and add them to other dishes. Or ask for a dish of sautéed vegetables.

5 **Take advantage of** the healthy bean curd (tofu). Always ask for sautéed bean curd, not deep-fried.

6 **Plan to take home leftovers**
Portions are often large. Stay healthy and save money: bring it home.

EATING OUT
ITALIAN

A single slice of pizza with vegetables is a fine choice, especially if it's made with a wholewheat and/or thin crust. A cup of pasta with marinara sauce is all right, too. The problem is, few of us stop there.

Ironically, southern Italian food, prepared the traditional way, is among the healthiest in the world. Unfortunately, Italian restaurants are often purveyors of mounds of overcooked pasta and pizza. Even before these arrive, you'll have ample opportunity to eat bread. So unless you want to overload on carbs and send your blood sugar soaring, tread carefully.

JUST SAY NO!

Garlic bread
Fried mozzarella sticks
Fried calamari
Pasta with alfredo or other cream sauces
Pasta carbonara
Aubergine, chicken or veal parmigiana
Any dish smothered with melted cheese
Tiramisu
Anything described as fritto (which means it has been fried)
Extra grated parmesan

YOUR GAME PLAN

1 **Ask the waiter/waitress** not to bring the breadbasket. Instead, order minestrone or another broth-based soup to fill up on while you await your main dish. *Pasta e fagioli*, an Italian classic, is a delicious bean/pasta soup that's also a good starter.

2 **If you want pasta,** order a dish from the starter section of the menu, or share. That's the traditional way – a small first course of pasta followed by simple grilled meat, poultry or fish and a side of sautéed greens. As for pasta sauces, opt for those based on tomatoes (marinara), vegetables, white wine and garlic – not cream. Watch out: pasta primavera is often made with lots of cream.

3 **If it's on the menu,** order simple grilled beef, veal, pork, chicken, fish or shellfish. Add a side order of sautéed spinach or broccoli rabe (a slightly bitter Italian version of broccoli). Finish with a mixed green salad with vinaigrette dressing.

4 **For dessert,** ask for fresh berries or fruit sorbet, if it's available, or a small plate of crunchy biscuits to share. Stay away from the custards and the cheesecake – and the tiramisu, dripping in cream.

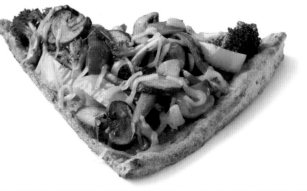

EATING OUT
MEXICAN

Ordering from a fast-food Tex-Mex place is about as big as a blood sugar challenge can get. Portions are generally enormous, the tortillas used for burritos are larger than your head and filled with mounds of white rice (blood sugar enemy number one), and the dishes tend to be loaded with cheese – and we don't mean the Magic low-fat variety.

Thread your way warily around these potholes, and you can arrive at a delicious, moderate-GL meal.

YOUR GAME PLAN

1 **Ask the waiter/waitress** to take away the tortilla chips. The Mexican equivalent of a big breadbasket is either a bowl of tortilla chips with salsa or nacho chips covered with cheese. Just say no.

2 **Order a healthy starter** instead. Look for ceviches (marinated raw fish or seafood); guacamole, which is full of 'good' fats (ask for soft tortillas instead of deep-fried chips to dip and don't eat too many); gazpacho, a spicy cold vegetable soup; black bean soup; and tortilla soup (chicken in broth with vegetables and thin fried tortilla chips). Ask for extra salsa for the table and eat it with a spoon rather than on chips.

3 **For the main dish,** look to fajitas. These are made with lean beef (or chicken or shrimp) grilled with onions and peppers. Other good choices are grilled chicken or fish dishes.

4 **Order tacos or burritos** without high-fat sour cream. Ask for extra salsa instead. Hard tacos are fried, so you're better off with soft tacos; soft tortillas are even better. A small tortilla is the equivalent of a slice of bread. If you're not eating rice, two or three soft tacos are fine, but stick to one or two if you are having rice. If you're getting a burrito, ask for no rice and more beans.

5 **As a side dish**, go for rice and beans instead of Mexican rice. Thanks to the beans, this dish has a lower GL than rice alone. But check first to be sure the beans aren't refried. Refried beans are loaded with fat.

6 **Have dessert at home** Desserts at Mexican restaurants, such as flan and fried ice cream, are usually high in calories and fat, so skip them and eat something healthier elsewhere.

EATING OUT
THAI

Thai food is a pretty good choice providing you stay away from dishes containing coconut milk, which is scarily high in saturated fat. Also avoid anything deep fried. Peanuts are a favourite ingredient in Thai dishes and they contain heart-healthy monounsaturates. The quantities used are generally small and so will not pile on the calories.

Thai menus usually offer a good choice of salads and simply cooked vegetable dishes, so make the most of these.

YOUR GAME PLAN

1 Tell the waiter/waitress to hold back the prawn crackers. They are often served and munched as you look through the menu, but they are full of fat, so avoid them. Ask for your drinks to be served instead. Better still, ask for a glass of water.

2 Avoid anything deep fried and that means the spring rolls and deep-fried prawns in batter. More healthy starters would be a soup such as tom yam or hot and sour; or chicken or beef satay. Thai fishcakes are usually reasonably low in fat and calories, too.

3 Be choosy with noodles When served with chicken, pork, fish or tofu and vegetables, noodle dishes are generally a good choice. The exception is Pad Thai, as the noodles are usually fried.

4 Jasmine rice, which is simply boiled rice that has been lightly fragranced with jasmine, is much better than coconut rice or fried rice. Remember your portion sizes – it is a good idea to share a portion of rice between two.

5 Go easy on the soy sauce This tasty, tangy accompaniment to Thai and Chinese food is laden with salt (1 tablespoon contains 2g, which is a third of the recommended daily allowance). You should also exercise control with the sweet chilli dipping sauce as this is packed with sugar (2 tablespoons containing the equivalent of 1 tablespoon of sugar).

6 Fresh pineapple makes a sweet yet healthy dessert. Avoid battered bananas in syrup or anything with coconut.

Lunch on the go

If you eat lunch on the go, you probably opt for a shop-bought sandwich or salad unless, of course, you're one of those incredibly organised and efficient types who makes lunch at home to take to work.

Be prepared: shop-bought sandwiches may look like a safe bet but they're not always as innocent as they seem. Before you buy, spend a few seconds checking the nutrition information on the pack – some sandwiches contain as many calories, fat and salt as a burger from McDonalds. Thankfully, most supermarkets and shops such as Boots offer a good selection of sandwiches between 300-400kcal, which is a sensible target.

Don't be seduced by the meal deal that some shops offer – you really don't need a packet of crisps and a soft drink at lunch; a fruit salad and a bottle of water are a much better option. If you buy your lunch from a shop which makes up sandwiches fresh this could be a problem, because you have no idea how many calories or how much fat you're consuming.

All you can do is follow a few general guidelines:
■ Choose lean fillings such as chicken or ham.
■ Prawns are another good choice providing they don't come swimming in mayo.
■ Cheese of any variety is probably best avoided.
■ Hummus and salad is another good choice.
■ Go for rye, granary or wholemeal bread rather than ciabatta or foccacia.
■ Ask for plenty of salad or vegetables to bulk out your sandwiches and look carefully at the portion size. If sandwiches are huge, try to share one with a friend.

Many sandwich chains such as Subway and Pret now publish nutritional information about their products on their websites. So if you usually use the same outlet, it's worth checking their website or contacting them to see if they can provide nutritional information.

As a healthy lunch option, you might be tempted by a salad. But choose wisely as salads are not automatically healthy or low in calories. Salad made from tuna, eggs, beans, pulses, bulghur wheat or brown rice are usually a good choice for better blood sugar control. Pasta salad often comes with a creamy dressing high in fat, so is best avoided unless you've made it yourself. Try to get a salad with a separate dressing, then you can control the amount you add.

A hidden hazard: coffee drinks

It's difficult to think of coffee as fattening but it can be if you choose some of the varieties now sold at outlets such as Starbucks, Costa Coffee and other high street coffee shops, which add cream, chocolate, caramel and sugar.

Consider the largest size of one 'Java chip' frappuccino with whipped cream. It has 520kcal and nearly 70g of sugar. As 10g of table sugar – about 2½ teaspoons – has a GL of 6, you could estimate that the sugar in this drink would provide a GL of around 40. And, since any food with a GL over 20 is high GL, this is very high. But this particular beverage also contributes almost 20g of fat, more than half of it saturated – the kind that not only clogs arteries but also contributes to insulin resistance. That single drink has more fat and saturated fat than you'd get in a McDonald's Quarter Pounder with Cheese. Are you still feeling thirsty?

You could do a little better with a mocha with whipped cream, but the largest size (with skimmed milk) still contains nearly 350kcal, more than 10g of fat and more than 40g of sugar. Consider as an alternative a cappuccino made with skimmed milk. Even the largest size has only 109kcal and about 14g of sugar (less than 4 teaspoons' worth, with a GL of 10).

Of course, freshly brewed black coffee has almost no calories at all. Consider a tall black coffee with 2 teaspoons of sugar. It has fewer than 40kcal. You'd have to drink more than 20 of them to get the same number of calories as in the Java chip frappuccino. Its GL is about 5. Even if you add 2 tablespoons of semi-skimmed milk, it has only 57kcal.

If you prefer a cold drink, ask for plain iced coffee (with skimmed milk if you like) and add your own sugar.

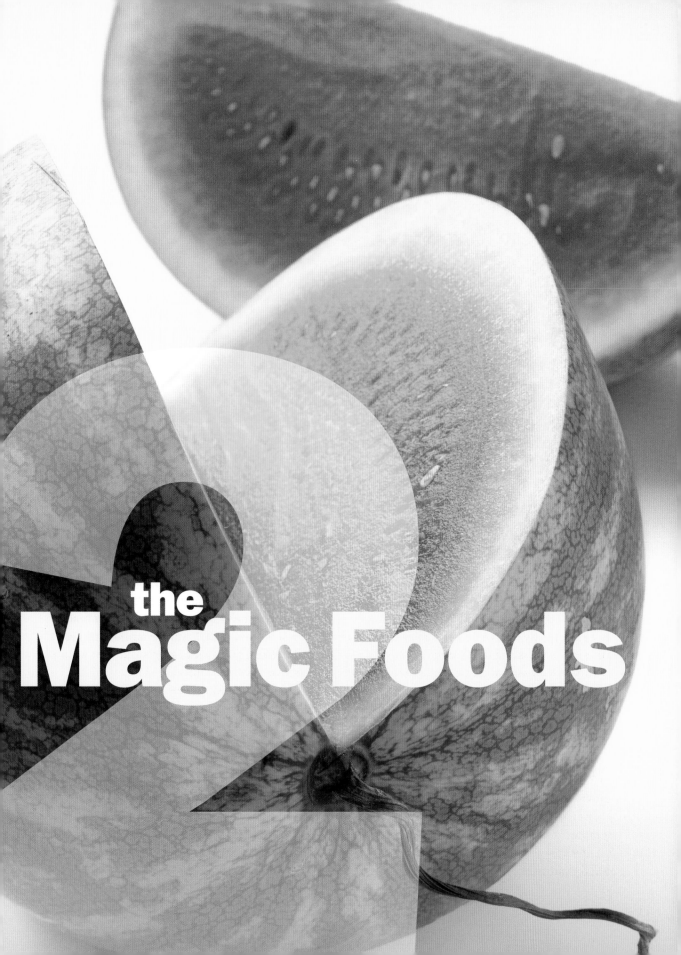

the Magic Foods

apples

Can eating an apple

a day really keep the doctor away? It can certainly help you to control your blood sugar and gain all the benefits that come with that control. In fact, researchers have discovered that women who eat at least one apple a day are 28 per cent less likely to develop Type 2 diabetes than those who don't eat apples. That's probably because apples, from tart Granny Smiths to juicy Golden Delicious, are loaded with soluble fibre – number one for blunting blood sugar swings. A medium apple dishes up an impressive 4g of fibre, mostly pectin, which is also known for its ability to lower cholesterol.

Looking to trim your tummy? (Remember, stomach fat is bad for blood sugar.) Try eating three small apples a day. A study from the State University of Rio de Janeiro found that doing so as part of a reduced-calorie diet not only helped women to lose more weight but also helped them to lower their blood sugar more than women who ate another food instead of apples.

To gain every bit of benefit from apples, opt for whole, unpeeled fruit. The apples with the lowest GL are Braeburns, which have more acid and less sugar than Golden Delicious. Next on the glycaemic scale is unsweetened apple sauce, which offers many of the same health benefits. But steer clear of apple juice; it's not much better than apple-flavoured liquid sugar.

Health bonus

Apples aren't particularly rich in vitamins or minerals, but that doesn't mean they're not good for you. In fact, they're packed with antioxidant compounds called flavonoids, believed to reduce the risk of cancer and heart disease. One study found that eating a small apple with its skin provided total antioxidant and anticancer activity equal to 1,500 mg of vitamin C.

Menu magic

■ **Add thinly sliced apples** to sandwiches for a bit of tang and crunch.
■ **Mix chopped apples** with low-fat yoghurt and wheatgerm (two other Magic foods) for a healthy midmorning snack.
■ **Make jarred salsa more healthy** by adding chopped apples, cucumbers, onions, jalapeño peppers and lime juice.
 Prepare apple sauce by cubing apples and simmering them in a small amount of water until desirably mushy. Add a sprinkling of cinnamon, a Magic spice.
■ **Snack on half** an apple with a smear of peanut butter (another Magic food).

Smart substitutions

Instead of raisins: try sliced or grated apples on your porridge or other cereal. Raisins have concentrated sugars that raise blood sugar more quickly than apples do.

Instead of oil: replace three-quarters of the butter or oil in biscuit, cake or scone recipes with unsweetened apple sauce.

Related recipes

Apple bran muffins 198
Chicken sauté with apples 246
Cranberry and apple crumble 301
Maple-walnut baked apples 296
Porridge with apple and flaxseeds 192

PERFECT PORTION: 1 apple

At about **80kcal** each, apples are the perfect **snack size** just the way Nature grew them.

aubergine

GL very low

Aubergine dishes

aren't exactly regulars on most of our tables, but they should be. Voluminous and almost meaty in texture, aubergine is a great addition to pasta because it lets you use less pasta, lowering the overall GL of the meal, and still fill your plate. It's also a fabulous filling for lasagna in place of meat, reducing calories and saturated fat.

When it's not deep fried (aubergine acts like a sponge, soaking up four times as much fat as chips), it's low in calories and carbs since it's almost 95 per cent water. Because its spongy flesh is also a good source of soluble fibre, aubergine makes the list of special foods that can help to lower both your blood sugar as well as your cholesterol.

Health bonus

While it's not a powerhouse of vitamins and minerals, aubergine is one of the richest plant sources of antioxidants you can find in the supermarket, ranking right up there with spinach and sweet potatoes.

Cooks' tips

Aubergines come in an unexpected variety of sizes, shapes and colours. Choose ones that are firm and heavy with shiny, smooth skins and avoid any that have brown patches as these will deteriorate quickly.

To limit the amount of oil aubergine soaks up, salt slices of aubergine and leave them in a colander over the sink for at least 15 minutes. Turn the slices, salt the other side and leave for at least another 15 minutes. Rinse off the excess salt, pat the slices dry and you're ready to go.

Menu magic

■ **As an appetiser,** whip up blood sugar-friendly baba ghanoush, a Middle Eastern dish made with puréed roasted aubergine, crushed garlic, tahini (sesame paste), lemon juice and olive oil. Serve it with a wholemeal pitta or wholemeal crackers. It's also good as a sandwich spread.

■ **For dinner,** make ratatouille, a hearty vegetable dish featuring aubergine and many other Magic foods, including onions, garlic, tomatoes and olive oil.

■ **Sauté aubergine** with onion and garlic and use it to replace some of the minced beef in beef dishes to cut fat and calories and add an antioxidant boost.

■ **Substitute aubergine** and mushrooms for minced beef the next time you make lasagna.

■ **For a quick,** easy side dish, grill small Japanese aubergines brushed with olive oil, crushed garlic, salt and pepper. There's nothing quite as good as grilled aubergine.

Related recipes

Caponata 201
Grilled aubergine sandwiches with red pepper
  and walnut sauce 227

DON'T fall for it...

Aubergines are members of the nightshade family, rumoured to aggravate arthritis symptoms. But according to the Arthritis Foundation, there is no clinical evidence that any member of the nightshade family has any effect on arthritis.

PERFECT PORTION: 80g

Since aubergine has **very few calories** *and a* **very low GL,** *feel free to eat more than this, especially if you don't add a lot of oil.*

avocado

Unlike virtually all

other fruits (yes, avocado is a fruit), these rich, creamy treats are full of fat – a whopping 25g to 30g each. Since fat has no impact on blood sugar, avocados are great additions to a low-GL diet if you eat them in moderation.

You may wonder about all that fat but there is a saving grace: most of it is monounsaturated fat, the same heart-healthy kind found in olive oil. Research suggests that diets rich in this type of fat may help to keep blood sugar in check. That's the main reason for secret number 5 of Magic eating: favour good fats. Add some avocado to a sandwich or anything else loaded with carbs, and the fat will slow digestion of the meal, thus making it easier on your blood sugar.

Unlike the saturated fats in butter and meat, monounsaturated fat won't increase insulin resistance, a condition that makes blood sugar control more difficult. In fact, the good fat in avocados (as well as in olive oil and nuts) may actually reverse insulin resistance, helping your body steady its blood sugar levels naturally. Avocados also contain more soluble fibre (which stabilises blood sugar and lowers cholesterol) and protein than any other fruit.

Of course, with fat come calories, so you don't want to start eating avocados with total abandon – though you probably wouldn't anyway, since a little avocado goes a long way.

PERFECT PORTION: 1/5 avocado

Cut an avocado into *five pieces* and have one piece for **55kcal**. If that sounds high to you, consider how it stacks up against a tablespoon of mayonnaise (100kcal), butter (also 100kcal) or salad dressing (about 75kcal). The avocado has fewer calories and more *healthy nutrients*.

Health bonus

Avocados are rich in sterols, compounds shown to lower cholesterol. They're also packed with vitamins and minerals, including vitamin E, magnesium, vitamin C, folate and zinc. Ounce for ounce, they provide more potassium than bananas!

Cooks' tips

To choose just the right avocado, try this: hold the pear-shaped fruit in your hand and press it gently, then roll it to the other side and press again. If it gives just a bit but pressure doesn't leave a permanent dent (an indication that it's too ripe), it's ready to eat.

Menu magic

■ **Guacamole is the classic** avocado dish. Add some curry powder for an Indian flair; hot bean sauce or oriental chilli paste for an Asian influence; or basil, sun-dried tomatoes and pine nuts for a taste of Italy.

■ **Mash some avocado** and use it as a spread on sandwiches (made with whole-grain bread, of course), bagels, or English muffins to lower the GL of your breakfast or lunch.

■ **Add chunks of avocado** to a side salad to lower the GL of the meal. Adding it to salads also increases your body's ability to absorb the good-for-you carotenoids found in salad greens.

Smart substitutions

Instead of cheese in your sandwich: add a slice of avocado. You'll swap good fats for bad ones.
Instead of cheese as a snack: have a slice of ripe avocado drizzled with lemon juice.

Related recipes

Spinach, grapefruit & avocado salad with
   poppy seed dressing 224
Turkey and bean chilli with avocado salsa 243

barley

If you've only encountered barley in soup, get ready to make friends with this underappreciated cereal grain. Whether pearled, hulled or quick cooking, this humble grain can help to transform your diet into a Magic one. In fact, think of barley as your new white rice.

Unlike white rice, which has a sky-high GL, barley's is low, thanks to its significant stash of soluble fibre. In fact, eating barley instead of white rice slashes the effect on your blood sugar by almost 70 per cent. Add it to soups, use it instead of Arborio rice (the worst rice offender of all) in risotto, and serve it as a nutty, flavourful side dish. The possibilities are endless.

Because its insoluble fibre slows the rate at which food leaves the stomach, barley also helps you to feel full on fewer calories.

Menu magic

While barley is a natural for soups, think outside the stockpot. Broaden your barley horizons and experiment.

■ **Instead of rice pilaf,** make barley pilaf to serve with any main dish.

■ **Add barley to casseroles** and use it as a base instead of rice in rice salads.

■ **Mix cooked barley** with onions, chopped fresh herbs and a beaten egg to make stuffing.

■ **Add cooked, chilled barley** to a bean salad for a filling lunch.

■ **Try corn and barley relish** Add canned or frozen corn to cooked barley along with olive oil, wine vinegar, chopped fresh basil, salt, pepper, chopped tomatoes, bell peppers and onions.

Related recipes

Barley-bean soup 229
Barley risotto with asparagus and lemon 272
Barley salad with mangetout and lemon
  dressing 216
Black bean and barley salad 216
Mushroom and barley pilaf 276

BARLEY glossary

Like oats, barley comes in different varieties determined by how the grain is processed. All forms are beneficial to blood sugar.

■ **Hulled barley (barley groats):** only the outer hull of the grain is removed; the bran is left intact. This is the least processed, most nutritious type.

■ **Pot or Scotch barley:** this is more processed than hulled barley but retains some of the bran layer.

■ **Pearl barley:** this is much more processed, with the outer hull and bran removed. Because the soluble fibre runs all the way through the grain, however, this type is still a smart choice.

■ **Quick-cooking barley:** similar to pearl barley in taste and nutrition, this is presteamed, so it takes only about 10 minutes to cook compared to an hour for other types.

■ **Barley flour:** this provides more than three times the fibre of refined white flour. For baking, combine it with wholemeal flour or it won't rise.

■ **Barley flakes:** made from steam-rolled and dried barley, these are cooked for hot cereal.

PERFECT PORTION: 80–100g cooked

This is a good amount for a side dish. For main dishes you can allow yourself a little more and still keep the GL in the 'low' category.

beans

GL low

You may remember a slightly naughty childhood rhyme that begins 'Beans, beans, they're good for your heart...' Well, they are. But these slow-acting foods, rich in complex carbohydrates, are also fantastic for your blood sugar and are surely one of the foods most deserving of special attention in your Magic diet.

All beans, canned or dried, from black to white and chickpeas to cannellini, can tame both insulin and blood sugar levels thanks to their high soluble fibre content. In a recent study, men and women who ate a meal that included about 170g of chickpeas had 40 per cent lower blood sugar an hour after eating than those who ate an equal amount of white bread with jam.

The soluble fibre in beans slows down digestion, leading to a slow, steady blood sugar rise rather than a sharp surge. Beans also contain loads of protein, which doesn't raise blood sugar and actually helps your body to process the carbohydrates in a meal more efficiently. Are they the perfect food for people with diabetes? Perhaps. Just make sure you stick to 100–125g (7–8 tablespoons) per meal, since beans do contain some carbohydrate.

If you're trying to lose weight, eat beans! Not only are they incredibly filling, they also pack a heap of nutrition in a relatively low-calorie package. Better still, some of the starch in beans is a type called resistant starch that the body can't even digest, so the calories don't count.

Beans are also full of folate, a B vitamin that may help to reduce some of the nasty consequences of diabetes by helping to keep arteries clean. Yet even with all these health benefits, the closest many of us get to including beans in our diet is the occasional tin of baked beans (often loaded with sugar and salt). We need to broaden our intake of beans.

Health bonus

Looking for antioxidants? Look no further. A recent study ranked beans among the top ten foods richest in these health protectors. And the same soluble fibre in beans that helps to stabilise blood sugar also helps to lower cholesterol.

Perfect pairings

Beans and rice is a classic dish, and for good reason, since together they make a complete protein (alone, each lacks certain amino acids, the building blocks of protein). While white rice has a high GL, combining it with beans – and therefore eating less rice – makes the GL of the dish much lower. To lower the GL of a pasta meal, use less pasta and top it with beans.

Cooks' tips

The only black mark for beans is the salt content of tinned beans. Cut it in half by rinsing the beans in cold water before using. Instead of buying regular baked beans, look for the brands now available that are low in salt and sugar.

Chickpeas can be ground into flour, allowing you to use less white flour and therefore lower the GL of your baking. Make some wholemeal bread with chickpea flour, and your blood sugar will be substantially lower a half hour after eating it than if you ate regular wholemeal bread, studies show.

> *Beans are your blood sugar's best friend, and since all you have to do to eat them is open a can, there's no excuse not to.*

Menu magic
■ **Serve bean dip** or hummus (made with chickpeas and tahini) with a toasted wholemeal pitta cut into wedges.
■ **Mash beans or chickpeas** to make a low-GL spread and serve on coarse-ground whole-grain bread.
■ **Use drained and rinsed** canned beans as the basis for quick and easy weeknight bean soups.
■ **Add canned kidney** beans (or any other kind) to green salads.
■ **Cook up a big pot** of black bean chilli at the weekend and freeze the leftovers.
■ **Mix mango, red pepper,** onion and black beans for a zesty summer salad.

Related recipes
Barley-bean soup 229
Black bean and barley salad 216
Black bean and sweet potato burritos 274
Black bean spread with Mexican flavours 209
Dahl with spinach 272
Hearty split pea soup with rye croutons 230
Lentil and bean chilli 273
Mediterranean split pea spread 208
Tuna and cannellini salad with lemon 218
Turkey and bean chilli with avocado salsa 252
Warm artichoke and bean dip 206
Wholemeal pasta with sausage, beans
   and greens 266

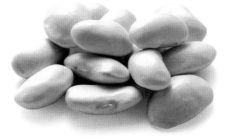

Silencing the 'MUSICAL FRUIT'

Beans can give you wind because they're rich in a specific type of indigestible carbohydrate that provides fodder for the bacteria that live in your intestinal tract and gas is the by-product. But there's no need to avoid a food that is so good for stabilising your blood sugar.

You can 'de-gas' beans by soaking them for at least 12 hours. Or boil them in water for 2 minutes, remove from the heat and let stand for 2 to 4 hours with the lid on. After either method, drain, then rinse twice and cover with fresh cold water before cooking.

If you don't eat beans often, your body will have to adapt to the extra work required to digest the complex sugars they contain. Start with small amounts and gradually increase your portions.

In general, the sweeter the bean, the easier it is to digest. Adzuki, black-eyed beans, lentils and mung beans top the list. The most indigestible include limas and whole cooked soya beans.

PERFECT PORTION: 100–125g cooked

This amount provides between 105 and 147kcal and keeps the GL low.

beef

Beef for dinner? It should be, as beef is an important source of protein, provided that you choose lean cuts and eat moderate portions (no giant T-bones or huge steaks), and there's no reason why it can't be part of a Magic diet. In fact, here's how important protein is to your blood sugar: a study at the University of Minnesota tested two different diets, one high in protein and one with only half as much. The fat content was the same in both diets. In the group that followed the high-protein diet (which was also lower in carbs), blood sugar levels were reduced by as much as if the participants had taken pills prescribed to lower blood sugar.

Your leanest choices are the 'skinny six': sirloin, fillet, silverside, top side, rump and tenderloin. The not-so-skinny cuts to trim from your diet include rib eye, prime rib, T-bone, and regular minced beef, which are all high in saturated fat. (To get the leanest minced beef for hamburgers or meat loaf, look for 'extra lean', or 93–95 per cent lean.) Saturated fat not only clogs your arteries, it can also contribute to insulin resistance, which makes it harder for your body to use insulin to get blood sugar out of the bloodstream and into cells.

Lean beef isn't just good for your blood sugar, it's even good for your waistline. Dieters tend to lose muscle along with fat, which slows their metabolisms, since muscle tissue burns more calories than fat tissue does. Eating protein helps you to hang on to that muscle mass and keep your metabolism burning on 'high'. We're not advocating a diet that is super-high in protein or super-low in carbs, which simply isn't healthy. (If you haven't already, read 'Why low-carb diets aren't the answer,' starting on page 34.) Aim to keep your protein intake at 20 to 30 per cent of the calories you eat.

Health bonus

Protein isn't the only selling point. Beef is also one of the best sources of zinc, a mineral that people often come up short on, especially if they're counting calories. Then there is vitamin B_{12}, which you can get only from eating animal foods such as eggs, milk and, of course, beef. Another beef bonus: its fat is rich in conjugated linoleic acid, or CLA, a fatty acid that helps to lower blood sugar.

Cooks' tips

Want to beef up the health benefits of beef? If you can find it, you may want to opt for grass-fed beef, which can have as much as 60 per cent more heart-healthy omega-3 fatty acids and about twice as much CLA as regular beef. But be prepared to pay: grass-fed beef can cost twice as much.

Menu magic

■ **Throw together fajitas** made with flank steak, peppers and onions for a quick weeknight meal.

■ **Toss hot grilled beef** with cold, crisp lettuce, lime juice and chopped onion for a refreshingly delicious Asian-inspired salad.

■ **When company comes,** serve up a nice (and lean) beef tenderloin.

■ **Stir-fry strips** of beef with lots of veggies for an easy way to have your beef and get your vegetables, too.

Lean beef is good for your blood sugar and even your waistline, so don't cross it off your shopping list.

- **Roast beef is not just for occasions** Cook a small joint mid week and use leftovers in sandwiches or a salad the next day.
- **Cook up three-bean chilli** with a small amount of extra-lean minced beef.
- **Make Asian kebabs** with beef marinated in soy sauce, sesame oil, crushed garlic and ginger. Serve over brown rice.
- **Create healthier meat loaf** with finely chopped spinach, onions and grated carrots and lean minced beef. Use oats as a binder.
- **Make any cut** of beef tastier by marinating it in balsamic vinegar, olive oil, basil, Dijon mustard and garlic.

Love me TENDER

While lean cuts of beef are better for you, they're also not as tender as fattier cuts (the fat is what makes a knife cut through a prime rib like butter). But there are ways to turn up the tenderness of healthier cuts.

- **Pound and flatten** the meat into thinner, more tender slices.
- **Use the juice** from a fresh pineapple or papaya as a marinade. It contains a powerful enzyme that breaks down the meat, tenderising it. (Canned juice won't work; the enzymes are destroyed during processing.)
- **Use a marinade** that contains vinegar, wine or citrus juice. The acid softens the tissues of meat, making it more tender and tastier.
- **Cook tenderised** beef either quickly at a high temperature or for an extended period with moist heat at a low to medium temperature.

Related recipes

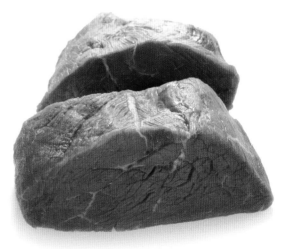

PERFECT PORTION: 85g

Forget the super-sized burgers with enough calories for breakfast, lunch and dinner. A **healthy serving** of lean beef is **85g cooked** (170g is okay if you eat meat only once a day). That's only about the size of a **deck of cards**. Fill the rest of your plate with low-GL vegetables and whole grains.

berries

From ruby-red strawberries to midnight-blue blueberries, berries may be heaven for your tastebuds, but they're Magic for your blood sugar. Their sweetness is deceptive. Fructose, the natural sugar found in most fruits, is sweeter than what's in your sugar bowl (sucrose), so it takes much less (with fewer calories) to get that sweet taste. And fructose is friendlier to blood sugar, causing a much slower rise than table sugar does.

Berries are full of fibre and red-blue plant compounds called anthocyanins that may help to keep your blood sugar in check. Scientists believe anthocyanins, also found in cherries, may help to lower blood sugar by boosting insulin production.

Opt for fresh or frozen berries over berry juices. While the juices are packed with the same phytonutrients as whole berries, they are concentrated sources of carbs, and they lack an important ingredient for blood sugar control – fibre.

What about that jar of jam in your fridge? Spread lightly. Even those whose labels say they're 100 per cent natural fruit usually contain either added sugar or added fruit juice and have higher GLs than whole fresh fruit. Still, a tablespoon is fine if you spread it on wholemeal toast or a wholemeal roll.

Health bonus

Berries, especially blueberries, have a well-earned reputation for being especially rich in powerful disease-fighting antioxidants. Studies show that if you make berries a daily indulgence, they can help to keep your eyes healthy, reduce your risk of heart disease and cancer, and even work to keep your brain and memory in tiptop shape. Strawberries are a surprisingly good source of heart-healthy vitamin C, giving even citrus fruits a run for their money. Weight for weight, strawberries contain more vitamin C than oranges. And studies show that people who eat a serving of strawberries a day tend to have lower blood pressure and higher blood levels of the B vitamin folate that helps to keep arteries clear.

Eating cranberries can help to fend off urinary tract infections. Experts say that about 45g of dried cranberries a day could do the trick. Researchers have discovered that blueberries contain some of the same infection-fighting compounds as cranberries.

Cooks' tips

Berries are nutrition powerhouses, but they're also fragile fruits. Choose berries that are plump and free of bruises or mold. The skin of blueberries should be smooth and not shrivelled. The hazy white coating you see on blueberries is a natural protective coating, so don't try to wash it off. Look for blackberries and raspberries that aren't leaking (if the small bumps that make up a berry burst, the juice inside leaks out, causing quicker spoilage). Always store berries in the fridge and rinse them just before serving; otherwise, they'll go off faster.

As strawberries are on a list – drawn up by the Pesticide Action Network Group UK (PAN UK) – of fruits and vegetables most likely to contain pesticide residues, it is best to buy organic when you can.

To feel the benefits of berries year round, buy them when they're in season and freeze them. Here are a few pointers.

Berries are full of fibre, which keeps blood sugar low, and antioxidants, which benefit every cell in your body.

■ **Blueberries and strawberries** freeze the best. Raspberries and blackberries are more delicate and freezing can change their texture.

■ **Wash the berries** in cold water and let them dry completely on a paper towel or in a colander.

■ **Spread the dry** berries out on a sheet of wax paper on a baking sheet and place in the freezer.

■ **Once they are** completely frozen, pack them in a tightly sealed freezer container and put them back in the freezer straightaway.

Menu magic

Berries can complement countless dishes, adding visual appeal as well as sweetness.

■ **Top your waffles,** pancakes, cereal and porridge with berries.

■ **Add berries** to muffin batter.

■ **Stir fresh or frozen** blueberries into plain yoghurt for a satisfying snack.

■ **Be adventurous** and make wild blueberry salsa (wild blueberries are smaller, so they work better) with diced onion, jalapeño pepper, red bell pepper, coriander leaves and lemon juice.

■ **Use whole strawberries** as edible garnishes at breakfast, lunch or dinner.

■ **Drizzle a tablespoon** of chocolate syrup over fresh strawberries for a decadent but healthy dessert.

■ **Spoon a generous** amount of fresh berries over a smallish serving of frozen yoghurt or ice cream.

■ **Sprinkle mixed fresh berries** over tossed green salads.

■ **Add dried cranberries** to green salads, muffins or grain side dishes.

■ **Make a very berry** smoothie with yoghurt, mixed berries (fresh or frozen), vanilla extract and orange juice.

Related recipes

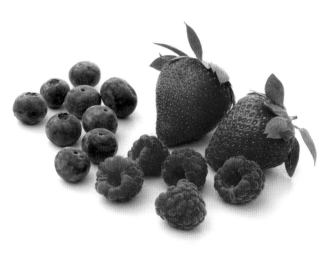

PERFECT PORTION: 80g (7 strawberries)

A *handful* of berries makes a perfect *low-calorie snack*.

bran

When you eat grains

– which should, of course, be a regular part of your diet – you can't do better than bran. In fact, a bowl of bran cereal has just a third of the GL of a bowl of cornflakes. (*See* 'How cereals rate' on the opposite page.) That means your blood sugar will go up only a third as much, so it doesn't have far to fall. (Remember, it's those precipitous drops that cause trouble and make you hungry again.)

There's really no better way to get one of the three daily servings of whole grains we recommend than starting your day with bran cereal. Top it with berries, and you've really hit your Magic eating stride.

Think of bran as the heavy 'overcoat' worn by kernels of whole-grain oats, wheat or rice. It contains the highest concentration of fibre of any part of the grain – 1 tablespoon (7g) of wheat bran contains 3.5g of fibre, while the same amount of oat bran contains 2g. As you know, fibre helps you to feel fuller on fewer calories, smoothing the way for weight loss.

Bran also helps to tame those wild blood sugar surges after meals. When researchers gave obese children either a sugar solution or a sugar solution plus 15g (about 4 tablespoons) of wheat bran, the youngsters' blood sugar levels were much lower when they ate the bran. If you add bran to your diet regularly, you could really lower your blood sugar over the long term – by as much as 22 per cent – a reduction experienced by people in one medical study who ate rice bran for two months as part of a heart-healthy diet.

Oat bran is high in soluble fibre, which gives it extra power over blood sugar. Adding oat bran to the mix – meaning pancake, muffin or cake mix – can significantly change the food's effect on your blood sugar. Researchers found that for each gram of beta-glucan (the type of soluble fibre found in oat bran) added to snack bars, the glycaemic index of the bar dropped by 4 points. A lower GI translates into a lower GL, which means a milder blood sugar response after you eat the bar. It takes only 30g of oat bran to provide 1.5 grams of beta-glucan.

As you can tell, we're big on bran!

Health bonus

Oat bran can bring down high cholesterol and reduce the risk of heart disease, and it has an FDA-approved health claim to prove it. In one study, men who consumed the most wheat bran (about 9g per day) were 30 per cent less likely to develop heart disease than those who consumed the least (not quite 2g per day).

Rice bran can also lower cholesterol, and early research in animals suggests it may help to tame high blood pressure as well. The natural oils in rice bran may be the Magic ingredient. Rice bran is also gluten-free, a real plus for people who have a sensitivity to gluten.

Wheat bran may help to reduce the risk of colon and breast cancer. And of course, bran helps to keep you regular.

Cooks' tips

Because bran contains oils that can become rancid, be sure to store it in the refrigerator or freezer once it's been opened. Many bran cereals, on the other hand, contain preservatives that will keep them fresh for several months in your kitchen cupboards.

DON'T fall for it ...

Bran muffins may appear to be a health food, but they're usually anything but. Most shop-bought muffins are full of sugar, fat and calories. Make your own for a much healthier treat (see the Apple bran muffins recipe on page 198).

How CEREALS rate

Some cereals are 'fast acting' and send blood sugar on a rollercoaster ride, while others are digested slowly – more like the speed of an old-fashioned merry-go-round. Bran is among the slowest-acting cereals of all.

CEREAL	SERVING	GLYCAEMIC LOAD
Oat Bran	30g	3
Bran Buds	30g	7
All-Bran	30g	9
Muesli	30g	9
Porridge (cooked)	250g	10
Raisin Bran	30g	12
Bran Flakes	30g	13
Instant porridge (cooked)	250g	13
Special K	30g	14
Corn Flakes	30g	24
Crispix	30g	22
Rice Krispies	30g	22

Menu magic

■ **Start your day** with plain bran cereal, hot or cold (look for Quaker and other brands). It's one of the lowest GL cereals you can choose.

■ **Use bran in muffin recipes** in place of half the flour for muffins that are high in fibre and loaded with nutrients. If you don't have bran flour on hand, try using bran cereal. Some brands have muffin recipes right on the box. Add fruit and nuts for truly Magic muffins.

■ **Make a meat loaf** more Magic by using oat bran or another bran as a binder instead of breadcrumbs. It will help to balance the effect of the mashed or boiled potatoes that you eat with it by lowering your blood sugar response to the entire meal.

■ **Make drop scones** or waffles with rice flour and rice bran or try adding different types of bran and experimenting with the taste and texture. Top with fresh blueberries to squeeze in a serving of fruit.

Smart substitution

Instead of a bowl of cornflakes: have a bowl of cooked bran cereal topped with dried cranberries or fresh strawberries.

Related recipes

Apple bran muffins 198
Chocolate fudge brownies 295

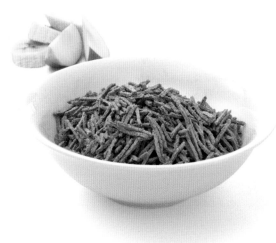

> **PERFECT PORTION: 2–3 tablespoons**
>
> *This much **bran cereal** should **fill** you up. Use less sprinkled over yoghurt and more when substituting for flour.*

broccoli

GL very low

Because it's big on volume and small on calories, broccoli is a great way to bulk up carb dishes (think pasta, casseroles and baked potatoes) to lower their GL.

Not only does broccoli have very little impact on your blood sugar, it's one of the best food sources of chromium, a mineral required for insulin to function normally (remember, insulin helps the body to use up blood sugar so there's less in the bloodstream). One serving (80g) of broccoli provides almost half of your daily chromium requirement.

Broccoli is also packed with vitamin C. One serving contains more than 100 per cent of its RDA. If you're fighting diabetes – or even if you already have it – that's important. A British population study found that people with the highest blood levels of vitamin C were less likely to have elevated levels of glycated haemoglobin, a long-term indicator of high blood sugar. Even if vitamin C can't protect you from diabetes – the jury is still out on this – like other antioxidants it can lower your risk of diabetes-related complications such as eye and nerve damage.

Health bonus

Broccoli is known for its cancer-fighting compounds. Numerous studies over the past 20 years have found that people who eat plenty of broccoli have a significantly lower risk of several cancers, including breast, colon, cervical, lung, prostate and bladder cancer. Broccoli's also a good source of calcium, which builds strong bones, protecting against osteoporosis in later life.

PERFECT PORTION: two florets (80g)

The GL of broccoli is based on a serving of two florets, but feel free to eat as much as you want.

Hate broccoli? blame it on **YOUR GENES**

Does the taste of broccoli make you recoil in disgust? You may be able to blame your genes. Researchers have discovered a gene that makes some people hypersensitive to bitter-tasting compounds in broccoli, Brussels sprouts and cabbage.

Cooks' tips

Don't overcook broccoli; it will turn pale and mushy and lose some of its nutrients.

Menu magic

■ **For creamy soup** without the cream, purée cooked broccoli, cauliflower and onion with a pinch of salt and white pepper. Add low-fat milk for a creamier texture.

■ **Add chopped broccoli** florets to omelettes, vegetable lasagna and pizza.

■ **For a super-low-GL** meal, make a beef and broccoli stir-fry and serve over a modest portion of brown rice.

■ **Whip up a broccoli** salad to take on your next picnic. Mix broccoli florets, sliced carrots, sliced green olives, diced pimentos and chopped walnuts and marinate in Italian dressing.

■ **Top steamed broccoli** with a spoonful of low-fat yoghurt dip or salsa and some slivered toasted almonds for a healthy side dish.

■ **Finely chop the thick stalks** of broccoli and use with white cabbage and carrot in coleslaw .

Related recipes

brown rice

GL medium

Brown rice doesn't have the wonderfully low GL of some other grains such as barley or oats. Nevertheless, it's a far better choice for your blood sugar than most white rice. So, if rice is on the menu, better make it brown.

As a nutrient-packed, fibre-rich whole-grain, brown rice has many of the good qualities you expect in a Magic food. Not only does it boast 4 times the fibre of white rice, it's packed with vitamins, minerals and natural plant compounds to protect your health. And, as a whole grain, brown rice is part of the formula for lowering your risk of diabetes and heart disease. Remember, we want you to aim to eat three servings a day of whole grains, which help to

protect against metabolic syndrome, diabetes, heart disease, stroke and cancer. A serving of brown rice is 50-70g uncooked rice.

Regular brown rice takes about 35 minutes to cook. When time is of the essence, don't opt for instant rice, whether it is white or brown; instant rice has been partially cooked and dehydrated and all types have a high GL. A better option – used in the USA but not yet readily available here – is converted rice, which has a GL similar to that of brown rice and many of the nutrients, too.

All rice starts off as brown rice. Only when it's been refined and the bran and germ have been removed is white rice born. Different types of rice vary in their GL depending on the type of starch they naturally contain (*see* 'Rice rankings'). Three rices to avoid: jasmine, Arborio (the kind used in risotto), and 'sticky rice' (the type found in sushi.

Health bonus

Brown rice offers more than just fibre. It's rich in the bone-building mineral magnesium, the immune-boosting antioxidant selenium, and manganese, a mineral important for keeping up the body's natural defences.

Cooks' tips

Because brown rice contains some fat naturally found in the whole grain, it won't stay fresh as long as white rice. You can store uncooked brown rice in the cupboard for up to 6 months. Always

Rice RANKINGS

There's much more to rice than just white or brown. And the different varieties vary as much in their effect on your blood sugar as they do in flavour. Take a look.

RICE	GLYCAEMIC LOAD per 150g cooked rice
Medium	
■ Brown rice	18
■ Wild rice	18
■ Cajun style rice mix	19
■ Long and wild rice blend	20
■ Mexican style rice mix	22
High	
■ Basmati rice	23
■ Long grain white rice	23
■ Long grain quick cooking	27
Very high	
■ Sticky rice (used in sushi rolls)	31
■ Arborio risotto rice	36
■ Jasmine rice	46

PERFECT PORTION: 50–70g raw rice

Stick to **one serving** per meal. You will need to measure this carefully at first. Rice is, after all, *a high-carb food.*

RICE glossary

Who knew rice could be so complicated? Here's a run-down of rice terms to help you through the rice maze.

 ■ Brown rice: still has the bran and the germ of the whole rice kernel, so it contains all the nutrition of a whole grain. Has a longer cooking time and a higher fibre content. Has a nutty flavour and a hearty texture.

■ Converted rice: the rice is steamed before it's husked, allowing the individual grains to absorb more nutrients. Takes about the same amount of time to cook as white rice, but less time than brown rice.

■ Wild rice: this is not a rice at all, but the seeds of a marsh grass. It's high in protein and fibre and several B vitamins. Has a pungent, earthy flavour.

 ■ Basmati rice: A long-grain, aromatic white rice grown in the Himalayas. It cooks up dry and fluffy. You can get brown or white basmati rice. The GL of brown basmati is lower – closer to that of brown rice.

■ Long-grain white rice: the most common rice used in cooking. The nutritious bran and germ have been processed out, taking fibre and natural plant compounds with them. As with most refined products, nutrients such as iron, thiamin, niacin and folate have been lost. Has a bland flavour.

■ Long-grain quick-cooking rice: the rice is completely cooked and dehydrated, so cooking time is short, usually 10 to 15 minutes. Comes as white or brown rice.

 ■ Sticky rice: also called glutinous rice, though it doesn't contain gluten, this is a short-grain, white, refined rice that sticks together. Though it's sometimes called 'sweet rice', it has a bland flavour like most white rice.

■ Arborio rice: a plump, refined, short-grain white rice that absorbs water without developing a mushy texture. Used in risotto and noted for its ability to absorb flavours.

■ Jasmine rice: long-grain white rice that has a subtle flower-like aroma.

keep it in an airtight container. You can store it in the refrigerator to make it last longer.

Menu magic

■ Substitute brown rice for white rice in casseroles, stir-fries and side dishes to lower the GL of a meal while adding a chewy texture and nutty flavour.

■ Make a batch of brown rice and store in the fridge for later use in salads and other dishes.

Related recipes

Brown rice pilaf with flaxseeds, lime and coriander 277

Brown rice pilaf with lemon and toasted flaxseeds 276

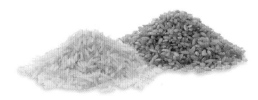

magic grains

Wholemeal bread

Whole grains

Don't blame GRAINS

– embrace them! The Magic grains
have a moderate glycaemic load and
are too good for you to exclude them
from your diet.

- barley
- bran
- brown rice
- bulghur
- oats
- pasta

- pumpernickel bread
- rye bread
- sourdough bread
- quinoa
- wheatgerm
- wholemeal bread

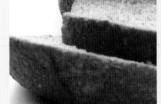

Oats

Wholemeal pasta

Brussels sprouts

GL very low

Like most vegetables, these mini-cabbages have a very low GL, which means they're kind to your blood sugar. But Brussels sprouts also have something special: soluble fibre (about 2g per 80g serving). This stuff forms a gel in your stomach that acts as a barrier between food and the enzymes that break it down, making your meal 'slow acting' instead of 'fast acting' when it comes to digestion. And that goes for everything in the meal – even the roll. Remember, where blood sugar is concerned, a slow rise is better.

One study found that women who ate cruciferous vegetables, including Brussels sprouts, appeared to reduce their risk of developing diabetes by as much as two-thirds compared to those who seldom ate cruciferous veggies.

Another surprising bonus: almost one-third of the calories in Brussels sprouts come from protein, meaning that even though they seem substantial, these veggies are blessedly low in carbs.

If you have diabetes or any other risk factor for heart disease, take note: Brussels sprouts are a top source of vitamin C (48mg per 80g serving), a must-have nutrient for keeping arteries healthy and fending off complications of diabetes. A large European study found that adults with the highest blood levels of vitamin C had only half the risk of dying from cardiovascular disease compared to those with the lowest levels.

Health bonus

Like their cousins cabbage and broccoli, Brussels sprouts are powerful anticancer foods. They're also rich in lutein and zeaxanthin, members of the carotenoid family that are celebrated for their ability to keep your eyesight sharp as you age. And sprouts are an underappreciated source of bone-building vitamin K.

Cooks' tips

Like cabbage, Brussels sprouts do not have a pleasant cooking smell. Cooking time equals odour intensity, so keep it short (steaming is a good option). Store leftovers in an airtight container, or else you'll smell the consequences when you open the fridge.

Menu magic

Brussels sprouts are one of those all-or-nothing foods; either you love 'em or you hate 'em. But before you decide once and for all, give these Brussels sprout dishes a try.

■ **Steam sprouts,** then sauté them in olive oil along with any or all of the following: crushed mustard seed, cumin, fennel seed, cayenne pepper, finely chopped ginger, fresh lime juice and salt. Top with flaked almonds.

■ **Get two Magic foods** in one dish by combining baby carrots and halved Brussels sprouts. Sauté them in olive oil (a third Magic food), then add chicken broth and simmer. Add some lemon juice (another!) and some chopped dill just before they're done.

■ **Pair the strong taste** of Brussels sprouts or other cruciferous vegetables with a sweet-tasting side dish such as apple sauce or sweet potatoes.

■ **To make Brussels sprouts** even more blood sugar-friendly, add vinegar. Marinate cooked sprouts overnight in vinegar (try tarragon vinegar), crushed garlic, minced onion, a pinch of salt and a spoonful of honey.

Related recipe

Sautéed Brussels sprouts with red pepper and caraway seeds 284

PERFECT PORTION: 80g

*A serving is about **8 sprouts**, but there's no reason not to eat **more.***

---

bulghur wheat

GL medium

If you're following the 'Seven secrets of Magic eating', you're trying to get three servings of whole grains a day. For a chewy texture and a slightly nutty taste, try bulghur wheat as a deliciously filling side dish or hot cereal. It can even be used to make stuffing. Best of all, it cooks quickly.

Bulghur wheat ranks alongside wholemeal bread and bran – all Magic foods and all forms of the same nutritious wheat grain. That's right, bulghur isn't an individual type of grain. It's wheat grain that's been partially cooked by boiling or steaming, then dried and cracked.

Eating more whole grains has been shown to cut diabetes risk by 35 per cent in men and women and reduce heart disease risk by 25 per cent in women and 18 per cent in men. Just six weeks on a whole-grain diet can markedly improve insulin sensitivity, according to one study.

Health bonus

As with all whole-grain foods, eating more translates into lower risk not only of diabetes and heart disease but also of certain cancers. In a Swedish study of more than 61,000 women, researchers found that those who ate at least $4\frac{1}{2}$ servings of whole grains a day had a 23 per cent lower risk of developing colon cancer compared to women who ate fewer than $1\frac{1}{2}$ servings a day. The lignans in bulghur may also help to protect against breast cancer.

Cooks' tips

You'll find bulghur wheat in different textures. Coarse bulghur is used for pilaf and rice dishes, medium is used as breakfast cereal and fine is used for tabbouleh (a Middle Eastern salad made with bulghur, chopped parsley, cucumbers, tomatoes, olive oil and lemon juice). The finer the grain, the quicker bulghur cooks up.

Menu magic

■ **Try bulghur pilaf** as a side dish. There are a million different recipes, some including dried fruit and some with vegetables and/or herbs. Grab a good cookbook and take your pick.
■ **Throw together** some tabbouleh as an excellent, portable summertime lunch salad or side dish. Toss in chopped vegetables such as tomatoes and cucumbers, and add some goat or feta cheese or chicken for extra protein.
■ **Add bulghur** to dishes such as spaghetti bolognese or chilli, to bulk out the meat.
■ **Stuff courgettes** with bulghur and extra-lean minced beef or pork.

Smart substitutions

Instead of rice: use cooked bulghur in stir-fries.
Instead of couscous: have bulghur as your accompaniment to stews and casseroles.

Related recipes

Bulghur wheat with ginger and orange 275

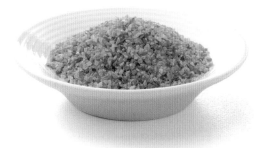

PERFECT PORTION: 90–100g cooked

A typical serving size is 100g, but you can have as much as 150g of cooked bulghur and the GL will still be in the medium range.

cabbage

GL very low

For centuries Russian peasants sustained themselves on this leafy vegetable. But even if your fridge is full of other foods, you should still consider eating cabbage. It's very low in calories (just 20kcal per 80g portion) and high in fibre. Together, these two attributes spell weight loss, which should benefit your blood sugar. Add to that the fact that cabbage is very low on the GL scale, and you've got a Magic winner. Eating cabbage doesn't mean spooning up a thin, unappetising stew; if you prepare it correctly, cabbage can be a culinary delight.

This veggie doesn't just help you to lose weight. Cabbage (especially the red variety) is also a surprisingly excellent source of vitamin C, which some experts believe may reduce the risk of developing diabetes. Red cabbage offers another bonus: it's rich in natural pigments called anthocyanins, which new research suggests may help to boost insulin production and lower blood sugar levels.

Finally, cabbage is often prepared with vinegar, which can help to lower the GL of your whole meal.

Health bonus

Cabbage contains sulphoraphane, which has anticancer properties. One study of women found that those who ate the most cabbage and other crucifers had a 45 per cent lower breast cancer risk than women who ate the least.

Cabbage may also help to guard against lung cancer. Fermented cabbage, also known as sauerkraut, may have even higher levels of anticancer compounds – a result of the fermentation process. Just be aware of sauerkraut's high salt content; always rinse it before heating and eating.

Cooks' tips

Overcook cabbage, and you'll regret it when the smell lingers. Overcooking also destroys cabbage's stores of vitamin C, which can't stand the heat. Steam cabbage until limp, stir-fry it quickly, or chop it raw for salads and slaws. Older cabbage or cabbage that's been in the fridge for a while may have a stronger smell. To minimise the odour, cook the cabbage quickly in an uncovered pan with as little water as possible. Try adding a tablespoon of vinegar to the cooking water to further cut the odour.

Menu magic

- **Enjoy cabbage** in coleslaw.
- **Add thinly sliced or chopped** cabbage to mashed potato.
- **Place sautéed cabbage** underneath a small serving of steak to add gourmet appeal.
- **Braise red cabbage** with chopped apples, walnuts and red wine.
- **Sauté cabbage** and onions to serve as a side dish.
- **Use shredded cabbage** in place of lettuce on sandwiches and burgers.
- **Combine cooked shredded** cabbage with low-fat yoghurt and caraway seed, then heat and serve as a side dish.
- **Wrap thick fish** fillets in cabbage leaves and steam over seasoned broth.

PERFECT PORTION: 80g

A serving is roughly ⅙ of a cabbage, but really **the sky's the limit** *with this* **low-calorie, nutritious** *food.*

Related recipes

Creamy coleslaw without mayonnaise 220
Oriental noodle hotpot 233
Pork chop and cabbage pan-fry 242

carrots

GL very low

Carrots perfectly

illustrate the difference between the glycaemic index (GI) and the glycaemic load (GL). When the GI first made waves among health enthusiasts, carrots got a bad rap for raising blood sugar. That's because the type of sugar they contain is transformed into blood sugar very rapidly – almost as fast as table sugar. But since the amount of sugar is low, carrots are still on the menu.

Thank goodness they are, because they're one of the richest sources of beta-carotene, which is linked to a lower risk of diabetes. One study found that people with the highest blood levels of beta-carotene had 32 per cent lower insulin levels (suggesting better blood sugar control) than those with the lowest beta-carotene levels. Carrots are also a good source of beneficial fibre.

Health bonus

Eating carrots won't mean that you can throw away your reading glasses, but they will help to protect against two sight-robbing conditions: macular degeneration and cataracts. They're also rich in soluble fibre, which lowers cholesterol.

Cooks' tips

Cut off the green carrot tops before storing, or they'll pull moisture from the carrots and make them wither.

Menu magic

■ **Add grated carrots** to sandwiches. For a decidedly different sandwich spread, mix finely grated carrots with low-fat cream cheese and add chopped green olives and grated onions.
■ **Munch on baby carrots** and hummus as a snack or with lunch.
■ **Cook baby carrots** with rosemary and thyme, olive oil, chopped onions and black pepper. Squeeze the juice of orange wedges over the top.

Don't fall for it ...

'Raw food' proponents would have you believe that all foods are most nutritious in their uncooked state. Not true. With raw and cooked carrots, you simply get different benefits. During cooking, the carrot's cell walls break down, releasing the beta-carotene inside. Raw carrots, on the other hand, contain more vitamin C.

■ **Mix up spicy carrot soup** by puréeing cooked carrots and adding them to sautéed onions and garlic along with vegetable broth and either soya milk or low-fat yoghurt.
■ **For a salad** with Middle Eastern flair, combine cooked sliced carrots, olive oil, chopped parsley, minced garlic, fresh lemon juice and salt. The lemon juice further reduces the GL of the dish.

Related recipes

Barley-bean soup 229
Creamy coleslaw without mayonnaise 220
Garden pasta salad 223
Moroccan spiced carrots 286
Oriental noodle hotpot 233
Pork chop and cabbage pan-fry 242
Savoury beef and vegetable loaf 239
Slow-cooker beef and red wine stew 238
Spring vegetable stir-fry with tofu 271
Tuna and carrot sandwich on rye 228
Wholemeal noodles with peanut sauce and chicken 220

PERFECT PORTION: 80g cooked

A serving is *3 heaped tablespoons* of cooked carrots or *1 tablespoon raw*. The GL of cooked is slightly higher.

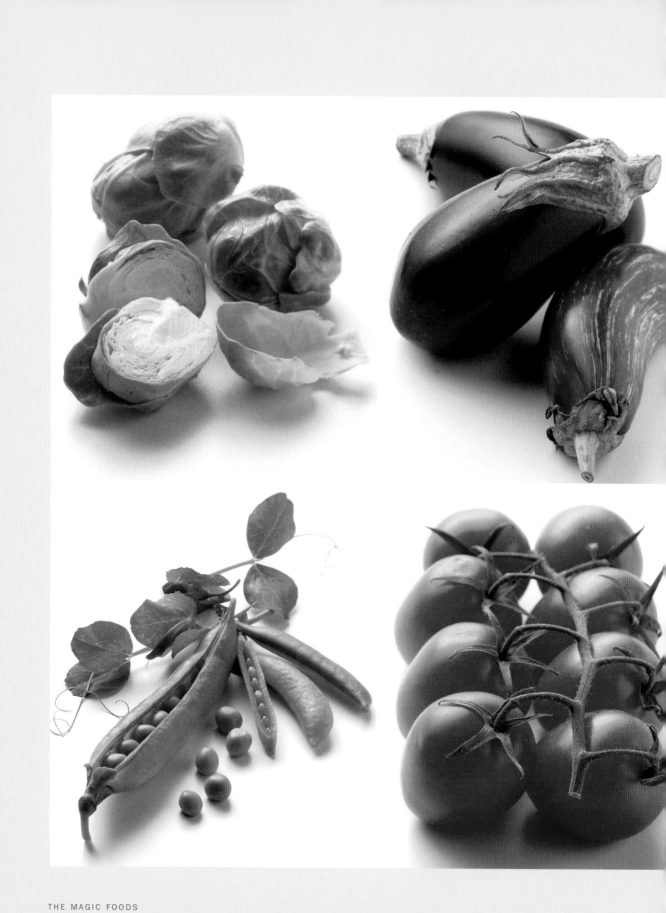

Magic vegetables

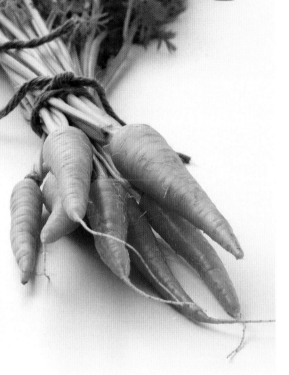

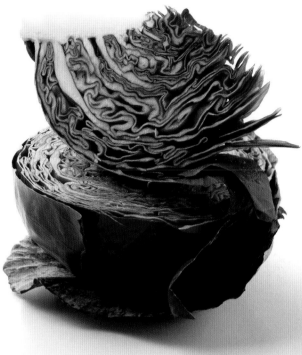

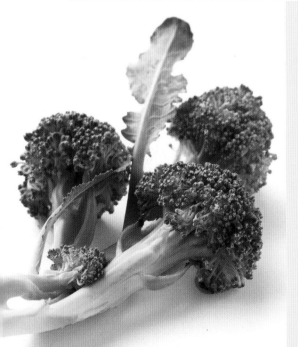

With low or **VERY LOW**

glycaemic loads, vegetables are one food group that won't play havoc with your blood sugar – and will help you to fight diabetes and weight gain. We've chosen these veggies as Magic foods because of their impressive nutritional profile, and in the case of aubergine, the ability to stand in for meat.

■ aubergine	■ cauliflower
■ broccoli	■ onion
■ Brussels sprouts	■ peas
■ cabbage	■ spinach
■ carrots	■ tomato

cauliflower

GL very low

Not many vegetables

are as filling and low in calories as cauliflower. While it's an acquired taste for some, cauliflower is perfect for your Magic diet if you like it, most obviously because it has so few calories, so much fibre, and so little carbohydrate. It's also good because, when cooked in the right way, it can be used as a substitute for mashed potatoes or even rice.

Cauliflower is packed with vitamin C: a single serving of cooked cauliflower supplies around 50 per cent of the RDA. That makes it an ideal food for protecting cells against damage from high blood sugar. One caveat: if cauliflower is swamped in a fatty cheese sauce, it's no longer a Magic food.

Health bonus

Cauliflower, like its cousins broccoli, cabbage and Brussels sprouts, is rich in anti-cancer compounds. A review of 80 studies found that people who ate the largest amounts of these foods had the lowest risk of all types of cancer, particularly lung, stomach, colon and rectal cancers. In a test-tube study, juice extracted from cauliflower blocked growth of breast cancer cells.

Cooks' tips

Cook cauliflower in an uncovered pan to avoid trapping its strong odour. Add a couple of tablespoons of lemon juice to preserve its colour. Overcooking not only intensifies the aroma, it also destroys much of the vitamin C.

PERFECT PORTION: 80g cooked

A serving of cauliflower, about *8 florets* cooked, provides a *slimline* *22kcal* and *2.5g of fibre*. Not a bad deal at all.

Menu magic

■ **Instead of mashed potatoes** try this tasty cauliflower purée. Boil a head of cauliflower cut into florets, one diced peeled potato and six peeled garlic cloves until tender. Drain and purée (in batches) in a food processor and thin with enough warm milk to make it velvety. Drizzle on olive oil and season with salt and pepper.

■ **Serve cauliflower** raw or lightly steamed with seasoned yoghurt dip or spicy tomato sauce.

■ **Combine cauliflower** with broccoli in quiches, omelettes and casseroles.

■ **Toss florets with** olive oil and garlic and roast in the oven.

■ **Bake a whole head** of cauliflower to serve with dinner. Place a trimmed and rinsed head in a steamer, cover and cook until firm but tender. Place in a baking dish and coat with a mixture of wholemeal breadcrumbs, olive oil, garlic powder, salt, dried oregano and crushed garlic. Sprinkle a bit of Parmesan cheese on top and bake for 10 to 15 minutes at 180°C.

■ **Stir-fry cauliflower** and broccoli florets with water chestnuts and season with a dash of soy sauce and sesame oil.

■ **Make a cauliflower** salad by combining florets with tarragon vinegar, Dijon mustard, salt, white pepper and olive oil. Cover and leave to marinate overnight.

Smart substitution

Instead of rice: shred cauliflower in a food processor until the texture is similar to rice. Lightly steam it and use in recipes that call for cooked rice.

Related recipes

cheese

With virtually zero

carbs and a lot of protein, cheese is certainly a 'better blood sugar' food because it won't move the blood sugar needle the slightest bit, and it will fill you up. Cheese is also an excellent source of calcium, and studies show that getting plenty of calcium from food may help to prevent insulin resistance, a harbinger of diabetes. According to a recent study, women who get plenty of calcium from dairy products also have a significantly lower risk of developing metabolic syndrome, which is linked to both diabetes and heart disease.

That doesn't mean you can eat as much full-fat cheese as you like, however. Cheese is packed not only with calories but also with its big 'design flaw' – saturated fat, the kind that clogs arteries and reduces your body's sensitivity to insulin. That's why it is important to choose, whenever possible, lower-fat cheeses, such as cottage cheese, fromage frais and soft goat's cheese. Otherwise, the drawbacks of cheese could easily outweigh its benefits. Weight for weight soft cheeses tend to have less fat than hard cheeses (usually about 6 or 7g per 30g instead of 8 or 9g.)

When you do use a hard cheese like cheddar, you'll want to eat less of it; you can choose a low-fat version (*see* 'The art of using low-fat cheese' on page 98). You probably won't want to snack on low-fat cheddar, though, so give another cheese a try for nibbling. We suggest goat's cheese

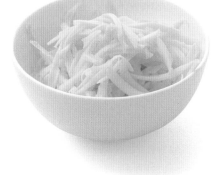

sprinkled with herbs and drizzled with lemon juice. The acidic juice offers an added benefit, since the acid has the power to lower blood sugar.

NUTRITIONAL value
of typical cheeses per 30g

	KCAL	FAT (g)	PROTEIN (g)	CALCIUM (mg)
Soft fresh cheeses				
■ Cottage cheese	30	1.2	3	22
■ Fromage frais (8%)	34	2.1	2	27
■ Mozzarella	87	6.6	8	177
■ Reduced-fat soft cheese	59	4.5	3.6	108
Semi-soft rinded cheeses				
■ Brie	96	7.8	5.8	162
Goat's and sheep's milk cheeses				
■ Feta	7.5	6	4.7	108
■ Goat's cheese (medium-fat)	102	8.5	3.5	56
Semi-hard and hard cheeses				
■ Cheddar (traditional)	124	10	7.8	216
■ Edam	100	7.8	7.8	231
■ Parmesan	136	9.8	11.82	360
Blue cheeses				
■ Danish blue	104	9	6	150
■ Stilton	124	10.8	6.6	96

PERFECT PORTION: 30g

A serving of cheese is a scant 30g.
For hard cheese, that's about the size of a small matchbox. *Cheese calorie counts range from a low of about 72 per serving for reduced-fat mozzarella to a high of about 130 per serving for Parmesan.*

cheese continued

Another way to cut cheese calories is to choose a strong-flavoured type such as Parmesan because a little goes a long way.

Cheese wouldn't be so bad if we didn't tend to use so much of it, as in lasagna or pizza that's often completely gooey with the stuff – but it's easy to remedy. When making lasagna, you can use the usual amount of ricotta (reduced fat) and Parmesan but only half the mozzarella (reduced fat). For pizza, you can ask for half the cheese at any pizzeria.

Health bonus

If you think milk is good for you, consider this: it takes about 4.5kg of milk to create 450g of cheese, making it a concentrated source of all the good stuff in milk, including phosphorus, zinc, vitamin A, riboflavin, vitamin B_{12} and calcium. Probably because of its calcium content, low-fat dairy food can also help to bring down high blood pressure. (If you're a cottage cheese fan, though, note that it's one type of cheese that's not high in calcium.) Cheese can even help to prevent cavities, if you eat it after meals.

Cooks' tips

To make cheese last longer in the fridge, wrap it tightly in aluminum foil to prevent it from drying out and change the wrapping each time you use it.

Menu magic

■ **Serve cheese and fruit** as an appetiser, a snack or even a dessert. Mix and match flavours and textures. Try cheddar with sliced apples, Brie with pears, shaved Parmesan with Asian pears, or cottage cheese with pineapple chunks.

■ **Add feta or goat's cheese** to a salad of seedless grapes, chopped pecans and chopped fresh basil. Serve with whole wheat crackers.

■ **Make an easy** toaster-oven pizza by topping a wholemeal pitta with tomato sauce, low-fat mozzarella, and a vegetable of your choice and cooking until the cheese melts.

Related recipes

All-new chicken cordon bleu 246
Cauliflower and spinach gratin 282
Cherry tomatoes filled with creamy
   pesto cheese 202
Chocolate and raspberry cheesecake 298
Greek lentil salad 223
Greek pasta and beef casserole 240
Lemony blueberry cheesecake bars 290
Macaroni cheese with spinach 264
Mediterranean salad with edamame 224
Penne with asparagus, ricotta and lemon 264
Quick spinach and sausage lasagna 267
Spinach and goat's cheese omelette 194
Courgette frittata 195

The art of using LOW-FAT CHEESE

At their worst, low-fat cheeses taste rather like cardboard. But used properly, they're perfectly good substitutes for their full-fat cousins.

■ **Low-fat cheeses are best** used as is (uncooked) for sandwiches and salads. They can be difficult to shred, so consider buying them shredded.

■ **Don't melt low-fat cheeses under the grill** or in a toaster oven. They tend to toughen and get rubbery under direct heat. They do work, however, in casseroles and heated sandwiches and burgers.

■ **To melt low-fat cheeses for sauces,** use a low heat and stir slowly in one direction. Cook for about 25 per cent longer than you would to melt full-fat cheese.

cherries

GL very low

Remember secret

number 3 of Magic eating: 'Eat more fruits and vegetables'? These foods from the produce aisle are full of disease-fighting plant compounds, and they barely budge your blood sugar thanks to their very low GL. Cherries may be an especially good choice. Besides plenty of sugar-lowering soluble fibre, they contain red pigments that may increase your body's insulin output, which ultimately lowers your blood sugar. And they're low in calories to boot.

When you get a snack attack, reach for a handful of cherries instead of higher-GL foods such as biscuits. At dessert time, pile them on a half portion of ice cream, and your bowl will look just as full but with far fewer calories.

Maraschino cherries, however, are far from Magic. These so-called cherries have been bleached, processed and injected with sugar and red dye, taking all the magic out of a once-healthy food. Also skip cherry juice, which is usually sweetened and lacks the fibre of whole cherries.

Health bonus

Cherries pack a real antioxidant punch, rivalling even oranges. Their stash of vitamin C and other antioxidants helps to fend off heart disease, cancer and complications of diabetes. One study found that the antioxidant compounds in cherries help to protect brain cells, while other plant compounds can put a dent in your cholesterol.

The type of soluble fibre cherries contain, called pectin, is also great at lowering cholesterol.

Cooks' tips

If chewing around the cherry pit and spitting it out is a little too messy for your taste, why not buy a cherry pitter? Some can pit olives as well. Instead of serve and spit, you'll pit and serve.

Caution: one bad cherry in a bag can truly spoil the whole bunch. Sort your cherries and pick out the bad ones before putting them in the fridge.

Menu magic
■ **Add finely chopped** cherries to minced meat; you'll cut the fat, boost the nutrition and add unexpected zip to meat loaf and burgers.
■ **Add frozen tart** cherries to your next smoothie.
■ **Add chopped** fresh cherries to low-fat yoghurt for a fantastic midday snack.

Smart substitution
Instead of hot fudge with ice cream: add cherries to your frozen treat.

Related recipe
Cherry clafoutis 300

PERFECT PORTION: 80g

The GL of cherries is based on a portion of around **14 cherries**, but since the GL and the **calorie count** are so **very low**, feel free to eat **more**.

chicken and turkey

Because chicken is full of all-important protein, low in fat, incredibly versatile and cooks quickly, we consider it the ultimate convenience food. Remember, protein foods don't raise blood sugar a bit. And chicken has the edge on beef in terms of fat and calories. An 85g serving of skinless chicken breast has 95 per cent less saturated fat – the stuff that hampers insulin sensitivity – than an equal serving of beef tenderloin. It also has 40 per cent fewer calories. (As you know, a wide waistline contributes to insulin resistance, which makes blood sugar control difficult.)

Because protein foods take a while to digest, they slow the digestion of the whole meal, including the carbs it contains (including the mashed potatoes on the plate with your roasted chicken breast and the bread holding your turkey sandwich fillings), making for a slower rise in blood sugar. Getting enough protein also helps you to feel full longer, which in turn helps with weight loss. The plan: serve up chicken as a main dish as often as you like, but also use it to add protein to salads and pasta.

Enjoy your chicken grilled, baked, sautéed, or grilled, but skip the fried chicken, or you'll be eating more fat than chicken. One extra-crispy fast-food chicken breast, for example, can contain close to half of a day's total recommended fat intake (28g), including a hefty 8g of saturated fat and 4.5g of trans fat – a virtual heart attack in a bucket. If you find yourself craving the taste of fried chicken, try our Oven-fried chicken recipe on page 249.

What about turkey? If you serve it only at Christmas, it's time to invite the big bird in more often. Turkey breast is actually lower in fat and cholesterol and higher in protein than chicken breast. Adding minced turkey is a great way to use less minced beef when making meat loaf, meatballs and chilli and thus lower the fat. Be sure to look for minced turkey breast, though; ordinary minced turkey is much higher in fat.

Health bonus

Chicken is a good source of the antioxidant mineral selenium. Low levels of selenium in the blood have been linked with poor blood sugar control and complications in people with diabetes, and selenium may offer some protection against the cell damage caused when blood sugar is out of control.

Chicken is also a good source of B vitamins, which play a role in preventing and treating many diseases, including asthma and nerve damage. They also support the immune system.

Got a cold? Homemade chicken soup really can help. Researchers have discovered that it can boost levels of immune cells that lessen inflammation, cutting short a cold.

Lean protein foods like chicken are at the crux of Magic eating, because they balance out the carbs in a meal and also make weight loss easier.

Cooks' tips

To keep chicken moist, cook it with the skin on, then remove it before serving.

Menu magic

A boneless chicken breast is like a blank canvas. Get as creative as you like. There are many possibilities, but here are a few easy suggestions.

■ **Marinate your chicken** in three other Magic foods – olive oil, lemon or lime juice and crushed garlic – to make it tasty and tender. Add chopped green chillies to take the flavour up a notch. Marinate for at least 2 hours, then grill or sauté.

■ **Sauté strips of fresh chicken** breast in olive oil and garlic and add to pizza.

■ **Keep grilled chicken** breast or turkey slices from the deli in the fridge so you can throw them over salad greens for an easy, high-protein lunch.

■ **Stir-fry or sauté** your chicken and add any of these other Magic foods: curry powder (its Magic ingredient is turmeric), broccoli, peaches, apples, almonds, peanuts, cashews, sesame seeds, spinach, tomatoes, onions and garlic.

■ **Whip up a tasty bowl** of chicken fried rice with cooked brown rice, chicken breast strips, egg, sliced scallions, chopped red pepper, soy sauce, ground ginger and crushed garlic. Quickly stir-fry in rapeseed oil.

■ **Make a light version** of chicken salad by using half low-fat mayonnaise and half low-fat yoghurt. Add scallions, dill, mustard and lemon juice and serve over fresh crunchy lettuce.

Smart substitutions

Instead of beef meatballs: make yours turkey meatballs, and you'll get great taste with fewer calories and less saturated fat.

Instead of beef chilli: Try turkey chilli.

Related recipes

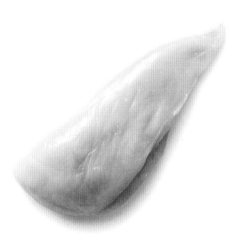

PERFECT PORTION: 85g

A serving of chicken is 85g if you eat it twice a day or 170g if you eat it once a day. For easy portion control, try what some supermarkets call 'mini fillets', small strips of skinless chicken breast perfect for stir-frying. Typically, two or three strips equal about one 85g serving. Bulk up your stir-fry with plenty of vegetables – and serve it over brown rice, of course.

cinnamon

When you think

of cinnamon, you might conjure up images of hot apple pie or warm-from-the-oven oatmeal biscuits. And of course, there wouldn't be cinnamon toast without it. You'd probably never imagine, though, that cinnamon has health benefits. In fact, researchers recently discovered that this warming spice can actually help to lower your blood sugar. Some of the natural compounds in cinnamon have the ability to mimic insulin, helping glucose to reach the cells, where it can be used for energy, and significantly lowering blood sugar in the process.

One study involving 60 men and women found that taking as little as $\frac{1}{4}$ to $\frac{1}{2}$ teaspoon of cinnamon a day lowered blood sugar by 18 to 29 per cent. It also reduced bad LDL cholesterol by 7 to 27 per cent in people with diabetes.

Cinnamon also contains the mineral manganese, which may improve the way your body uses blood sugar. Just 2 teaspoons can set you up with more than a third of the manganese you need for the day.

Health bonus

The natural chemicals in cinnamon can help to prevent blood platelets from clumping together and forming dangerous clots that can trigger a heart attack. And studies show that the spice has an unexpected effect on the brain: a mere whiff of cinnamon can boost brain activity and improve concentration.

PERFECT PORTION: $\frac{1}{2}$ teaspoon

Just $\frac{1}{2}$ teaspoon a day can benefit your health. If you like cinnamon, go ahead and eat a couple of teaspoons a day, but don't go overboard. Cinnamon contains natural compounds that can be toxic in high doses.

Menu magic

There are more ways than you can imagine to sprinkle cinnamon into your diet.

■ **Add cinnamon** to apple sauce as the apples are cooking or use it to spice up baked apples.

■ **Shake it on** whole-grain toast or whole-grain English muffins.

■ **Add a half teaspoon** or so of cinnamon to ground coffee before starting the pot. You can also add it to tea or drink chai, which contains cinnamon and other spices.

■ **Mix it into hot cereals,** especially porridge.

■ **Sprinkle a little cinnamon** on top of ice cream or frozen yoghurt or add it to plain yoghurt along with a little honey.

■ **Mix some with** low-fat cream cheese for a tasty spread.

■ **Add a cinnamon stick** or a pinch of ground cinnamon to minced beef dishes or stews.

■ **Flavour winter squash** or sweet potatoes with cinnamon.

Related recipes

citrus fruits

Are you in the mood for a sweet snack? Whether you grab an orange, a tangerine, or half a grapefruit, citrus fruits have an amazing ability when it comes to steadying your blood sugar.

First, they're packed with pectin, a type of soluble fibre that helps to keep blood sugar – and cholesterol – low. Pectin, like most types of fibre, also leaves you feeling full longer, taming the temptation to overeat at your next meal. How high in soluble fibre are these fruits? Out of the 20 most-eaten fruits and vegetables, oranges and grapefruit come out on top.

Citrus fruits are naturally low in calories (80 for an orange, 41 for half a grapefruit and 45 for a tangerine). And speaking of calories, it seems we may have misjudged the much-maligned 'Grapefruit Diet'. Apparently, grapefruit really can help you to lose weight. A study at the Scripps Clinic in San Diego looked at 100 obese people and found that those who ate half a grapefruit or drank grapefruit juice before each meal lost an average of 1.5 to 1.6kg over 12 weeks compared to a loss of only 225g by the people who didn't have the fruit. Grapefruit probably works by reducing insulin surges after meals. (The smaller the rise in insulin, the better your body is able to process sugar.) Obviously, eating grapefruit before a meal also dampens your appetite a little so you eat less of the higher-calorie main dish.

Citrus fruits are most renowned for their vitamin C, an antioxidant that can help to fight heart disease and complications of diabetes, such as nerve damage and damage to the retina of the eye. You'll get more than a whole day's vitamin C requirement in a single orange; half a grapefruit will give you 78 per cent.

Now, a few words about fruit juice. First, while it's much more nutritious than fizzy pop, you'll need to pour yourself a small glass. About 125 to 180ml is appropriate – that's why they make juice glasses. Without the fibre found in the whole fruit, fruit juice contains a lot more calories, and it has a greater effect on your blood sugar. The GL of a whole orange, for example, is very low at 5. The GL of 125ml of orange juice, however, is a much higher 12 – and most of us drink more than that.

Don't think that orange juice with pulp contains more fibre; it doesn't. Freshly squeezed juice, however, may be higher in fibre than high-pulp juice, since the fruit's membranes go into the juice.

If you choose grapefruit juice, check the label to be sure you're buying an unsweetened brand. Too bitter for you? Stick to red or pink grapefruit juice for a naturally sweeter taste.

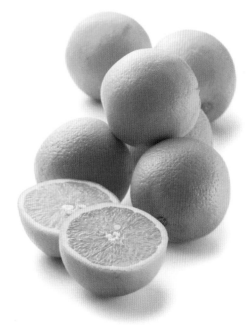

PERFECT PORTION: 1 medium orange

If you're eating a grapefruit, a serving is half of one fruit.

citrus fruits continued

Health bonus

Because citrus fruits can help to lower your cholesterol, they deserve a starring role in your diet. You'll get some cancer protection, too, for your effort. Research shows that compounds in citrus fruits can help to prevent cancerous changes from occurring in colon cells. Pink and red grapefruits contain lycopene, which studies show may help to reduce the risk of developing breast and prostate cancer.

Cooks' tips

Do you shun grapefruit because it's tricky to prepare? Make it easy on yourself and buy a grapefruit knife or special tool for citrus sectioning. This gadget looks like a cross between salad scissors and a pizza cutter and lets you remove sections or leave them in place (it works for oranges, too). A grapefruit spoon, the kind with serrated edges, is handy, too.

At the supermarket, don't judge an orange by its colour. That bright hue that looks so appealing may be due to dye rather than ripeness. Instead, look for fruit that's firm and heavy for its size.

Menu magic

■ **Start breakfast** with half a grapefruit.
■ **Add grapefruit** or orange sections to jazz up a green salad.
■ **For a refreshing dessert** set orange or grapefruit segments in sugar-free jelly.

Grapefruit and drugs MAY NOT MIX

If you take prescription medication, watch your grapefruit intake or discuss it with your doctor. Researchers have found that the natural compounds in grapefruit can interfere with the action of some prescription drugs, making them either stronger or weaker than they're supposed to be. For example, grapefruit and grapefruit juice can increase the action of statins, cholesterol-lowering drugs commonly prescribed for people with diabetes. The result? An increased risk of developing toxic side effects from the medication.

■ **Whip up an orange** smoothie with peeled, seeded oranges, low-fat plain yoghurt, frozen strawberries and vanilla. Blend and pour.

Related recipes

Grilled chicken salad with orange 214
Orange and pomegranate compote 292
Pink grapefruit brulée 288
Spinach, grapefruit & avocado salad
with poppy seed dressing 216

You know oranges are loaded with vitamin C, but they also offer antioxidants called flavonoids that guard against heart disease.

coffee

Health experts have

debated the coffee issue for decades – is it bad for you or good for you? Our answer: in moderation, coffee, especially decaf, may have beneficial effects on your blood sugar. A study from Finland, which boasts the highest coffee consumption in the world, found that the risk of developing Type 2 diabetes went down as coffee consumption went up. The biggest benefits were to people who drank a massive six cups a day (although we don't recommend that you follow suit). And a recent study from the Harvard School of Public Health found that among more than 88,000 women, drinking just one cup of coffee a day (caffeinated or decaffeinated) was associated with a 13 per cent lower risk of developing Type 2 diabetes compared with non–coffee drinkers; drinking two to three cups a day was associated with a 32 per cent lower risk.

Coffee contains a long list of natural plant compounds, including polyphenol antioxidants called chlorogenic acids, that may contribute to its beneficial effect on blood sugar.

That said, caffeine does tend to cause blood sugar to surge, not to mention giving you the jitters. One clinical study found that among nine people who drank a single large cup of caffeinated coffee after an overnight fast, blood sugar was significantly higher for half an hour afterwards than it was after drinking a sugar solution; not so after drinking decaffeinated coffee. The answer: switch to decaf.

Coffee's not only our morning wakeup call, it's also a significant source of antioxidants in our diets, outpacing even cranberries and red grapes, according to a recent study. Mind you, cranberries, grapes and other fruits and vegetables are much higher in antioxidants than coffee is, but we don't consume them the way we do coffee – too bad for us.

Health bonus

Several studies show that the antioxidants in coffee offer protection against diseases of the liver and colon and Parkinson's disease. And a recent Canadian study found that as coffee drinking increased, the risk of developing Alzheimer's disease decreased.

Menu magic

A cup of coffee with your breakfast or after dinner, especially if it's decaf, is a good alternative to fizzy drinks and may even reduce your craving for a sugary doughnut or dessert if you add a little flavour twist. Here are but a few.

■ **In the summer** swap your steaming cup of decaf for iced coffee made with low-fat milk.

■ **Create a delicious** drink by adding cloves, nutmeg, cinnamon, grated lemon and orange zest to coffee. Add skimmed or semi-skimmed milk and lightly sweeten.

■ **Mix strong coffee** and sugar-free hot chocolate. Add a dash of cinnamon and grated orange peel.

Related recipe
Iced coffee frappé 213

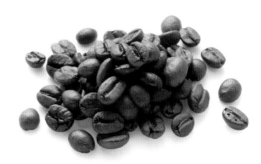

PERFECT PORTION: 1 mug

Always choose decaf for better blood sugar.

eggs

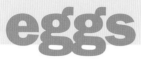

If there's one food

that's developed an undeserved reputation over the years for being bad for your health, it's eggs. Let's reveal the realities.

Eggs are an excellent, inexpensive source of high-quality protein – so high, in fact, that egg protein is the gold standard nutritionists use to rank all other proteins. What makes the protein in eggs so superior? It contains all of the essential amino acids (the ones your body can't make on its own) in just the right proportions.

Because they're all protein and fat, eggs have no impact on your blood sugar, making them a much better breakfast choice than, say, a stack of white-flour pancakes. And like all protein foods, they may help to control your appetite by keeping you full longer. One study found that women who ate two eggs with toast at breakfast felt less hungry before lunch and ate significantly fewer calories during the rest of the day than those who ate a bagel and cream cheese that provided the same number of calories.

Now, about eggs and cholesterol. Yes, it's true, eggs have a lot of it – about 230mg in a medium egg – all in the yolk. It's also true that if you have diabetes, your heart health should be a top

Designer eggs: WORTH THE PRICE?

Environmental and ethical issues of chicken housing and feeding aside, eggs vary little in nutrition from one brand to the next. But there is one exception: eggs fortified with heart-smart omega-3 fatty acids. Usually, this is accomplished by adding flaxseed to the chickens' feed. Each egg typically provides 150–200mg of omega-3s. This is a small fraction of the amount you'd get from eating a piece of fish, but some is better than none.

priority. But dozens of studies have found that it's saturated fat, not cholesterol, that has the greatest effect on blood cholesterol, so eating eggs in moderation is just fine.

For people with elevated cholesterol or those who are especially sensitive to the cholesterol in foods (for some people, cholesterol levels do rise after eating a cholesterol-rich meal), experts recommend eating no more than three or four egg yolks a week. Egg whites, which contain no cholesterol, don't count.

Health bonus

Egg yolks are one of the few foods naturally rich in vitamin D, a much-needed vitamin that few of us get enough of. Vitamin D helps the body to absorb calcium and has recently been linked with lower risks of various cancers to boot. Eggs are also a surprisingly good source of bone-building vitamin K. Plus, they're loaded with lutein (the chickens get it from their feed), which helps to protect against macular degeneration, a

---

PERFECT PORTION: 1 medium egg

A *medium egg* contains about **90kcal** and **7g of fat**, about **2g of it saturated.** The fat and cholesterol are all in the **yolk**. You can enjoy a two-egg omelette with a piece of whole-grain toast, and your breakfast will still be reasonably low in calories as long as you don't load it up with butter and cheese. Studies find that even **two eggs** a day have **no effect on cholesterol** in most people. Replace one with two egg whites if you like.

(continues on page 108)

Magic proteins

Eggs

Soya

Lean PROTEIN

sources make the grade because they benefit blood sugar without clogging arteries.

- beans
- beef
- low-fat cheese
- chicken
- eggs
- fish
- lamb
- lentils
- low-fat milk
- nuts
- peanut butter
- pork
- shellfish
- soya
- yoghurt

Beans

Fish

eggs continued

leading cause of blindness in older people. Eggs also contain choline, a compound that animal studies suggest could help to improve your memory as you age. Some studies found that giving extra choline to pregnant rats created better-functioning brain cells in their babies.

Cooks' tips

If you have an egg tray in your refrigerator door, ignore it. Eggs stay fresh best if you keep them in their original container, pointed ends down. Keeping the eggs in the carton they came in helps to prevent the eggs from losing moisture and absorbing smells from other foods. But do keep the carton in the fridge as eggs age much faster when stored at room temperature. To tell if an egg is fresh, place it in a large bowl of salted water. If it sinks it's fresh; if it floats throw it out.

Eating raw or undercooked eggs carries a small risk of salmonella poisoning, though the the Food Standards Agency (FSA) classed it as 'very low' after a 2004 survey of 28,500 eggs which showed that contamination had been cut by a third since 1995-1996. At least 80 per cent of UK laying hens are vaccinated against Salmonella Enteritidis. But the FSA advises that the elderly, pregnant women, children and anyone who is unwell should eat only eggs that have been well-cooked.

Scrambled, poached, or hard boiled, eggs keep your blood sugar steady and provide many vitamins and minerals.

Menu magic

Like the chickens they come from, eggs are one of Nature's most versatile foods. And they're not just for breakfast.

■ **Keep hard-boiled** eggs in the fridge for a perfect protein-rich snack.

■ **For lunch, have an** egg salad sandwich (made with low-fat mayonnaise) on wholemeal bread. Add chopped pickles to lower the glycaemic effect of the bread. Or sprinkle on some turmeric, another Magic food (also good on scrambled eggs).

■ **Serve a frittata** for dinner (think of it as Italian egg pie). We provide one recipe on page 195, but you can add almost anything to your frittata, such as lean ham, diced tomato, spinach and goat's cheese.

■ **Prepare devilled** eggs with low-fat mayonnaise, chopped pickles, chilli powder or paprika and mustard powder.

■ **Grill some French** toast for breakfast. Dip wholemeal bread in a mixture of egg, cinnamon (another Magic food), vanilla and milk, then spray the skillet with oil, add the bread, and cook. The protein and fat in the egg will help to reduce the blood sugar impact of the bread.

■ **For a quick and easy lunch** serve Spanish eggs. Spoon some spicy tomato sauce into a shallow heatproof dish, make a well in the sauce then crack a large egg into the well. Bake in a medium hot oven until the egg is cooked.

Related recipes

Lemony blueberry cheesecake bars 290
Pumpkin custards 292
Spinach and goat's cheese omelette 194
Courgette frittata 195

fenugreek

GL very low

This pungent spice

is not only an important ingredient in strongly flavoured dishes such as curries, it's also proven to tame blood sugar. In fact, fenugreek supplements are sold for that reason. Here's why fenugreek works: new research suggests it has a knack for mimicking insulin, which brings down blood sugar.

The yellowish brown seeds, which smell like celery but taste more bitter, also pack a soluble-fibre punch, and you know by now that this type of fibre helps to lower blood sugar. One study in animals even suggested that fenugreek could help to prevent weight gain, in part by preventing the absorption of fat calories – a definite plus for lowering your diabetes risk. Added together these facts make fenugreek seeds a sweet prospect.

Fenugreek leaves are used in traditional Indian dishes. Like the seeds, they're packed with healthy plant compounds, but they haven't been studied as much as the seeds for their ability to lower blood sugar.

Health bonus

Fenugreek seeds are a fabulous source of cholesterol-lowering soluble fibre. Plus, the natural antioxidant compounds they contain may help to counteract some of the damaging effects of diabetes.

Cooks' tips

For milder flavour, roast fenugreek seeds before grinding them (a coffee bean or spice grinder works well) for recipes. Don't overcook them, or they'll turn bitter.

Menu magic

Because of fenugreek's penetrating, some might say peculiar, flavour, the spice won't work with all your favourite recipes. But there are some dishes in which fenugreek adds a certain pungent lift, enhancing the overall flavour.

■ **Add ground seed** to bread dough to make a spicy loaf.

■ **Sprinkle ground seed** into eggs along with coriander, garlic, cardamom and cumin for a taste of India in your omelette.

■ **Stir seeds into** lentil dishes. Dahl is an Indian lentil or split-pea dish that wouldn't be complete without fenugreek.

■ **Find a favourite** curry recipe; fenugreek is a common ingredient, either in the curry or in Indian spice mixes.

■ **Use a combination** of fenugreek, cinnamon, ginger and cumin as a spice rub for chicken. You could also add turmeric, another Magic food, or celery seeds. Store the mixture in an airtight container in a dark, cool place.

■ **Make an after-dinner** drink using ½ teaspoon fenugreek seeds. Steep for 5 to 10 minutes in freshly boiled water, then strain.

Related recipes

Crushed curried butternut squash 282
Dahl with spinach 272

PERFECT PORTION: 30g

*It takes only about ½ **teaspoon** of fenugreek seeds a day to make a big difference in blood sugar. In one study, people with **diabetes** were even able to cut back on their blood sugar–lowering medications by consuming this amount.*

fish

GL very low

The Greenland Inuit

eat an incredibly high-fat diet with few vegetables, yet their rate of heart disease is stunningly low. The key may be all the fatty fish they eat: the staple food in their diet is fish naturally rich in omega-3 fatty acids. You've probably heard by now that omega-3s fend off heart disease – something that could be right around the corner if your blood sugar is stuck in overdrive. It's no wonder fish makes our list of Magic foods.

A study at the Harvard School of Public Health found that women with diabetes who ate fish just once a week had a 40 per cent lower risk of dying from heart disease than did women with diabetes who ate fish less than once a month.

But omega-3s do more than protect your heart. They also quell inflammation in the body, a major contributor to numerous chronic diseases of ageing, including insulin resistance and diabetes. Some researchers think that it may even play a role in brain diseases such as Alzheimer's as well as certain cancers.

Of course, fish is also a protein food, and protein foods have virtually no impact on blood sugar. We suggest that you aim to eat fish for dinner once or twice a week when you might otherwise have chicken or beef. But sure that it is baked, grilled, pan-fried in a minimum of fat or poached. Avoid deep fried fish in a batter, such as fish and chips or scampi. Packed with bad-for-you fats, they give fish a bad name. One study concluded that eating fried fish offered no heart benefits at all.

All fish contain some omega-3s, but fatty types such as salmon, mackerel, herring and sardines are richest in them (*see* table, right).

Health bonus

While the strongest proof of the health benefits of fish points to the heart, there's also plenty of research showing that food with fins can cut the risk of prostate cancer and help to maintain brain power as you age. There's also evidence that oil-rich fish may help to protect against depression.

Cooks' tips

One of the keys to successful fish dishes is buying the freshest fish possible. Here's what you should look for whether you're shopping at a high street fishmonger's or supermarket.

FOR WHOLE FISH

■ **Shop at a busy** fish counter. Lots of customers mean lots of turnover and fresher fish.
■ **The fish's eyes** should be clear, not cloudy.
■ **The inside of the gills** should be bright red, not greyish or even pink.
■ **It shouldn't smell** bad. Fish should have a moist, almost musky smell like a cucumber or melon.

Fishing for omega-3s

Some fish are naturally richer in heart-healthy omega-3 fatty acids than others. See for yourself.

FISH	OMEGA-3s g per 100g
Cod	0.25
Haddock	0.15
Herring	1.8
Mackerel	2.8
Kippers	3.4
Pilchard (canned in tomato sauce)	2.8
Sardines (canned in tomato sauce)	2.0
Fresh tuna	1.6
Tuna (canned in brine)	0.17
Salmon (fresh)	2.5
Salmon (canned)	1.8
Trout	1.2

FOR FISH FILLETS

- **They should be** moist and firm.
- **If there are gaps** or separations in the flesh, it's not fresh.
- **They shouldn't smell fishy.** Fresh fish will keep in the fridge for a day or two, but cook it as soon as possible or freeze it for up to six months.
- **Don't bypass frozen fillets.** Vacuum-packed fish fillets are the next best thing to fresh.

Menu magic

Fish makes a perfect weeknight meal because it's done before you know it.

- **Turn on the grill;** almost any type of fish tastes fabulous grilled, especially salmon. Brush it with a little olive oil to keep it from sticking.

Throw some courgette strips on the grill, too, and you have a blood sugar-friendly meal.

- **Wrap trout** in foil with lemon slices, dill, thyme, salt and pepper and bake. Serve over quinoa.
- **Squeeze fresh lemon** juice over fish seasoned with rosemary and sautéed on the stove. Serve with brown rice pilaf.
- **Stuff a tomato** with tuna salad made with low-fat mayonnaise or plain yoghurt, hard-boiled eggs, chopped apples, celery and onion. Serve with wholemeal crackers.
- **If you're a fan** of sardines, try this: sauté some onion and garlic in olive oil, then add sardines canned in tomato sauce. When thoroughly heated, pour the mixture over wholemeal pasta and toss. Top with lemon juice and grated Parmesan.
- **Pickled herring** is another acquired taste, but it may be worth acquiring – check out its extraordinarily high omega-3 content in the chart on the facing page. As an appetiser, try pickled herring on squares of whole-grain rye toast, sprinkled with chopped parsley and paprika.

Safer SALMON

Salmon and other oil-rich fish, such as tuna and swordfish, have a tendency to store environmental pollutants such as mercury by absorbing them into their fat tissue. Experts have debated whether the benefits of eating these fish outweigh the risks and whether it is better to opt for wild or farmed fish.

A recent analysis by a handful of researchers from different institutions came to the conclusion that you should, whenever possible, choose wild salmon over farmed salmon, which is generally higher in several chemical contaminants. But farmed salmon has higher levels of omega-3s and is usually cheaper and, based on current knowledge, most experts agree that the benefits of eating salmon and fish far outweigh any risks. Canned salmon happens to come from wild varieties, making it a safe choice.

Related recipes

PERFECT PORTION: 35g

If you are having fish as your **main meal** *of the day,* **a serving of up to 170g** *is acceptable.*

flaxseed (linseed)

GL very low Teeny-tiny, shiny brown flaxseeds (also known as linseeds) are a godsend to your blood sugar as well as your heart, so if you haven't tried them yet, it's time you did. Buy ground flaxseed or grind it yourself in a food processor or coffee grinder. If you don't see it in your supermarket, look in a healthfood shop. Using flaxseed may be a mystery to you now, but it's simple once you know how. It has a pleasant, nutty flavour.

Flaxseed is rich in both protein and fibre (more than 2g per tablespoon of ground seeds). It's also a good source of magnesium, a mineral that's key to good blood sugar control because it helps cells to use insulin. Several large studies have found that the risk of developing Type 2 diabetes skyrockets when magnesium intake is low, so get your fill. Even if you already have diabetes, getting plenty of magnesium can help.

Don't eat enough fish? Eat plenty of flaxseeds. It's rich in alpha linolenic acid (ALA), which the body uses to make the same type of omega-3 fatty acids you get from fish. Like fish, flaxseed keeps your heart healthy by lowering cholesterol, keeping your heart pumping normally, and preventing dangerous blood clots from forming. Also like fish, it guards against inflammation in the body, which is linked to many age-related disorders, including insulin resistance and diabetes.

Health bonus

Because flaxseed protects against inflammation in the body, it also has a protective effect against inflammatory conditions such as rheumatoid arthritis, asthma, Crohn's disease, eczema and psoriasis.

The omega-3 fats in flaxseed may help to prevent and even treat breast cancer as well, thanks to hormone-like plant compounds called lignans. In the body, these turn into compounds that are similar to the body's own oestrogen but have much weaker activity. By occupying oestrogen receptors on cells, they block the effects of natural oestrogen and thus may provide protection against hormone-fuelled cancers such as breast cancer. Flaxseed has several hundred times more lignans than any other plant food.

Like fish, flaxseed may also offer protection from Alzheimer's and depression.

Constipated? Flaxseed should do the trick. (Eat too much, and you'll quickly discover the laxative effects.)

Cooks' tips

The lignans in flaxseed are much better absorbed by the body if the seeds are eaten ground or crushed. (Whole seeds tend to pass right through your body undigested.) But because of its high fat content, flaxseed will spoil if you grind it but don't use it straightaway. The solution: buy whole seeds in bulk and grind them only as you need them. Whole seeds will last up to a year stored at room temperature. If you buy ground flaxseed, keep it in the fridge.

Especially if you don't eat fish, make a point of adding heart-smart, cancer-fighting flaxseed to your diet.

Menu magic

You can easily make ground flaxseed part of almost any meal.

- **Sprinkle on hot** or cold cereal.
- **Stir into yoghurt** or add to muesli.
- **Add a tablespoon** or two to doughs and batters for pancakes, muffins and breads. Just keep an eye on anything you bake in the oven; the flaxseed could make it brown more quickly than usual.
- **Add to meatballs,** burgers and casseroles.
- **Use as a topping** for ice cream or frozen yoghurt.
- **Add to smoothies.**
- **Use to replace** a quarter of the flour in muffin or pancake batter.
- **Add to cooked fruit** desserts such as baked apples or blueberry compote.
- **Sprinkle in your favourite** sandwich filling, such as tuna or chicken salad.
- **Add to cream cheese** or sprinkle on a soft cheese and enjoy with some whole-grain crackers for a blood sugar–friendly snack.

Related recipes

Berry and flaxseed smoothie 212
Brown rice pilaf with flaxseeds, lime
   and coriander 277
Brown rice pilaf with toasted flaxseeds 276
Porridge with apple and
   flaxseeds 193
Wholemeal flaxseed
   bread 196

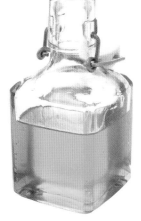

what about FLAXSEED OIL?

Flaxseed oil provides the omega-3 fatty acids of whole flaxseeds, but not the fibre or lignans. If heart health is your main concern, you may want to consider taking either flaxseed oil or fish oil daily to get more 'good fats' into your diet. Because flax thins the blood, talk to your doctor before taking it if you're on aspirin therapy or taking blood-thinning medication. Dosages range from 1 teaspoon to 1 table-spoon once or twice a day.

The oil goes rancid easily, so keep it refrigerated. Use it in salad dressings, add it to steamed vegetables after cooking, or sprinkle it over grain dishes. But don't cook with it as heat destroys its nutrients.

PERFECT PORTION: 1 to 2 tablespoons

A tablespoon or two a day, ground and blended into other foods, could do wonders for your **blood sugar** *control and overall good health. You can also mix 1 or 2 tablespoons of ground flaxseed into a* **glass of water** *and drink it.*

garlic

GL very low

You probably know garlic is good for your cholesterol. And if you like garlic, you wouldn't even think of making your favourite recipes without it, which is a good thing because this pungent herb may also be beneficial for your blood sugar.

According to early research with animals, garlic may increase insulin secretion, which would lower blood sugar and improve insulin sensitivity, in effect helping to reverse diabetes. Since supplements show no blood-sugar benefits, enjoy garlic the old-fashioned, tasty way. A recent animal study found that high doses of raw garlic significantly reduced blood sugar levels.

'The stinking rose' offers other health benefits as well. Study after study shows it can help to keep cholesterol under control by lowering 'bad' cholesterol (LDL) and boosting 'good' (HDL). In an analysis of five trials in which participants received either garlic supplements or placebos, the authors concluded that you could lower your total cholesterol by about 9 per cent with the equivalent of 1½ to 3 cloves of garlic daily for two to six months. Garlic also thins the blood, making it less likely to form artery-clogging clots.

Health bonus

A diet rich in garlic could mean a lower risk of several types of cancer, including cancer of the stomach and colon. Garlic also has the ability to bring down high blood pressure.

Cooks' tips

Unless you enjoy chopping, buy a garlic press. Keep your garlic in a cool, dark place, either in a cup in your larder or in a fancier garlic keeper – the kind made of terracotta or pottery with a lid to keep light out and holes in the sides to let air in. Don't keep it in the fridge, or it will sprout quickly.

To peel garlic with minimal hassle, bang the side of the clove with the side of a large knife. The peel will practically slip off at that point.

Menu magic

■ **Add sautéed garlic** to just about any chicken, fish, beef or tofu dish.
■ **Use roasted garlic** as a spread for bread instead of butter or add it to mashed potatoes or pasta. To roast, break the heads into cloves but don't peel them. Spread them on a baking sheet, drizzle with a little olive oil, sprinkle with salt and bake at 190°C/gas 5, shaking the pan occasionally, until tender, for about 30 minutes. Then simply squeeze the cloves out of their skins.
■ **Add crushed garlic** to rice or other grain dishes before cooking.
■ **Add crushed garlic** to vinaigrette dressing.
■ **Make a garlic/mustard** marinade for beef by mixing spicy mustard, olive oil, balsamic vinegar, black pepper and chopped garlic. Add the beef and refrigerate for at least 2 hours.
■ **At a barbecue,** add the whole garlic bulb to the grill. Turn it so all sides are exposed to the heat. It's ready to eat when the skin is dark brown and peels easily.

Related recipes

Barley-bean soup 229
Broccoli with lemon vinaigrette 287
Caponata 201
Cherry tomatoes filled with creamy pesto cheese 202
Mediterranean split pea spread 208
Oriental peanut dip 206
Penne with tomato and aubergine sauce 262
Prawn and orzo casserole 260
Spiced cauliflower with peas 284
Spring vegetable stir-fry with tofu 271

PERFECT PORTION: no limits

The more, the better.

jerusalem artichokes

GL very low

This Magic food is

unusual in more ways than one. Not only does it have no connection with Jerusalem or artichokes (it's actually related to the sunflower), it looks like a small gnarly potato and, like potatoes, it grows underground. But, unlike potatoes, Jerusalem artichokes (which are crunchy and slightly sweet) have an amazingly beneficial effect on your blood sugar. That's because the starches they contain, called fructans (specifically types of fructans called inulin and oligofructose), aren't readily digested the way typical carbs are. In fact, they're barely digested at all.

Because these starches can't be broken down by enzymes in the small intestine, they travel to the large intestine (colon), where they are digested by intestinal bacteria and eventually excreted. In the end, they supply less than 40 per cent as many calories as regular carbohydrates.

As well as being a low-GL food, Jerusalem artichokes may have another advantage. Foods that contain inulin, as artichokes do, may help to smooth out blood sugar and insulin levels after a meal. Preliminary studies are investigating whether higher doses of inulin may also increase fullness and so help to cut calorie intake.

Health bonus

Jerusalem artichokes may improve the health of your colon, too. The fructans they contain act as prebiotics, meaning that they provide fodder for beneficial bacteria in the intestinal tract. Fructans also increase the amount of water and bacteria in the stool, helping to relieve constipation.

Looking to boost your heart health? Jerusalem artichokes can help there, as well. The same indigestible carbs that help to regulate blood sugar and relieve constipation may direct the liver to produce fewer triglycerides and fatty acids that can clog your arteries.

Cooks' tips

In the UK, Jerusalem artichokes are fairly seasonal and generally available only in the autumn. Look for firm artichokes with a smooth, unblemished surface, and avoid those that feel soft, look dried out, or have sprouts. Scrub them well with a vegetable brush to get rid of any grit and dirt. Peeling is optional. You can drizzle on a little lemon juice or vinegar so that the flesh retains its white colour.

A note of caution: start with small servings; inulin can cause flatulence.

Menu magic

- **Boil and mash** a Jerusalem artichoke just like a potato; or if you prefer, add to regular mashed potatoes to decrease the GL.
- **Toss thin raw slices** into salads.
- **Slice an artichoke** and use in place of water chestnuts in stir-fries.
- **Steam cubes or slices,** then drizzle with olive oil and lemon juice.
- **Grate** into a vegetable coleslaw.
- **Slice and serve** with a dip, along with other vegetable crudités.

Smart substitutions

Instead of grated potatoes: use grated in potato pancake recipes.

Instead of puréed potatoes: use as a thickener in soups.

Related recipe

Jerusalem artichoke drop scones 281

PERFECT PORTION: 80g

One serving of artichoke contains only **152kcal** *and few blood sugar-raising carbs.*

---

lamb

GL very low

Lamb, probably the first meat humans ate from animals they had reared rather than hunted, has become a staple food in many parts of the world. If you choose the right cuts, lamb is a Magic source of protein, just as beef is.

The leg – the classic spring roast – is the leanest of all, especially if you buy the shank as opposed to the sirloin. (Actually, the foreshank is even slightly leaner but must be tenderised, usually by cooking in liquid for hours.) Loin chops are a bit fattier and the shoulder is a bit fattier still. The ribs (rack of lamb) are the fattiest cuts of all, along with minced lamb. Some supermarkets do stock lean minced lamb, but you may need to ask the butcher to make mince from one of the leaner cuts.

Fortunately, lamb isn't marbled the way beef is; most of the fat is on the outside and is easily trimmed away.

Health bonus

Like beef, lamb is rich in B vitamins, iron and zinc. Zinc is essential for a healthy immune system. A shortfall of iron can sap your energy and concentration. As for the B vitamins, they help to improve cholesterol ratios and lower levels of homocysteine, an amino acid linked with increased risk of heart attack, stroke and Alzheimer's disease.

Cooks' tips

Lamb is meat from sheep less than a year old, so it's generally moist and tender. Get the most for your money by purchasing fine-textured, pink meat with a minimum of firm white fat. Always trim off visible fat from fresh lamb and remove any pieces of 'fell', a papery membrane that covers surface fat. Meat from sheep more than a year old is called mutton and has a stronger taste. It tends to be leaner, though less tender, than lamb. To keep it tender, cook it slowly over medium heat.

Menu magic

Lamb stew, lamb chops, lamb curry, leg of lamb … there are so many different, delicious ways to enjoy this Magic food.

■ **Make a big pot** of lamb stew at the weekend and freeze the leftovers or enjoy them during the week. Include plenty of vegetables, such as carrots, squash, onions, peas and sweet potatoes.

■ **Make some lamb kebabs** by alternating chunks of uncooked lamb and vegetables such as red peppers, tomatoes and onions on skewers. Grill and serve over wholemeal couscous.

■ **Braise lamb shanks** slowly (2 to 3 hours) in a combination of red wine, crushed garlic and rosemary. You'll want to brown the shanks before braising.

■ **Serve roasted** or grilled lamb with a spoonful of mint yoghurt sauce made with low-fat plain yoghurt, chopped mint leaves, crushed garlic and a pinch of cayenne pepper.

Related recipes

Lamb stew with spring vegetables 239
Mustard-crusted lamb chops 241

> **PERFECT PORTION: 85g**
>
> *If this is your **main meat** for the day, a serving of **up to 170g** is appropriate.*

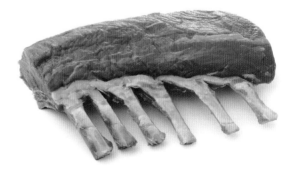

lemons

GL very low

When lemons are around, eat them and don't let their sourness put you off. Lemon juice helps to lower blood sugar, because of its acidity (*see* Chapter 2 in Part 1 for details of the acid effect). Having even a small amount of lemon juice with a meal can lower the meal's GL. Lime juice should have a similar effect.

Health bonus

Four tablespoons of lemon juice will give you almost half the vitamin C you need for the day. Remember, antioxidants such as vitamin C make cholesterol less likely to stick to your artery walls. Lemons are also packed with a natural disease-preventing compound called limonene that may help to lower cholesterol and is even being studied for potential anti-cancer properties.

The citric acid in lemon juice also helps to stave off kidney stones by reducing the excretion of calcium in the urine. Lemon rind is rich in a compound called rutin, which strengthens the walls of veins and capillaries, potentially reducing the pain and severity of varicose veins.

Cooks' tips

Looking for a juicy lemon? Give it a squeeze. The softer the lemon, the thinner the skin and the juicier the fruit is. To maximise juice output, bring lemons to room temperature and roll them firmly back and forth on the counter a few times with the palm of your hand before cutting.

Menu magic

■ **Use lemon juice** in salad dressings.
■ **Serve plenty of** lemon slices alongside fish, which wouldn't be the same without them.
■ **Add the juice to tuna** next time you make yourself a tuna sandwich.
■ **Soak chicken pieces** in lemon juice before you grill or pan-fry them. Slipping half a lemon inside a roast chicken keeps the meat moist, too.

■ **Add a squirt of lemon juice** to flavour water or seltzer (possibly encouraging you to drink more water) to lessen the blood-sugar impact of whatever you're eating.
■ **Use lemon juice** in marinades for meat or poultry. Combine lemon juice, balsamic vinegar, olive oil, fresh rosemary and crushed garlic, then add the meat and refrigerate overnight.
■ **Squeeze fresh lemon juice** on vegetables, pasta, soups, rice and stews. It will add so much flavour, you'll be able to cut back on salt.

Related recipes

Barley risotto with asparagus and lemon 272
Barley salad with mangetout and lemon dressing 216
Black bean spread with Mexican flavours 209
Blueberry and melon compote with green tea and lime 288
Broccoli with lemon vinaigrette 287
Greek lentil salad 223
Grilled chicken salad with orange 214
Lemony blueberry cheesecake bars 290
Mediterranean split pea spread 208
Penne with asparagus, ricotta and lemon 264
Moroccan-style chicken thighs with butternut squash and baby onions 247
Smoked salmon canapés 205
Tuna and cannellini salad with lemon 218
Wholemeal noodles with peanut sauce and chicken 220

> **PERFECT PORTION: 1 to 2 tablespoons**
>
> *If the effects of* lemon juice *are anything like those of* vinegar – *and we think they are – 1 to 2 tablespoons should be enough to* lower the blood sugar impact *of a meal by as much as* 30 per cent.

lentils

GL very low

Lentils are the perfect slow-acting food, with an ideal mix of slow-digesting protein and complex carbohydrates. And since they cook quickly – no presoaking required – there's little excuse not to use them in soups, salads and main dishes even on weeknights. If you add them to rice dishes, you'll be able to use less rice and significantly lower the GL of the dish.

Their secret weapon against blood sugar surges is soluble fibre, and plenty of it. A portion of lentils carries 8g of fibre, most of it the soluble type. Of course, soluble fibre is also the stuff that lowers cholesterol. It's little wonder that lentils are a staple in the Mediterranean diet, famous for protecting the heart.

Lentils are also a good source of protein (8–10g per portion), which makes them wonderfully filling and weight-loss friendly.

Health bonus

One recent study found that women who included lentils or beans in their diets at least twice a week had a 25 per cent lower risk of breast cancer compared to women who ate them less than once a month. Lentils are also unusually rich in folate, a B vitamin proven to lower blood levels of homocysteine, an amino acid linked with an increased risk of heart disease and dementia. The fibre in lentils also helps to keep you regular.

Cooks' tips

Stored in a cool, dry, dark place, lentils will keep for up to six months. Hang on to them any longer and they'll dry out. Don't mix new lentils with older ones, since the older ones will take longer to cook.

Menu magic

■ **Add cooked lentils** to green salads or pasta dishes.

■ **Mash cooked lentils** and blend with fresh salsa or with crushed garlic, yoghurt and lemon juice for an easy and healthy dip or spread.

■ **Cook a pot** – or open a can – of lentil soup. Interesting options include red lentil and tomato soup, lentil-barley soup, lentil and Swiss chard soup with lemon (chock full of Magic foods) and chicken and lentil stew.

■ **Make lentils** a main dish by cooking them with smoked turkey sausage, onion, tomatoes and herbs.

■ **Reinvent rice by** adding lentils. Cook and season a variety of coloured lentils and serve over brown or converted rice.

■ **Keep a few tins of lentils handy** You can use them if really pushed for time – they will only need reheating.

Related recipes

Curried red lentil soup 230
Dahl with spinach 272
Greek lentil salad 223
Lentil and bean chilli 273
Mustard-glazed salmon with lentils 257

PERFECT PORTION: 100g (cooked)

Since the GL *is* very low, *and lentils are among the most nutritious plant foods around, you can enjoy a bit* more.

melons

GL
very low

Despite their mouthwatering sweetness, melons are surprisingly blood-sugar friendly, making them perfect with breakfast, as snacks, or in fruit salads and even salsas. Yes, the sugar they contain is quickly converted to glucose, or blood sugar, but melons are mostly water (as much as 90 per cent), so they don't contain as much sugar as you'd think. Because of their water content, melons are also remarkably low in calories.

Watermelon perfectly illustrates the difference between the glycaemic index (GI) and the glycaemic load (GL). Because the sugar it contains is fast acting, it has a sky-high GI – but since you get very little sugar when you eat a serving of watermelon, its GL is low.

The vitamin C in melons (cantaloupes are the richest source) makes them excellent for preventing some of the damage high blood sugar can cause to cells as well as to arteries and blood vessels. And melons' potassium helps to guard against high blood pressure, a real risk of diabetes. As one of the richest sources of lycopene, it may also help to keep heart disease at bay, which is important since the risk of developing heart disease is high for people with diabetes.

Health bonus

Lycopene-rich foods such as watermelon may offer protection against certain kinds of cancer, including prostate, breast, endometrial, lung and colon cancers. The strongest evidence has been for prostate cancer. One study of 47,000 men found that those who ate two to four servings of tomatoes (another lycopene-rich food) a week had a 26 per cent reduced risk of prostate cancer compared to those who ate none.

Remember the old wartime advice that eating carrots helps you to see in the dark? Well it turns out that there in some truth in it after all: it's the beta-carotene in carrots that makes them good for your eyes. And cantaloupe is rich in this nutrient, too.

Cooks' tips

If only melons came with tags indicating how ripe they were, you'd never pick a bad one again. They don't, but you can use these clues.
Watermelon: thump it to see if it's ripe. If it sounds a bit hollow, it should be ready. You can also shake it to see if the seeds are loose, an indication of ripeness.
Cantaloupe: if it smells too sweet and musky, it's past its prime. Unlike watermelon, cantaloupe will continue to ripen at room temperature, so if you buy one that's not quite ripe, keep it on the worktop until it's ready.
Honeydew: look for a smooth outer peel and softness at the stem end of the melon (press it with your thumb).

Be sure to rinse melons well before you cut them. Since melons are grown on vines that lie on the ground, they come in contact with all kinds of bacteria from dirt, water and animals.

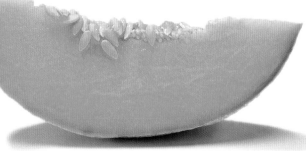

PERFECT PORTION: 30g (5cm wide slice)

As melons are mostly water*, there's no harm in having a little* more*.*

When you slice through the peel, you could move that bacteria from the outside to the inside on the knife.

Consider buying a melon baller. These come in various sizes and make it easy to serve melon as an appetising snack or dessert. They're also useful for coring pears and apples.

Menu magic

■ **Make melons** part of any fruit salad. Use a scooped-out watermelon shell to serve the salad at a picnic.

■ **Try a salad** with watermelon chunks and feta cheese, topped with fresh mint leaves and, if you like, some toasted pumpkin seeds or toasted pine nuts.

■ **Make a refreshing dessert** by mixing cubed watermelon and ice in the blender. Drizzle on a little honey.

■ **Garnish plates** with a slice of watermelon – and eat it!

■ **Serve honeydew** with vanilla ice cream.

■ **Mix small melon** cubes with chicken or seafood salad.

■ **Make watermelon** salsa by blending watermelon, sweet onions, black beans, jalapeños, chopped coriander leaves, crushed garlic and salt.

■ **Keep melon cubes** or balls in the fridge for handy, refreshing snacks.

■ **Blend cantaloupe,** orange juice, lime juice and cinnamon for a cold soup appetiser.

■ **Make a melon** smoothie with cantaloupe, honeydew, lime juice and a little honey.

■ **Place chunks or balls** of different types of melon on skewers for a colourful appetiser.

■ **Eat thinly sliced** cantaloupe or honeydew on top of Swiss cheese for an attractive snack.

Related recipe

Blueberry and melon compote with green tea and lime 288

Bitter melon — more like MEDICINE

Bitter melon, also part of the melon clan, is anything but sweet. As its name implies, this light green vegetable (yes, all melons are vegetables), which looks more like a warty cucumber than a melon, has a very bitter taste due to a high quinine content. Animal research shows that the natural compounds in bitter melon can lower blood sugar levels as much as some prescription drugs, possibly by boosting insulin secretion, improving the ability of cells to absorb glucose, blocking the absorption of sugar in the intestine and hindering the release of glucose from the liver.

One of the largest studies of bitter melon in people with Type 2 diabetes lasted only two days, but it showed significant reductions in blood sugar levels for 100 participants within hours of drinking a liquid containing suspended pulp from the melon. A number of smaller but longer trials have had similar results.

Most people who try bitter melon use supplements, but if you want to eat the melon itself (it's very much an acquired taste), cut the white fibrous seed core in half and remove the seeds. Don't eat them, as the red seed covering can be toxic. Blanching the melon before cooking will reduce the bitter flavour. It can then be used in soups or stir-fries.

milk

GL very low

There's something rather mysterious about milk in relation to blood sugar. It moves the needle only a smidge, which isn't surprising since it's fairly low in carbohydrates and rich in protein (a perfect combination for steadying blood sugar). But researchers think there's some natural component in milk that may directly help to protect against insulin resistance, a forerunner of Type 2 diabetes.

Two Harvard studies found that people who made dairy foods part of their daily diets were 21 per cent less likely to develop insulin resistance and 9 per cent less likely to develop Type 2 diabetes for each daily serving of dairy foods they had. This is pretty impressive (yet some websites still suggest that milk causes diabetes).

Choose skimmed milk rather than whole or even semi-skimmed, which still has a fair amount of saturated fat, the kind that increases insulin resistance and clogs arteries.

Health bonus

Milk is, of course, rich in calcium and vitamin D, both important for healthy bones. Fat-free milk actually has more calcium than whole, and it's also virtually the only good source of vitamin D you're likely to find in your kitchen. D is a 'don't miss' vitamin: experts are realising not only that our needs for it are higher than previously thought – and our blood levels woefully low – but also that it may play a key role in preventing certain cancers if we get enough.

Low-fat dairy foods such as skimmed milk are also included in some medically-approved diets for controlling high blood pressure.

Cooks' tips

If you don't really like skimmed milk because it's too thin, you might want to try ultra-pasteurised skimmed milk, also called UHT (ultra-high temperature). It tends to have a creamier taste and texture than regular skimmed milk but has roughly the same amount of fat and calories.

Menu magic

■ **Pretend you're a child** again and drink a cold glass of skimmed milk with lunch or dinner.
■ **Make yourself a** banana-strawberry smoothie with frozen strawberries, a frozen banana, skimmed milk and ¼ teaspoon of vanilla extract.
■ **Create 'cream' of carrot** or tomato soup using skimmed milk. Thicken it with a small amount of flour.
■ **Enjoy a soothing** cup of chai (spicy, milky tea) once in a while instead of coffee.

Related recipes

Cauliflower and spinach gratin 282
Chai 210
Cherry clafoutis 300
Greek pasta and beef casserole 240
Macaroni cheese with spinach 264
Plaice florentine 255
Porridge with apples and flaxseeds 192

PERFECT PORTION: 200ml

Three 200ml servings a day of low-fat milk or other *dairy* products, such as *yoghurt*, may help to tame insulin resistance and also provide much of the *calcium* you need.

nuts

GL very low

There's a good reason why people take a nut mixture with them when they're hiking. Nuts provide sustained energy because, thanks to their mix of fat and protein, they're a 'slow-burning' food. For the same reason, they're friendly to your blood sugar. In fact, Harvard researchers discovered that women who regularly ate nuts (about a handful five times a week) were 20 per cent less likely to develop Type 2 diabetes than those who didn't eat them as often.

Yes, nuts are high in fat – but it's mostly 'good' fat. Remember secret number 5 of Magic eating: 'Favour good fats'? Good fat may reduce insulin resistance, and in the case of most nuts, 85 per cent of their fat is this kind.

Good fats, of course, also improve heart health, even boosting levels of 'good' HDL cholesterol. In studies, people who ate as few as 150g of nuts a week as part of an overall heart-healthy diet lowered their risk of developing heart disease by 35 per cent compared to those who ate nuts less than once a month. (This doesn't apply to macadamia nuts, though, because of their high saturated fat content.) In fact, one study found that a diet that includes unsaturated fats from almonds and walnuts may have 10 per cent more cholesterol-lowering power than a more traditional cholesterol-lowering diet.

If you eat nuts frequently, you may also be damping down chronic inflammation in your body, which can help to reduce your risk of both diabetes and heart disease. And the protein in most nuts is unusually rich in the amino acid arginine, which may help to relax blood vessels, making a heart attack less likely.

Some nuts, including peanuts, walnuts and almonds, also contain plant sterols, which have been shown to lower cholesterol. They also contain a natural compound called resveratrol, the same one found in red wine and shown to

How many NUTS in a serving?

NUT	SERVING SIZE 30g
Almonds	20–24
Brazil nuts	9 or 10
Cashews	16–18
Hazelnuts	18–20
Peanuts	40
Pine nuts	150–157
Pistachios	45–47
Walnuts	8–11 halves

lower the risk of heart disease. Like fish, walnuts are a good source of omega-3 fats, another shot in the arm against heart disease.

Peanuts aren't technically nuts at all, but legumes. Unlike nuts that grow on trees, they grow underground, but in terms of health benefits, they rank right up there with all the above-ground nuts (*see* Peanut butter on page 136).

Health bonus

Nuts provide vitamin E, an important antioxidant that may help to fight prostate and lung cancers. Brazil nuts are selenium superstars, providing a massive 200 times more of the mineral than any other nut. Selenium has been linked to prevention of both cancer and heart disease. Almonds provide bone-building calcium. Hazelnuts and cashews boast the most copper, a vital nutrient for people with diabetes.

Cooks' tips

To squirrel away nuts, store them in an airtight container in the fridge for up to six months; in the freezer, they'll last for up to a year. Roasting nuts brings out their flavour. Preheat the oven to

150°C/gas 5. Place 75g of shelled nuts on a baking sheet in a single layer and roast for 7–10 minutes. Check near the end of the roasting time to make sure they don't burn.

Menu magic

Pick a dish, almost any dish – adding nuts can make it really special in terms of both taste and nutrition. Here are but a few simple suggestions to take your recipes to the next level.

■ **Stir chopped walnuts** or pecans into rice dishes.

■ **Add pistachios to** chicken salad.

■ **Mix pine nuts** or chopped walnuts into pasta dishes along with olive oil, basil and some chopped sun-dried tomatoes.

■ **Create your own** mixture to snack on with dried fruit, high-fibre cereal and a selection of your favourite nuts.

■ **Top off pumpkin,** squash, or tomato soup with chopped roasted nuts.

■ **Sprinkle your favourite** chopped nuts and some dried cranberries on green salads.

■ **For better-tasting** pancakes and muffins, add chopped nuts to the batter.

■ **For a single-serving,** low-GL snack in place of crisps or crackers, place 30g of nuts in a self-sealing bag to carry with you.

■ **Sprinkle pecans** into unsweetened apple sauce.

■ **Stir nuts into** stir-fry dishes.

Smart substitution

Instead of white flour: use ground nuts to replace some of the white stuff called for in a crust or cake batter.

Related recipes

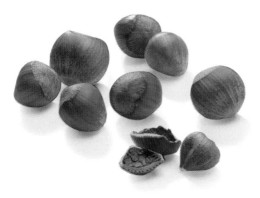

PERFECT PORTION: 30g

Nuts are **high in calories**, *so a* **serving is small**. *Because nuts come in all shapes and sizes, the number that equals a serving varies quite a bit (see 'How many nuts in a serving?' on opposite page).* **Macadamia nuts** *contain a whopping 925kcal per 125g, so* **indulge sparingly**.

oats

GL medium

A steaming bowl of porridge – sprinkled with Magic cinnamon, of course – is more than comfort food. Studies show that oats can reduce postmeal blood sugar and insulin levels in people with and without diabetes.

Soluble fibre is the reason porridge is top-notch for steady blood sugar. This type of fibre turns into a gel in your stomach, slowing the digestive process and blunting the rise in blood sugar that normally goes with it. Oats are also an excellent source of the mineral manganese, which plays a role in blood sugar metabolism.

Dozens of studies have concluded that eating porridge five or six times a week can reduce your risk of developing Type 2 diabetes by 39 per cent. And, since oatmeal's a whole grain, starting your day with a bowl will take you one step closer to living the second secret of Magic eating: 'Make three of your carb servings whole grains.'

Oats also fight heart disease, as it says on the packet. This has been proven beyond a shadow of a doubt in more than 40 studies over 30 years of research. It's largely because of the special type of soluble fibre, called beta-glucan, found in porridge.

One more benefit of this flaky food: it fills you up and keeps you full. In one study, people who ate porridge for breakfast consumed a third fewer calories at lunch than those who ate a sugared flaked cereal. (The bran of the oat is just as good for your blood sugar as flakes, so be sure to read the bran entry on page 84.)

Health bonus

The soluble fibre called beta-glucan not only helps to tame blood sugar and cholesterol, it may also boost your immune system's ability to fight off infection, as well as reduce high blood pressure. Oats are also a good source of natural plant compounds that may help to reduce the risk of breast cancer by mimicking oestrogen and preventing the natural hormone from triggering the growth of cancer cells. And they're packed with powerful disease-fighting antioxidants called polyphenols and saponins.

Cooks' tips

Don't substitute instant oats in a recipe that calls for quick-cooking or old-fashioned oats. The texture is different, and instant oats usually have other flavours added.

Menu magic

■ **Grind oats in** the blender and use them to coat fish and chicken.
■ **Make a batch of** oat-bran muffins and keep them to hand for tasty breakfast treats.
■ **Next time you** make pancakes or waffles, replace up to a third of the flour in the batter with oats ground to a fine powder in the blender.
■ **Make fresh oat** biscuits.
■ **Use oat flour** as a thickener for stews and soups.

Are some oats better than OTHERS?

Some oats have been processed more or less than others. On the 'less' end of the scale are steel-cut oats (see the 'Oats glossary' on the facing page). The GL of less processed oats is about 20 per cent lower than that of more processed forms, but even instant oats are a good source of fibre and have a moderate GL. Shop carefully for instant porridge, though; most brands have added sugar – as much as 4 teaspoons per packet. Generally, only plain (unflavoured) instant porridge is sugar free.

OATS glossary

While all oats have the power to tame your blood sugar, there are differences in taste and texture among the various types.

- **Rolled (old–fashioned) oats:** oats that have been steamed, rolled, resteamed and toasted. They take about 15 minutes to cook.
- **Instant oats:** these are prepared the same way as rolled oats but cut into smaller pieces so they cook faster. No actual cooking is required; just pour boiling water over them, stir and they are ready to eat.
- **Oat flour:** flour made by grinding groats and separating out the bran.
- **Oat bran:** this is made by grinding oat groats and separating the bran from the flour. It's higher in insoluble fibre than whole oats and can be prepared as a hot cereal like porridge.

- **Bake up a tray** of oatmeal biscuits (using wholemeal flour in place of one-third of the white flour) and include a teaspoon of Magic cinnamon, of course!

Smart substitutions

Instead of sugary cereal: have steel-cut or old-fashioned porridge with raisins and walnuts for a hearty and filling breakfast.

Instead of bread crumbs: use oatbran in meat loaf, nutroast and meatballs.

Instead of wheat flour: substitute oat flour for a third of the wheat flour in baked goods.

Instead of cheese crackers: serve oatcakes with the cheeseboard or with soups.

Related recipes

Blueberry and oat muffins 198
Cranberry and apple crumble 301
Multi-Grain griddle cakes or waffles 192
Oat and peanut butter bars 210
Porridge with apples and flaxseeds 192
Turkey meatballs in tomato sauce 254

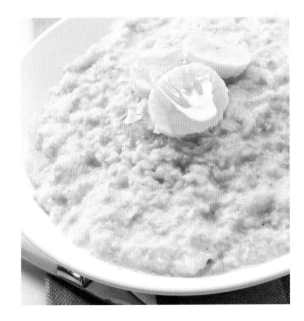

PERFECT PORTION: 150g

Oats are *slow-acting carbs* that are good for your blood sugar – if you keep the portion size reasonable. Eat more than a small bowl, and the GL moves into the high range. Fill up the rest of your bowl with *fresh fruit* and a sprinkling of *nuts*.

olive oil

It's a wonder olive oil isn't more expensive, because in the world of Magic eating, it's liquid gold. Remember secret number 5 of Magic eating, 'Favour good fats'? Well, olive oil is the flagship of the good-fats fleet. In fact, we recommend using olive or rapeseed oil (when you need a neutral-tasting oil) most of the time instead of other oils.

Good fats such as those in olive oil work miracles for your blood sugar – and your health in general. Unlike butter, these unsaturated fats don't increase insulin resistance and may even help to reverse it, helping your body to steady its blood sugar.

Olive oil also helps you to avoid sudden blood sugar surges by slowing digestion so carbs take longer to break down into blood sugar. Simply tossing your salad with olive oil and vinegar will help to blunt the blood sugar impact of whatever else you're eating (*see* page 159 to find out why the vinegar's also important).

One recent Australian study found that when six men were given either olive oil, water or a mixture of water and oil before a high-carb meal,

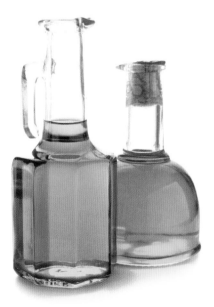

Olives: MAGIC FRUITS

Olive oil comes from olives – the motherlode of good-for-you fats. So consider olives a Magic food, too. For the best olive taste, buy fresh ones from the deli section, not canned. (Once you get used to them, you'll never go back to canned.) If you use quality, flavourful olives, a little will go a long way.

Like olive oil, olives pack a lot of calories (about 6 per medium black olive), so try to use them in place of other fats in your diet, not in addition to them.

it took almost three times as long for their stomachs to begin emptying – significantly delaying the subsequent rise in blood sugar – when they had the olive oil. You may also remember from the first chapter that meals that raise blood sugar quickly result in feeling hungrier before the next meal. Slower rises in blood sugar equal feeling full longer, which in turn equals weight loss!

As for heart health, eating generous amounts of olive oil is one of the main reasons that people who follow the Mediterranean diet have less heart disease and far fewer heart attacks.

One study found that when 28 men and women added 2 tablespoons of extra-virgin olive oil a day to their usual diets for six weeks, they experienced a 12 per cent drop in total cholesterol and a 16 per cent drop in LDL ('bad') cholesterol. Numerous studies over the years have shown that olive oil not only lowers LDL but also raises HDL, the good kind. Olive oil is also rich in antioxidants called phenols, which help to protect artery walls from cholesterol buildup.

Health bonus

Olive oil contains an anti-inflammatory component so strong that researchers liken it to aspirin. This may be another reason that people who follow the Mediterranean diet have such low rates of heart disease, which is linked to inflammation. So, by the way, is Type 2 diabetes, not to mention other chronic diseases such as Alzheimer's.

In contrast, a diet heavy in corn, safflower, and sunflower oils can actually promote inflammation in the body, which can damage arteries and lead to heart disease and other health problems. We do not recommend using any of these types as your main cooking oil.

Olive oil also contains natural compounds called lignans, which may reduce the risk of cancers of the colon, breast, prostate, pancreas and endometrium.

Cooks' tips

Olive oil isn't like wine; it doesn't improve with age. In fact, it can become rancid. Store it in a tightly sealed dark container in a cool place.

Menu magic

Good cooks use olive oil in most dishes. Use it when you can in place of other vegetable oils, margarine or butter. Here are a few suggestions.

■ **Serve a dish** of good olive oil seasoned with cracked black pepper for dipping fresh bread (whole-grain, of course).

■ **Instead of using** butter on bread or mashed potatoes, try olive oil mixed with roasted garlic (*see* the garlic entry for tips on roasting).

■ **Use it as a base** for marinades for beef, chicken, fish or pork.

■ **Dice olives into** sauces, especially tomato-based types.

■ **Add it to pasta,** chopped tomatoes, crumbled feta cheese, chopped fresh basil and capers for a fast and oh-so-simple supper.

■ **Use it to replace** the smoked meats and sausage typically used to flavour bean soups.

■ **In recipes that call** for butter or margarine, use ¾ teaspoon olive oil in place of 1 teaspoon butter or margarine.

■ **Top your pizza** with olives along with other vegetables of your choice.

■ **Add olives to** green salads, pasta salads and tuna sandwiches.

Related recipes

PERFECT PORTION: 30g

Use olive oil whenever you can in place of other oils, but **pour lightly.** *At* **99kcal per tablespoon,** *those* **healthy calories** *could easily turn into* **unhealthy pounds.**

onions

Though onions may make your eyes water and give you 'onion breath', we want you to embrace them. They're essential to cooks for their unique flavour and, what's more, they're very good for you. It's true that these underground vegetables don't offer many nutrients, but what they do have in bulk are powerful sulphur-containing compounds, which are responsible for their pungent odour and many of their health benefits.

According to several studies, onions may help to bring down high blood sugar in diabetic animals. In one Egyptian study of diabetic rats, onion juice reduced blood sugar levels by an amazing 70 per cent. One of few published studies in humans, from India, dates back some 30 years, but it found that people with diabetes who ate 60g of onions a day experienced a significant drop in blood sugar levels.

Researchers credit these effects to the sulphur compounds in onions as well as their flavonoids. These powerful antioxidant compounds also help to fight some of the side effects of high blood sugar, not to mention heart disease.

Onions even seem to boost HDL, the 'good' cholesterol. One study found that people who ate the most onions, along with other foods rich in flavonoids, had a 20 per cent lower risk of heart disease. Thanks to their sulphur compounds, onions, like aspirin, also help to prevent dangerous blood clots. And they're known to help to lower high blood pressure.

Finally, onions are one of the richest food sources of chromium, a trace mineral that improves the body's ability to respond to insulin.

Health bonus

Onions' sulphur compounds and flavonoids may help to fend off several forms of cancer. One Chinese study found that men who ate at least 1 tablespoon of chopped onions and other related vegetables (garlic, spring onions, chives and leeks) a day had about half the risk of developing prostate cancer compared to men who ate less than ¼ tablespoon of these veggies daily. There's also a link between a high intake of flavonoids and reduced risk of lung cancer.

Evidence suggests that onions may help to preserve bone and prevent osteoporosis. And because the sulphur compounds are strongly anti-inflammatory, onions may also help to relieve the pain and swelling of arthritis.

The green tops of spring onions are rich in vitamin C and beta-carotene.

Cooks' tips

The more tears they cause, the more health benefits onions tend to have. To stop your eyes from watering while you're chopping them, try chilling onions for about half an hour before peeling and cutting, and slice them from the top,

Antioxidant-rich ONIONS

There are many different varieties of onion – from pungent red onions to the mild Spanish variety – and each has its own unique flavour. The nutritional value and antioxidant capacity of onions varies slightly according to the variety. To reap the most benefit from onions, choose the varieties that contain the most antioxidants, which tend to be the stronger tasting ones.

TYPES OF ONION	OXIDANT RATING
Shallots	Highest
Red onions	
Yellow skin onions	
Spring onions	
Spanish onions	Lowest

leaving the root end intact; it is this part of the onion that has the strongest concentration of eye-burning compounds.

Wash onions before chopping, especially if you're going to eat them raw. Onions grow underground and can harbour bacteria. Store onions in a cool, dry place, not in the fridge, and not near potatoes. Potatoes give off moisture and a gas that causes onions to spoil faster.

Menu magic

Like garlic, onions can be added to just about anything. Here are just a few suggestions.
- **Add onions** to almost any stew or stir-fry.
- **To get a bit of** raw onion into your diet, combine chopped onions, tomatoes, avocado and jalapeño peppers for a blood sugar–friendly dip. Finish with a splash of lime juice.
- **Sauté chopped onions** in olive oil and add to corn, potatoes or peas.
- **Add chopped spring onions** to rice dishes.
- **Add sliced mild onions** to green salads.
- **Use chopped red onions** to add crunch and flavour to any sandwich salad, such as chicken, tuna or egg salad.
- **Make fruit chutney** with peaches, mangos,

pears, apples or apricots and plenty of chopped onion. Serve with meals as a condiment that won't upset your blood sugar balance.
- **Use caramelised onions** to add flavour to any vegetable and pasta dish. To caramelise an onion, thinly slice the onion, then heat 1 tablespoon olive oil in a heavy skillet over medium heat. Add onion and cook, covered, for 10 minutes, stirring often. Remove cover and cook for 10 more minutes, stirring occasionally.
- **Enjoy French onion** soup, but go easy on the bread and cheese topping. Try adding a few whole-grain croutons instead.

Related recipes

Crushed curried butternut squash 282
Curried red lentil soup 230
Greek pasta and beef casserole 240
Hearty split pea soup with rye croutons 230
Jerusalem artichoke drop scones 281
Lamb stew with spring vegetables 239
Moroccan-style chicken thighs with butternut
　squash and baby onions 247
Orange beef stir-fry with broccoli and
　red pepper 234
Pork chop and cabbage pan-fry 242
Pork stew with Mexican flavours 239
Sautéed Brussels sprouts with red pepper
　and caraway seeds 284
Slow-cooker beef and red wine stew 238
Spinach with pine nuts and currants 286
Turkey and bean chilli with avocado salsa 252

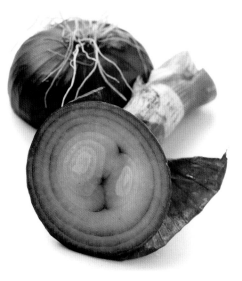

PERFECT PORTION: 80g

Onions have **very few calories**, *so add them to as many dishes as you can think of. Finely chopped* **raw onions** *offer the greatest health benefits.*

pasta

You might think there's nothing worse for your blood sugar than a bowl of pasta. Surprisingly, you'd be wrong. As it turns out, pasta has only a moderate effect on blood sugar levels. (The Italian bread you may eat with your pasta, however, is a different story.)

Yes, pasta is high in carbs. But the type of wheat it's made from (durum wheat) appears to be digested more slowly than similar white flours used to make bread. You can also thank the special protein structure of the dough for pasta's moderate GL. It's a protein 'latticework' that traps the starch molecules so it takes more time for your stomach's digestive enzymes to get to them and turn them into blood sugar. (Want to know more? You'll need a degree in food chemistry.) The more thoroughly you cook pasta, though, the easier it is for your body to break it down, so if you like your pasta *al dente* – or slightly firm – all the better.

Choose wholemeal pasta instead of regular white pasta, and you'll have a serving or two of whole grain – and about three times as much fibre per serving. Remember, you're aiming to make three of your daily carb servings whole grains, which will lower your risk of diabetes.

Pasta is just about as good – or as bad – for you as what you eat with it. Pile on vegetables such as tomatoes and spinach or steamed broccoli, add a little olive oil and garlic, and you've got a terrific low-GL meal. Drown your pasta in cream sauce, and you might as well eat cheesecake. If you're watching your cholesterol, you might go a little easy with egg noodles. It's no secret that they're made with eggs, and since eggs contain cholesterol, so do the noodles. (As we pointed out in the egg entry on page 106, though, dietary cholesterol isn't the main contributor to high cholesterol levels.) Another option? Look out for eggless noodles.

Health bonus

By law, all white flour in the UK and Europe is fortified with iron, calcium and B vitamins, which means that all white pasta has these benefits, too (wholemeal flour already contains these nutrients). Pasta also contains some protein, but it's not a complete protein source, meaning that it's missing some of the amino acids that make up a complete protein. You can remedy this by sprinkling a little grated cheese on your pasta.

Cooks' tips

Pasta can last for up to three years. Store it in an airtight container so you can easily toss it into boiling water at short notice. When it is ready, (taste it; it should be firm when you bite it), drain it immediately or it will continue to cook.

Menu magic

Pasta has to be one of the most versatile foods ever invented. All you need to do is pick your pasta; for toppings, the sky's the limit. Think herbs, sautéed vegetables, beans, chicken, perhaps a bit of olive oil and a sprinkling of Parmesan cheese. If you include garlic and onions, you could get as many as six Magic foods on one plate!

■ **Grab a bag** of frozen vegetables, cook them, and toss them with hot pasta, some olive oil, sautéed garlic, and a bit of cheese for a healthy dinner in no time at all.

■ **Cook any vegetable** you like and purée it. Serve on hot pasta topped with herbs.

■ **Top pasta with** meatballs made with minced turkey breast or extra-lean minced beef and some low sugar, low salt tomato sauce. Serve with a big green salad.

■ **Add pine nuts** or toasted pumpkin seeds to your pasta dish. Remember, nuts and seeds are Magic, too.

■ **Add beans, chickpeas,** or lentils to a modest portion of pasta to fill up your plate and lower the GL of the meal. You'll also get more protein.

Smart substitution

Instead of mashed potatoes: make pasta with olive oil and courgettes as a side dish to have with dinner.

Related recipes

Garden pasta salad 223
Greek pasta and beef casserole 240
Macaroni and cheese with spinach 264
Oriental noodle hotpot 233
Penne with asparagus, ricotta and lemon 264
Penne with tomato and aubergine sauce 262
Prawn and orzo casserole 260
Quick spinach and sausage lasagna 267
Turkey and pasta with spinach 251
Wholemeal noodles with peanut sauce
  and chicken 220
Wholemeal pasta with sausage, beans
  and greens 266

PERFECT PORTION: 75–100g (cooked)

Serve *150g* of pasta as a *main dish* or *75g* as a *side dish* to keep the GL within the medium range.

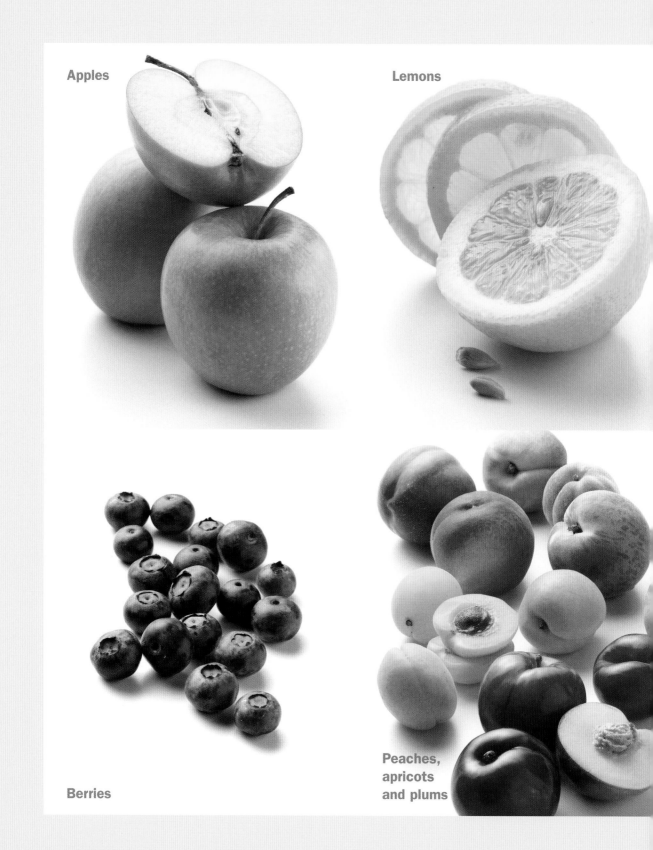

Apples

Lemons

Berries

Peaches,
apricots
and plums

Magic fruits

Citrus fruits

Cherries

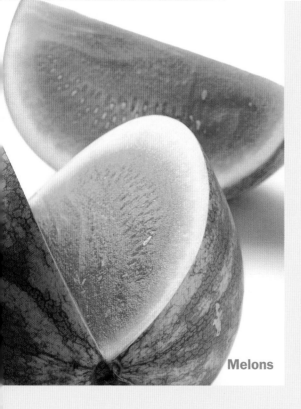

Melons

Despite their
SWEETNESS,

most fruits have a low glycaemic load and fit in perfectly with a Magic diet. Lemons even directly lower blood sugar.

- **apples**
- **citrus fruits**
- **berries**
- **melons**
- **lemons**
- **cherries**
- **peaches, apricots, plums**

peaches, apricots and plums

GL very low Apricots, peaches and plums make perfect low-calorie snacks and sweet desserts. Known as stone fruits because of the stone-like seed inside, they owe their low GLs to their high water content and their stash of blood sugar-taming, cholesterol-busting soluble fibre.

Peaches boast the most fibre of the three. Apricots, which are close cousins to peaches, are richest in beta-carotene, linked with protection from heart disease and cancer. Plums are packed with several disease-fighting antioxidants. Prunes outrank more than 20 other popular fruits and vegetables in antioxidant power, which is important for staving off heart disease and preventing damage caused by high blood sugar.

Fruit you bite into is generally healthier for you than fruit you spoon from a can. A fresh peach contains only 35kcal, whereas a 125g serving of peaches in heavy syrup has 66kcal. If you must buy canned peaches, look for those packed in their own juice.

You may as well cross peach and apricot fruit juice blends off your shopping list. They usually contain a lot of added sugar or high-fructose corn syrup and little or no fibre – a devastating combo that could send your blood sugar through the roof. If you like drinking these fruit juices, dilute them with an equal amount of fizzy water. (Why not try our Peachy iced tea on page 213? It serves eight people and has only 30kcal per glass – which makes it highly preferable to sugary fruit drinks.)

Health bonus

Stone fruits contain compounds that may help to keep your eyes crystal clear and free of cataracts. And study after study has concluded that people who eat more fruits and vegetables are healthier in general, with less diabetes, heart disease, cancer and obesity. Stone fruits also offer potassium, a mineral that protects against high blood pressure and stroke. And while we are at it, let's not forget the unique intestinal benefits of dried plums (or prune juice) – both help to combat constipation.

Cooks tips

Apricots are delicious raw but, when they're cooked, their beta-carotene and soluble fibre are made more available to the body. For a savoury accompaniment to grilled meat or poultry, pit and quarter fresh apricots and gently sauté them in olive oil with a touch of crushed garlic.

Menu magic

■ **Top whole-grain** pancakes and waffles with peach slices.

■ **Give chicken** dishes or stews an exotic taste of the Middle East by adding a handful of diced dried apricots or plums.

■ **Poach plums** in red wine and sprinkle with grated lemon zest for a healthy dessert.

■ **Sprinkle a little cinnamon** and nutmeg onto sliced peaches and mix them into low-fat yoghurt.

■ **Sauté sliced, peeled** peaches in a small amount of cholesterol-lowering margarine (and some ginger, if you like) and serve alone or as a dessert topper.

■ **Blend up a peach** smoothie with low-fat vanilla yoghurt, diced peaches, frozen strawberries and vanilla.

■ **Add diced peaches** to chicken salad for a sweet twist.

■ **Add chopped dried** plums to poultry stuffing.

■ **Top porridge** with sliced peaches, dried plums or diced apricots.

■ **Add chopped dried** apricots to cold cereal.

Stone fruits make delectable snacks that just happen to benefit your blood sugar thanks to their stash of soluble fibre.

What's in a **NAME?**

Have you ever heard of plumcots or pluots? Both fruits were hybridised in the USA – the plumcot is a cross between a plum and an apricot and the pluot is a cross between a plum and a plumcot. Some hybrids, such as nectarines – a peach/plum cross – are hugely popular; others, such as the peacharine (a peach/nectarine cross) are seldom seen.

Did you know that the plum sauce in some Chinese foods is actually made from a type of Japanese apricot?

Finally, take note that in future it may be harder to find a packet of 'prunes'. Producers are apparently remarketing them as 'dried plums' in a bid to improve their image.

■ **Dip dried apricots** in dark chocolate for a decadent but relatively healthy treat (provided that you keep portions small).

■ **Add chopped dried apricots** to wild rice before cooking.

■ **Create your own** trail mix with nuts, pieces of bran cereal and chopped dried apricots.

■ **Make plum sauce** by blending juice-packed plums with cinnamon and spices. Pour over grilled chicken breast or pork tenderloin.

DON'T fall for it ...

Have you sworn off dried fruit because you've heard it will send your blood sugar skyrocketing? Better rethink that decision. While the glycaemic index (GI) of dried fruit is high, the glycaemic load (GL), which takes serving size into account, is low. For the record, a serving of dried fruit is about 60g – not a whole packet.

Related recipes

Chicken fillets with peaches and ginger 244
Nectarine, plum and mixed berry soup 289
Orange-glazed roasted plums 296
Peachy iced tea 213
Plum and walnut crumble 302
Spice-crusted pork tenderloin with peach salsa 243
Upside-down nectarine muffins 200

PERFECT PORTION: 1 peach

Because apricots and plums are smaller, you can consider two of them as one serving.

peanut butter

GL very low

You probably think that peanut butter is just for children. Well, perhaps the classic peanut butter on sticky white bread is best left as part of childhood, but don't abandon it altogether. Peanut butter is a sensible addition to a Magic diet, and it makes perfect sense because peanuts are a Magic food, too.

Peanut butter is doubly effective against blood sugar surges: protein and 'good' (unsaturated) fat. In fact, the prestigious Nurses' Health Study in the USA found that women who ate peanut butter at least five times a week were up to 30 per cent less likely to develop diabetes.

On a related note, you may have heard of the peanut butter diet. It's not quite as crazy as it sounds because peanut butter is quite filling as well as healthy, with its winning combination of good fat, protein and fibre. A study at Purdue University found that eating it can dampen the appetite for up to 2 hours longer than a low-fibre, high-carb snack. (*See* page 210 for our Oat and peanut butter bars.)

Like nuts, peanut butter can also protect your heart. Its good fat helps to tame high cholesterol – after all, it's the same type of fat found in olive oil. One study found that diets taking most of their monounsaturated fat from peanut butter reduced heart disease risk by almost as much as diets that got most of their mono-unsaturated fats from olive oil.

Peanut butter is rich in plant compounds called sterols, one of the top proven cholesterol busters. (In fact, sterols are added to some cholesterol-lowering margarines.) Plus, it has a gram of fibre per tablespoon. You really couldn't pack many more benefits into something you can spoon out of a jar.

The good news SPREADS

Peanut butter doesn't stand alone when it comes to health benefits. Other nut butters, such as almond, walnut and pistachio butters, are healthy choices, too. (Cashew and macadamia nut butters are higher in saturated fat.) They are expensive, but a little goes a long way. Seed butters, including sunflower seed and pumpkin seed butter, fit the better-blood-sugar bill as well. You will find the more unusual varieties in health-food shops and online stores.

Be careful which brand you buy, though. Some are sweetened with corn syrup or sugar – as much as $\frac{1}{2}$ teaspoon per 2 tablespoons of peanut butter. There's little excuse for this as ground peanuts taste great on their own. Wholefood and organic brands generally have no added sugar and less salt than regular brands.

Health bonus

The sterols in peanut butter not only help to control cholesterol, it is believed that they may also help to fend off colon, prostate and breast cancers. Peanut butter is also a rich source of the heart-healthy antioxidant compound resveratrol, that is, the antioxidant for which red wine is most acclaimed. Wholefood brands of peanut butter generally contain more resveratrol than other types.

Eating peanut butter (or nuts) several times a week is a proven way to keep high blood pressure under

Packed with protein and 'good' fat, peanut butter serves your heart, your waistline, and, oh yes, your blood sugar.

control. And peanut butter ranks right up there with most nuts for its stash of vitamin E, which is important for a healthy immune system.

Could peanut butter be good for your bones? Yes indeed. It's one of the top sources of the bone-building mineral boron.

Finally, eat peanut butter and/or nuts at least five times a week, and you could lower your risk of developing gallstones, according to one study.

Cooks' tips
Some natural peanut butters do not contain preservatives and need to be refrigerated after you open them (check the label). If the oil separates, let the jar come to room temperature, then stir it up. Most brands can be sealed tightly and stored in the larder.

Menu magic
■ **For a nibble** that won't make your blood sugar soar, spread peanut butter on wholemeal crackers, wedges of toasted wholemeal pitta bread or oatcakes.
■ **For an even lower-GL** snack that will stave off hunger longer, spread peanut butter on apple slices, celery sticks or carrots.
■ **Be adventurous and** try different types of nut butters with different types of fruit and vegetables.

Smart substitution
Instead of jam: spread peanut butter on your wholemeal toast or crispbread. You'll get more calories but also more hunger-satisfying protein and less sugar.

Related recipes
Oriental peanut dip 206
Oat and peanut butter bars 210
Peanut and chicken soup 232
Wholemeal noodles with peanut sauce
  and chicken 220

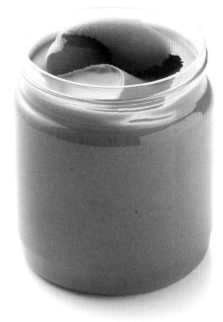

PERFECT PORTION: 1 tablespoon

Peanut butter won't raise your blood sugar, but it does contain almost **100kcal per tablespoon**. *When you're spreading bread, a cracker, or a crispbread, be sure you* **control your portion size.**

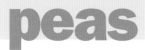

peas

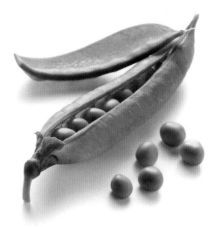

GL very low

Eat up your peas.

Being on the starchy side as far as vegetables go, they may seem like a bad idea for blood sugar. But this is not true. Peas are a super source of protein, which one reason that they don't make blood sugar soar. A serving of 80g contains an impressive 4.5g of protein and only 55kcal. Peas also have a low GL thanks in part to their soluble fibre content, the kind that lowers blood sugar. At almost 4.5g of total fibre per 80g (about a third of which is soluble), a small serving of peas will help you to reach the recommended target of 24g of fibre per day.

For heart protection, you can't beat these legumes. The type of soluble fibre they contain, pectin, is top-notch at lowering cholesterol. Peas also contain potassium, which helps to lower high blood pressure, and they serve up quite a bit of the B vitamin folate, which experts think may play a role in keeping arteries clear.

Health bonus

Green peas are an outstanding source of lutein and zeaxanthin. These members of the carotene family are thought to lower the risk of cataracts and macular degeneration, the leading cause of blindness in older adults.

Cooks' tips

Frozen peas are handy, but avoid tinned peas, which sometimes contain added salt and have much less flavour.

■ **Cook peas** until just tender, to retain their nutrients. Use a steamer for the best results.

PERFECT PORTION: 80g

Though a portion is about **3 heaped tablespoons,** *peas are firmly in the very low GL category, so don't be too concerned about eating a little more.*

Menu magic

■ **Serve up a** classic peas-and-carrots side dish.
■ **Add peas to any** soup with noodles or other grain products in it. Peas are a complete protein when combined with grains.
■ **Top salads** with a sprinkling of peas.
■ **Make peas part** of just about any stew or casserole. You can add them to mince dishes such as spaghetti bolognese or shepherd's pie.
■ **Mix up a cold green pea salad** for your next picnic. Try mixing frozen young peas, chopped pimientos, chopped spring onions, a small amount of low-fat sour cream, chopped apple, lemon juice, salt and pepper. Or mix peas with toasted almonds, spring onions, feta cheese, low-fat mayonnaise and balsamic vinegar.
■ **Toss peas into** wholemeal pasta.
■ **Snack on mangetout** – sometimes known as sugar-snap peas. The pods give you more fibre, although the peas contain less protein than more mature, out-of-the-pod types.

Related recipes

Barley salad with mangetout and
  lemon dressing 216
Chicken pot pie with a wholemeal crust 248
Spiced cauliflower with peas 284

pork

GL very low

People tend to associate pork with fat and think it unhealthy but the truth is that eating pork – like other protein foods – will not raise your blood sugar a bit. And the leanest cuts, such as tenderloin, are almost as low in fat as chicken. In the USA advertisers often market pork as 'the other white meat', although it is in fact red meat.

Over the past 20 years, changes in feeding and breeding practices have produced much leaner cuts of pork, making them appropriate in a Magic diet. Less fat means fewer calories, which means less excess weight and better blood sugar control.

Health bonus

Like all other animal foods, including beef and eggs, pork is a good source of vitamins B_6 and B_{12}, which help to keep homocysteine in check. High levels of this amino acid raise the risk of heart disease and dementia. Pork is also a good source of riboflavin (vitamin B_2), important for metabolising carbohydrates and for producing red blood cells.

Cooks' tips

To keep pork as lean as possible, trim off any excess fat before you cook it. One of the biggest mistakes made with pork is overcooking it. That's a recipe for a tough, dried-out dish. To keep lean cuts moist during roasting and to bring the GL of the meal even lower, try using a marinade that contains vinegar, wine or citrus juice. The acid from the marinade will soften the meat, making it juicier and tastier.

Years ago, people worried about getting intestinal parasites (trichina) from eating pork. Today, because of changes in the way animals are fed and raised, it's much less of a concern. And as was the case all along, cooking pork properly – to an internal temperature of at least 75°C – will kill any trichina parasites that may be lurking.

Menu magic

Think of using pork just as you would beef or chicken, and the possibilities are endless.

■ **Use pork strips** or cubes in stir-fries along with plenty of vegetables.

■ **Try pork tenderloin** on the grill.

■ **Create hearty pork** and wild rice soup with cubed pork loin, white beans, chickpeas, cooked wild rice, chopped onion, chicken stock, olive oil, cumin, chopped parsley and coriander.

■ **Make pork and** black bean chilli with cubed pork, black beans, chopped red peppers, diced tomatoes, chunky salsa, crushed garlic, chopped onion and chilli powder. Cook in a slow cooker for 7 hours.

■ **Throw a lean pork** chop on the grill along with sliced summer squash and halved tomatoes.

■ **Use extra-lean** minced pork (labelled 97 per cent lean) in place of regular or even extra-lean minced beef for meat loaf, meatballs or burgers. You may have to go to a health food shop to get such lean pork, or order it online, but it's worth the effort since it's significantly lower in fat than pork labelled 'lean' (and often lower than minced pork whose label says 'extra lean' but doesn't include an actual figure).

■ **Use pork in** kebabs, along with cherry tomatoes and wedges of onion and chopped yellow bell pepper.

Related recipes

Pork chop and cabbage pan-fry 242
Spice-crusted pork tenderloin with
    peach salsa 243

PERFECT PORTION: 85g

If this is your only meat of the day, up to 170g is appropriate. Be sure to choose a lean cut.

---

pumpernickel bread

GL low

Made with coarsely ground rye flour (and perhaps some wheat flour) and fermented with a sourdough starter, traditional pumpernickel bread combines the benefits of two other Magic foods: rye bread and sourdough bread. The acetic acid from the starter (*see* Sourdough bread on page 147) and the soluble fibre in rye (*see* Rye bread, opposite) keep the GL of pumpernickel bread low – much lower than that of white or even wholemeal bread.

One Canadian study found that pumpernickel bread had four to eight times as much resistant starch as breads made with wheat or barley. Resistant starch benefits blood sugar because it doesn't digest easily. Like dietary fibre, it travels right past the stomach and small intestine and settles in the colon, where it's broken down by bacteria and eventually expelled.

Not all shop-bought pumpernickels have the same benefits as traditional German pumpernickel, though. Many get their dark colour from molasses, not from whole rye kernels and a special baking process that takes many hours. These types usually contain more wheat flour than rye, and some are made using yeast instead of sourdough starter.

Your best bet is to shop at specialist bakeries, which tend to use more traditional pumpernickel recipes. If the bread feels heavy for its size, it's probably the real thing. There are brands available of traditionally made pumpernickel – you will need to check the labels. Better still make your own.

Health bonus

As with rye bread, pumpernickel loads you up with lignans – plant compounds that may help to reduce the risk of breast and prostate cancers.

Cooks' tips

If you buy traditional pumpernickel bread from the bakery or make it yourself, it will be preservative free, so you'll need to store it in a plastic bag and use it within a few days.

Menu magic

■ **For a tasty starter,** top small squares of pumpernickel bread with cream cheese, sliced onion and tomato.

■ **Serve strong-flavoured** sandwich fillings, such as mature cheese, on pumpernickel.

■ **Mustard goes well** with pumpernickel, so spread this Magic food on your next ham and Swiss cheese pumpernickel sandwich.

■ **Serve a slice** of pumpernickel as a satisfying accompaniment to soup or chilli.

Related recipes

Salmon sandwiches with wasabi mayonnaise 226
Smoked salmon canapés 205

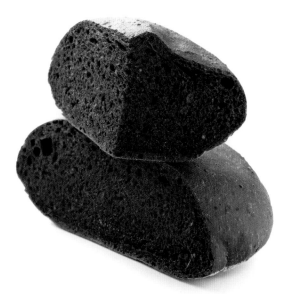

PERFECT PORTION: 30g

A serving is about the size of a small slice. *Obviously, you'll need two servings to make a sandwich.*

rye bread

GL low

Why rye? Because research shows that unlike white bread, which is one of the worst foods for your blood sugar, whole-grain rye bread (or whole-grain rye crackers or cereal) can help to smooth out blood sugar swings and actually reduce the risk of developing Type 2 diabetes. Proper rye bread is even superior to wholemeal bread when it comes to keeping blood sugar levels steady.

In one study, on days when women ate whole-rye bread, their blood sugar levels were 10 per cent lower than on days when they didn't eat it. Another study found that eating rye bread reduced the release of insulin compared to eating refined wheat bread, meaning that less insulin was needed to keep blood sugar in check. That's a good thing, because when the body regularly pumps out a lot of insulin, the risk of insulin resistance goes up (and so does the risk of diabetes).

A third study found that men who ate whole-grain rye bread, crackers and cereal (they got 18g of fibre a day from rye) for four weeks saw a drop in blood sugar of up to 19 per cent compared to their levels at the start of the study.

What's so special about rye? The structure and size of the starch particles in the bread certainly play a role. Another explanation: rye contains about three times as much soluble fibre as wheat, which lowers high cholesterol.

There's one note of caution. By 'rye' bread, we mean bread made from whole rye flour. Most of the rye breads you find on the supermarket shelves contain a combination of refined rye and wheat flour, so they don't have the same fibre content or health benefits. Get out the magnifying glass if you have to and look for 'whole grain rye flour' at the top of the ingredients list on the label. Real rye bread feels heavy for its size and bears little resemblance to white sandwich bread.

Health bonus

Rye is loaded with lignans, plant compounds that may help to reduce the risk of breast and prostate cancers. And researchers have found that some of the unique plant compounds in whole-grain rye are helpful for intestinal health. One study from Finland, where rye is very popular, found that people who ate 4½ slices of whole-grain rye bread a day had 26 per cent lower levels of compounds linked to colon cancer.

Cooks' tips

If you feel a baking spree coming on, and you want to make your own whole-grain rye bread, visit your local health food store or shop online for whole-grain rye flour.

Menu magic

■ **Serve your favourite** sandwich fillings on whole-grain rye bread.
■ **When you reach** for cheese and crackers, make the crackers whole-grain rye.
■ **Try whole-grain** rye rolls at dinner instead of white rolls, if you can find (or make) them.
■ **For something** different at breakfast, try a multi whole-grain hot cereal that contains rye. Health food shops have the widest selection.

Related recipes

Hearty split pea soup with rye croutons 230
Smoked salmon canapés 204
Tuna and carrot sandwich on rye 228

PERFECT PORTION: 30g

A serving works out at one slice but rye bread is healthy enough to allow yourself two for a sandwich.

seeds

GL very low

Like nuts, seeds have recnetly emerged as nutritional superstars. Packed with protein, 'good' fat and fibre, they're just what the doctor ordered for levelling your blood sugar, whether you add them to dishes or eat them between meals as snacks.

Although seeds are indeed high in fat – about 12–14g in a 30g serving – almost all of that fat is the heart-healthy monounsaturated and polyunsaturated kinds. Another advantage is that seeds pack plenty of protein, to the tune of 4–9g in 30g. For the same weight, you'll also get up to 10g of fibre (pumpkin seeds have the most).

Break open that packet of sesame seeds and sprinkle them on. When you do, you may also lower your cholesterol. Seeds are rich in the natural plant compounds called sterols, which are proven cholesterol busters. (Sterols derived from other sources are even added to some cholesterol-lowering margarines.)

One recent study found that when people with high levels of 'bad' LDL cholesterol ate about 40g of sesame seeds a day for four weeks as part of an already heart-healthy diet, their LDL levels dropped by almost 10 per cent more than when they followed the same diet without sesame seeds. Not surprisingly, their LDL levels went back up after they stopped eating the sesame seeds.

Researchers in another study tested 27 varieties of nuts and seeds and found that sesame seeds had the highest sterol content. Sunflower seeds also ranked high in sterols. So be sure to make sesame and sunflower seeds a regular part of your diet.

PERFECT PORTION: 30g

A typical serving is **1 tablespoonful,** *which contains* **175kcal.**

How to roast SEEDS PERFECTLY

You can make your own roasted seeds once you've eaten your fill of squash, pumpkin or watermelon. Here's how.

Separate the seeds from the flesh and strings, wash them well, and let them dry. Then mix them in a bowl with a small amount of vegetable oil and salt. Spread them in a single layer on an ungreased baking sheet and sprinkle on some seasonings (take your pick of cumin, celery salt, cinnamon, paprika or chilli powder). Place the baking sheet in a preheated oven at 150°C/gas mark 2 for about 45 minutes, shaking the seeds from time to time to prevent burning.

Health bonus

By weight, both pumpkin and sesame seeds have more iron than liver does. And a tablespoon of sesame seeds has almost as much calcium as a glass of milk. Sunflower seeds serve up selenium, a mineral that's been linked to a lower risk of both heart disease and cancer. Most seeds are also great sources of vitamin E. Sunflower seeds, for example, provide most of the day's needs for vitamin E, a nutrient that helps to protect against everything from cataracts to cancer. Seeds are also good sources of immune-boosting zinc.

Pumpkin seeds are a traditional home remedy for prostate enlargement, and research suggests there may be good reason. Their zinc, vitamin E, selenium and sterol content probably all help towards this end. The nutrients in seeds may even protect against prostate cancers.

(continues on page 144)

Magic fats

Olive oil

Avocado

The 'good' FATS

in these foods are essential to Magic eating. They steady blood sugar and may even boost insulin sensitivity.

- avocados
- nuts
- peanut butter
- flaxseeds (linseeds)
- olive oil
- seeds

Nuts

Peanut butter

seeds continued

Smart substitution
Instead of crisps: when you crave a crunchy, salty snack, reach for a handful of roasted and seasoned seeds. Your blood sugar and your arteries will thank you.

Cooks' tips
Seeds can go rancid if you store them too long. To keep them fresh for several months, store them in an airtight container away from heat.

A note of caution: although peanut allergies are better known, reactions to sesame seeds are among the fastest-growing allergies. They are still relatively rare, but if you notice a rash, swelling or trouble breathing after eating the seeds, you may be allergic.

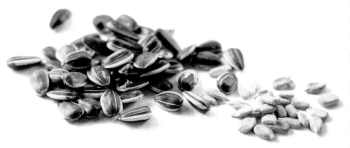

Menu magic
■ **Add seeds to** steamed or sautéed vegetables.

■ **Sprinkle sesame** seeds over brown rice.

■ **Coat thin fish** fillets or chicken cutlets with a mixture of crushed sunflower and pumpkin seeds, then pan fry.

■ **Chop pumpkin** or sunflower seeds and add to hot or cold cereal.

■ **Add toasted sesame** seeds to minced meat for meatballs. They add crunch as well as boosting the nutrition in your meal.

■ **Toss some sesame** seeds into bread dough, cake mixes or pancake batter. You can also add them to pastry.

■ **Spread tahini** (ground sesame paste) on toasted whole-grain bread.

■ **Top off your favourite** salad greens with pumpkin seeds.

■ **Add sunflower seed** kernels to tuna salad.

■ **Blend sunflower seeds** into scrambled eggs or a vegetable omelette.

■ **Sprinkle your favourite** seeds on top of tomato, carrot or squash soup.

■ **Add sesame seeds** to fruit salad for crunch.

Related recipes
Creamy coleslaw without mayonnaise 220
Oven-fried chicken 249
Quinoa with chillies and coriander 278
Salmon sandwiches with wasabi
   mayonnaise 226
Sautéed Brussels sprouts with red pepper
   and caraway seeds 284
Sautéed spinach with ginger and soy sauce 287
Spinach, grapefruit & avocado salad
   with poppy seed dressing 224

shellfish

GL very low

When it comes to

Magic eating, fish are fabulous. It's not just food with fins that benefit your blood sugar; prawns, lobster, crabs and clams all count, too. They're rich in protein and low in calories, which undoubtedly qualifies them as Magic foods.

Prawns and lobster are almost completely devoid of saturated fat, and they provide useful amounts of omega-3 fats. These are the same heart-smart fats found in oil-rich fish and renowned for their ability to reduce the risk of heart disease, a goal that's at the top of the list for anyone with diabetes. It's true these crustaceans are relatively high in cholesterol, but as we explained in the eggs entry (page 106), it's saturated fat, more than dietary cholesterol, that raises levels of cholesterol in the body. An average serving of shellfish has about a third the cholesterol found in one egg, so moderate consumption generally isn't a problem. In fact, shellfish helps to protect against heart disease.

Lobster, the upper crust of the crustacean world, happens to be a particularly rich source of a little-known mineral called vanadium, which some studies suggest may enhance insulin's effect in the body, helping to keep an anchor on blood sugar. (In human studies at Harvard's Joslin Diabetes Center, vanadium improved insulin sensitivity and lowered cholesterol, too. In another study, at Temple University in Philadelphia, vanadium supplements were shown to lower blood sugar.)

Despite how rich it tastes, lobster is low in fat – as long as you don't plunge it into a pool of melted butter. It's lower in fat than beef, pork and even chicken.

Health bonus

Most shellfish are rich in copper and zinc, both important for your immune system to function at its peak. They also pack an astounding amount of vitamin B_{12}, which may help to ward off depression, heart disease and even Alzheimer's. And they're super sources of selenium, an anti-cancer mineral.

Clams also contain sterols, the beneficial cholesterol-lowering compounds we've mentioned elsewhere.

Cooks' tips

Clams, oysters, mussels and scallops should be alive when you buy them. That means the shells will be tightly closed or should close when you tap them. You can store them in the fridge in a container covered loosely with a damp cloth, but don't store them in water. The shells will open during cooking (discard any that don't). Steam for 4–9 minutes or boil for 3–5 minutes after the shells open.

Eating shellfish raw (think oysters on the half shell) or less than well done is risky business. They may harbour bacteria, viruses and parasites, all of which are killed by cooking.

Many large supermarkets now carry large bags of frozen prawns, so stock your freezer. Thaw them according to package directions and you have the makings of a fast, high-protein meal, such as stir-fried prawns.

Menu magic

Keep it simple. Too often, shellfish are battered and deep fried or served in a creamy sauce. A generous squeeze of lemon juice (another Magic food) will usually suffice, especially if you don't overcook the shellfish (which makes them dry).

PERFECT PORTION: 85g

If shellfish are part of your main meal of the day, up to 170g is an appropriate serving.

shellfish continued

■ **Serve cooked prawns** with a low-fat cocktail sauce as a healthy party appetiser.

■ **Use prawns in** stir fries instead of chicken or beef. Add the prawns during the last 5 minutes to avoid overcooking them.

■ **Add cooked prawns,** clams or mussels to your favourite pasta sauce.

■ **Chop some cooked** prawns and sprinkle over a green salad to add low-fat protein. Use a lemony dressing.

■ **Make crab salad** by mixing crabmeat (tinned is fine) with vinaigrette dressing. Serve over mixed lettuce leaves and cucumber.

■ **Top pizza with** minced cooked clams.

■ **Place a cooked** large prawn, some small chunks of avocado and tomato, and a bit of salsa onto a lettuce leaf. Roll it up and eat.

■ **Toss some prawns,** scallops if you have them, and even fish chunks with olive oil and lemon juice, skewer them, pop them on the grill, and you're ready to eat in 5 minutes.

■ **Put together** prawn tacos by combining prawns, lettuce, tomato, a bit of shredded cheese and green salsa in a corn taco shell.

■ **Instead of creamy,** high-fat clam sauce like you'd get at a restaurant, make linguini with clams using tinned clams (minced), garlic, olive oil, chopped hot peppers and chopped tomatoes.

Related recipes

Prawn and orzo casserole 260
Prawn and scallop stew 259

Shellfish by the **NUMBERS**

Because shellfish are virtually devoid of carbohydrates, their GL is virtually zero. All shellfish are low in saturated fat, but different types offer slightly different nutritional advantages, as you'll see below.

SHELLFISH (100g)	CALORIES (kcal)	PROTEIN (g)	TOTAL FAT (g)	CHOLESTEROL (mg)	VITAMINS AND MINERALS
Clams	77	16	0.6	67	Contains useful amounts of iron and potassium.
Crab (white meat)	77	18	0.5	72	Good source of copper, zinc and selenium.
Lobster	103	22	1.6	110	Excellent source of vitamin B_{12}. Good source of zinc.
Mussels	104	17	2.7	58	Contains useful amounts of iron.
Oysters	65	11	1.3	57	Contains iron, zinc and selenium
Scallops	118	23	1.4	47	Good source of vitamin B_{12}.
Prawns	76	17	0.6	195	Fair source of various vitamins and minerals and omega-3 fatty acids.

sourdough bread

GL low

This is one white bread that won't adversely affect your blood sugar. Even though it's made from white flour (typically a no-no for Magic eating), sourdough bread has a relatively mild effect on blood sugar compared to other types of white bread.

Sourdough is an ancient type of bread with thousands of years of bread-making history behind it. It has a distinctive taste, the result of lactic acid produced by bacteria used to ferment the dough. A sourdough 'starter' is made from a combination of yeast and bacteria growing in a paste of flour and water. Some is used for making a loaf, and the rest is saved to grow and use in future baking.

It's the acid produced by the bacterial culture that makes a poor blood-sugar choice into a better one. One small Swedish study involving 12 healthy people found that when the volunteers ate a breakfast that included bread with added lactic acid in an amount found in sourdough bread, the rise in their blood sugar was 27 per cent less after $1\frac{1}{2}$ hours than it was when they ate the same breakfast but with a bread made with a combination of whole-grain flour and processed white flour.

Health bonus

One study using sourdough bread made with specific strains of bacteria found that it could reduce gluten intolerance in people sensitive to wheat gluten. While that doesn't mean that people diagnosed with gluten intolerance can eat sourdough bread with impunity, it does suggest that the bread is more easily digested than other breads made with wheat flour.

Cooks' tips

You can either make your own sourdough bread using a sourdough starter or buy a loaf at the local bakery. Note that all rye breads made with whole-grain rye are by nature sourdough. (For bread to rise, yeast reacts with the gluten in the wheat. Rye doesn't contain enough gluten to rise with yeast, so the sourdough starter is used to achieve the same effect.)

Some breads are called sour breads because they have sour flavouring agents added. While it's possible that they could have a beneficial effect on blood sugar (say, if the souring agent is vinegar), they haven't been studied in the same depth that sourdough bread has.

Menu magic

Sourdough bread has a distinctive sharp taste, but you can use it whenever you might use regular bread. Try it for sandwiches and hamburgers and as a crunchy accompaniment to any type of soup.

Related recipe

Grilled aubergine sandwiches
with red pepper and walnut sauce 227

PERFECT PORTION: 30g

A serving is about the size of ONE small slice, depending on the brand. Eat two slices, as you would in a sandwich, and the bread becomes a medium-GL food – still reasonable.

soya foods

If you've already turned to this entry, it probably means you've already discovered soya foods and want to know more about their health benefits. At the very least it means you have an open mind and are willing to try them. That's good news – because soya is so beneficial.

For a start soya has more protein, by volume, than beef and almost none of the saturated fat. This immediately earns it a secure spot on the list of Magic foods. Soya beans have an extraordinarily low GL of 1, which means that foods made from them (*see* 'Soya glossary' below) should be in your Magic diet.

Studies suggest that soya may have special power that helps to lower blood sugar, beyond its low glycaemic load. In a recent study involving overweight people who regularly consumed meal-replacement drinks, those using soya-based drinks lost slightly more weight than those using milk-based drinks. The participants on soya milk also saw their blood sugar levels drop (the milk-drinking group didn't). This result may be thanks to the type of protein in soya. When Swedish researchers fed study subjects meals containing protein from fish (cod), milk (cottage cheese) and soya, they discovered that the soya-protein meal was the friendliest to blood sugar.

Like many other foods, soya beans are best enjoyed in their most unadulterated forms. Products such as soya protein bars and flavoured soya milk often contain far too much added sugar or fat to be considered as healthy eating.

Health bonus

Soya is good for your heart. Its cholesterol-lowering powers may not be quite as strong as was once thought, but soya is still good for overall heart health thanks to its 'good' fats, its fibre and its cholesterol-lowering plant sterols.

Eating soya can also help to reduce the risk of a serious diabetes complication: kidney disease. In a study of people with Type 2 diabetes and kidney disease, those who took a third of their protein as soya protein saw their urinary albumin excretion (UAE) drop by 9.5 per cent, a sure sign that their kidneys were functioning better.

Population studies suggest that soya can lower the risk of several kinds of cancer, including prostate, breast and endometrial

SOYA glossary

Soya is a bean, but out of that bean come many different products.

■ **Edamame:** fresh green soya beans, available shelled or in the pod. You can eat them raw, but most people prefer them steamed with a bit of salt. You don't eat the pods.

■ **Mature soya beans:** you can buy these canned. Just rinse them before adding to casseroles, soups or chilli.

■ **Soya nuts:** roasted mature soya beans, usually eaten as a snack.

■ **Tofu:** as one manufacturer put it, tofu is to the soya bean as cheese is to milk. Cheese is made when milk separates into curds and whey. Soya beans produce soya milk, which can also be separated into curds and whey; tofu is the bean curd. It comes in different textures, with silken tofu being the very softest and extra-firm the firmest.

■ **Tempeh:** made from fermented soya beans and formed into a chewy cake, tempeh is used as a meat substitute in recipes.

■ **Miso:** fermented soya bean paste, used as a seasoning or soup base.

■ **Soya milk:** the creamy liquid that's pressed out of soaked, cooked soya beans.

cancers, probably as a result of soya's oestrogen-like compounds, called isoflavones. More research is needed before any specific recommendations on soya intake can be made.

Cooks' tips

Keep tofu and tempeh refrigerated and use them within two or three days of opening. Opened tofu should be stored in water that is changed daily. Miso will last in the refrigerator for several months. Fresh edamame should be eaten within a day or two. Roasted soya nuts can be kept in a cool, dry place for up to six months.

Menu magic

Soya products are a mystery to many people, but once you get to know them, you'll find they're easy to use and quite handy.

EDAMAME

■ **Steam edamame** in their pods, then shell them. Add the beans to grain or vegetable salads.
■ **Keep a bag** of frozen edamame in the freezer and steam some for a high-protein Magic snack.

SOYA NUTS

■ **Snack on these** or sprinkle them into stir fries. They have less fat and more fibre than true nuts (but they're still high in calories, so watch your portion size).

SOYA BURGERS

■ **Crumble and add them** to pasta sauces in place of meat.

SILKEN TOFU

■ **Stir into low-fat** sour cream for vegetable dip.
■ **Replace all** or some of the cream in cream soups with silken tofu.
■ **Blend silken** tofu with banana and peaches and a touch of honey to make a delicious protein-rich smoothie.

TOFU

■ **Marinate tofu** in low-sugar barbecue sauce and cook it on the grill.
■ **Mash it with** cottage cheese and seasonings to use as a spread on whole grain rye crackers.
■ **Use extra-firm** tofu instead of beef in stews.
■ **For Asian stir-fry** dishes, use extra-firm tofu with red bell pepper strips, carrot strips and snow peas.
■ **Make a tofu** salad with cubes of firm tofu stir-fried in rapeseed oil. Add to Romaine lettuce, corn, sliced avocado, sliced tomatoes and chopped coriander leaves. Top with roasted pumpkin seeds and a squeeze of lime juice.
■ **Create a tofu** curry with stir-fried tofu, red bell pepper strips, chickpeas, vegetable oil, curry powder (it contains turmeric, a Magic spice) and sesame seeds. Serve over brown rice.

SOYA MILK

■ **If you like** soya milk, use it in place of regular milk in smoothies, on cereal and in recipes. Buy the low-fat, unsweetened variety.

Related recipes

PERFECT PORTION: 125g tofu

If you're eating raw *soya beans, a serving is* 60g *shelled. For* dry-roasted *soya beans, which are higher in calories, a serving is* 40g.

spinach and other dark greens

GL very low If everyone ate more spinach, it's probable that far fewer people would suffer from diabetes, not to mention diseases such as heart disease and cancer. Spinach doesn't have any particular power to lower your blood sugar. Its virtue stems from the fact that it's a vegetable and like almost all vegetables, it has little impact on your blood sugar. We already know that the more fruits and vegetables we eat, the lower the risk of being overweight and of developing diabetes. It's that simple (remember secret number 3 of Magic eating: 'Eat more fruits and vegetables). Spinach is an all-round good-for-you food, packed with nutrients and low in calories. This makes it a must for a Magic diet.

Despite what Popeye may have thought, spinach is not a very good source of iron. That's because the iron it contains isn't absorbed very well by the body. But spinach is full of other nutrients that can help to stave off or treat just about every health concern, especially if you have diabetes or any of the risk factors for it.

Because spinach contains a lot of potassium and magnesium, it (and other dark greens) can help to keep blood pressure in check. Thanks to its store of carotenoids, it's one of the most antioxidant-rich vegetables on Earth. These antioxidants are powerful weapons against diabetes-related complications, including heart disease and nerve damage, not to mention cancer.

Spinach is a surprisingly good source of the antioxidant vitamin C. Just 50g of raw leaves (enough for a good-sized salad) provides a third of your recommended daily allowance for just 14kcal. With such a small calorie count, spinach can help to lower the overall calories of any dish you add it to.

Health bonus

Spinach-eaters may also be protecting themselves against cancer. Several studies have found that people who eat a lot of green, leafy vegetables, including spinach, have a lower risk of developing cancer than people who eat little.

Researchers have identified at least a dozen antioxidant compounds in spinach that may have anti-cancer activity. Lutein and beta-carotene are two at the top of the list. Known as carotenoids, they've been linked time and again with a reduced risk of several kinds of cancer, including colon and prostate cancers, lower risk of heart disease and better eye health.

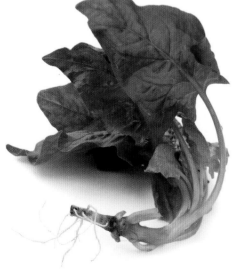

The more fruit and vegetables you eat, the lower your risk of being overweight or developing diabetes, so save room for spinach on your plate.

Spinach and other dark green leafy vegetables such as kale are also some of the richest sources of lutein, which research shows may help to protect against cataracts and age-related macular degeneration, two conditions most likely to rob you of your sight as you age. Another fact to consider: a single serving of spinach offers a full day's supply of vitamin K, which researchers now know is needed for a strong skeleton.

Are you having too many 'senior moments'? Eat more spinach. Some US studies found that feeding middle-aged rats a spinach extract prevented some of the loss of long-term memory and learning ability that rats normally experience. Researchers attribute this to the antioxidant compounds in spinach – and it may work for humans, too.

Cooks' tips

Wash fresh spinach thoroughly with cold water – twice. In addition to washing off any bacteria that may be lurking in the leaves, you want to get rid of the dirt that can make spinach gritty. If you buy bagged spinach leaves to save time, it's still a good idea to rinse them well before eating. Remove the stems, at least the larger, thicker ones, before cooking.

Menu magic

Look for any and every opportunity to consume dark green leafy vegetables, from spinach salad to these ideas.

■ **For a super-nutritious** side dish, sauté spinach (Swiss chard or kale works well, too) and sliced onions in olive oil. Sprinkle with sesame seeds, another Magic food.

■ **Stir steamed spinach** into mashed potatoes so you get less potato and a lower GL with every bite. Top with sliced spring onions.

■ **Top pizza** with spinach.

■ **Steam spinach,** then purée with parsley and a squirt of lemon juice and use as a sauce for chicken or pasta.

■ **Make spinach pesto.** Purée raw spinach with almonds, garlic, olive oil and a bit of Parmesan cheese, then toss with whole grain pasta and chickpeas.

■ **'Beef' up lasagna** with spinach instead of minced meat.

■ **Serve spinach** with garlic and olive oil over pasta cooked *al dente*. Sprinkle with sesame seeds.

■ **For a quick** soup, purée steamed spinach with garlic and low-fat plain yoghurt.

Related recipes

Barley-bean soup 229
Cauliflower and spinach gratin 282
Dahl with spinach 272
Greek lentil salad 223
Macaroni cheese with spinach 264
Penne with asparagus, ricotta and lemon 264
Plaice florentine 255
Quick spinach and sausage lasagne 267
Salmon sandwiches with wasabi
    mayonnaise 226
Sautéed spinach with ginger and soy sauce 287
Spinach and goat's cheese omelette 194
Spinach, grapefruit & avocado salad
    with poppy seed dressing 224
Spinach with pine nuts and currants 286
Tuna and cannellini salad with lemon 218
Turkey and pasta bake with spinach 251
Wholemeal pasta with sausage, beans
    and greens 266

PERFECT PORTION: 80g (cooked)

Because spinach shrinks so much, the raw leaves for one serving will start off filling a cereal bowl. *But since spinach is so good for you and so low in calories, the* more the better. *Pile your plate.*

sweet potatoes

GL medium

These sweet-tasting potatoes are surprisingly healthy. If you eat a baked sweet potato instead of a baked white potato, your blood sugar will rise about 30 per cent less. Compared to standard white potatoes, sweet potatoes rank relatively low on the GL scale. And the fact that they're packed with nutrients and disease-fighting fibre (almost 40 per cent of which is soluble fibre, the kind that helps to lower blood sugar and cholesterol) makes them an eminently healthy and also a delicious choice.

Sweet potatoes are extraordinarily rich in carotenoids, orange and yellow pigments that play a role in helping the body to respond to insulin. And, as unlikely as it may seem, coffee (another Magic food) and sweet potatoes have something in common: they're both rich in the natural plant compound chlorogenic acid, which may help to reduce insulin resistance.

You may not think of vitamin C when you think of sweet potatoes, but they're actually an excellent source. That's important when you're battling high blood sugar, because the vitamin's antioxidant powers may help to protect arteries from damage. Vitamin C may also help to fight heart disease and complications of diabetes, such as nerve and eye damage.

Health bonus

A recent study found that among almost 2,000 men studied, those whose diets were richest in beta-carotene and vitamin C – two nutrients plentiful in sweet potatoes – were more likely to survive prostate cancer than those whose diets contained little of the two nutrients. The respected Nurses' Health Study at Harvard Medical School found that women who ate lots of foods rich in beta-carotene, such as sweet potatoes, reduced their risk of breast cancer by as much as 25 per cent.

Eating sweet potatoes is a smart move for you if you have high blood pressure. That's because they're rich in potassium, a mineral known for bringing blood pressure down. You'll get more potassium from a sweet potato than you will from a banana.

And YAMS?

Is there a difference between sweet potatoes and yams? You bet. What you see in the supermarket is most likely one of two popular varieties of sweet potato. One has orange flesh and is moist and sweet; the other is yellow fleshed, drier, and not as sweet. Unless you're shopping at a market that specialises in ethnic foods, you're unlikely to find yams, which are native to Central America. Much larger than sweet potatoes, they have ivory-coloured flesh and aren't particularly sweet.

Sweet potatoes raise blood sugar about 30 per cent less than white potatoes do, thanks to their soluble fibre and plant compounds that help cells use insulin.

Cooks' tips

Choose sweet potatoes that are heavy for their size, with intact peels (no decay). If you're going to cook them whole, buy potatoes that are similar in size so the cooking time will be the same. Peel or scrub thoroughly before cooking. They'll keep for a month if you keep them cool but not cold (don't put them in the fridge).

Menu magic

Steer clear of tinned sweet potatoes. These processed sweets are usually packed in sugary starch. The fresh variety cook quickly enough in a steamer. Our suggestions show you just how versatile they can be. You'll soon be adding sweet potatoes to your weekly shopping list.

■ **Bake a sweet** potato just as you would a white potato and serve alongside your favourite protein dish (beef, chicken, fish, pork or lamb).

■ **If you're hooked** on regular mashed potatoes, try using half regular potatoes and half sweets.

■ **Top mashed sweet potatoes** with healthy, cholesterol-lowering margarine, season with cinnamon and sprinkle with chopped pecans.

■ **Grill sweet potato** slices to serve with pork loin chops.

■ **Place sweet potato** slices on top of your next casserole. Cover with foil to keep them moist and bake as usual.

■ **Add sweet potato** cubes to soups and stews 30 to 45 minutes before the dish is done.

■ **Cube cooked sweet** potatoes and use them in stir fries.

■ **Make roasted sweet** potatoes seasoned with thyme for a savoury side dish. Combine olive oil, minced garlic, thyme, salt and coarsely ground black pepper in a bowl. Arrange peeled, sliced sweet potatoes in a single layer on a baking sheet and brush with the mixture. Bake at 220°C until tender and slightly brown.

Related recipes

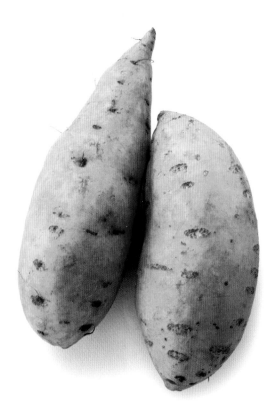

> **PERFECT PORTION: 1 medium**
>
> A *medium-sized* sweet potato (about *140g*) is big enough to satisfy your appetite without tipping the blood sugar scales.

tea

GL very low

Put the kettle on,

because after reading this entry, you'll be ready for a healthy cup of tea. Laboratory studies show that tea can boost insulin activity more than 15-fold. The research, carried out by the US Department of Agriculture, found that all types of tea – green, black and oolong – have the ability to enhance insulin activity, which of course means lower blood sugar. Almost all of that power comes from the antioxidant compound EGCG (epigallocatechin gallate) found naturally in tea.

Leave out the milk, though. Adding milk may decrease this insulin-activating power by as much as 90 per cent. It's not that milk is bad for you, it's just that it binds with the EGCG, making it unavailable to the body.

Drinking tea could even benefit people already being treated for diabetes. In a Taiwanese study of 20 people with Type 2 diabetes, all of whom were taking glucose-lowering medication, drinking a lot of oolong tea – about six 250ml glasses a day was linked with a 29 per cent drop in blood sugar. Most of us won't want to drink that much (tea has a diuretic effect), but even a cup or two should benefit you.

Some research suggests that tea may even speed up the body's metabolism and help to control weight, which by itself could lower your risk of insulin resistance and Type 2 diabetes. In a group of 10 healthy men, a green tea extract that provided the active compounds found in about 2 cups of green tea increased the number

DON'T fall for it …

Rumour has it that only green tea packs a big enough antioxidant punch to make a difference to your health. Not so. Tea is one of the most researched drinks around, and studies have found that while the exact types and amounts of antioxidant compounds vary from one tea type to the next, all types pack a healthy dose of these natural compounds.

of calories burned in a 24-hour period by 4 per cent. Another study found that people who drank tea at least once a week for more than 10 years had almost 20 per cent lower body fat than people who seldom drank tea, even after taking into account other lifestyle factors such as diet and exercise.

Want to make tea even better for your blood sugar? Brew a cup of chai, which combines tea with spices such as cinnamon, another Magic food. Watch out for the chai lattes you get at coffee shops like Starbucks, though. They're usually made with premixed liquids that include milk and are generously sweetened. Ask for a chai tea bag instead, and don't add anything (or just one packet of sugar, if you must).

If you're worried about your caffeine intake, you'll be pleased to know that a cup of tea has about half the caffeine of a cup of coffee.

Health bonus

Tea outranks even the best vegetables in terms of antioxidant power. Remember that antioxidants protect against everything from cancer to stroke to heart disease. In a controlled study, 15 men and women who drank five 180ml cups of black

---

PERFECT PORTION: unlimited

Tea has zero carbs and virtually no calories, so you can have **several cups** *a day as long as you* **don't add sugar.** *If you're sensitive to caffeine, just have one cup in the morning.*

(continues on page 156)

Magic leaves, herbs & spices

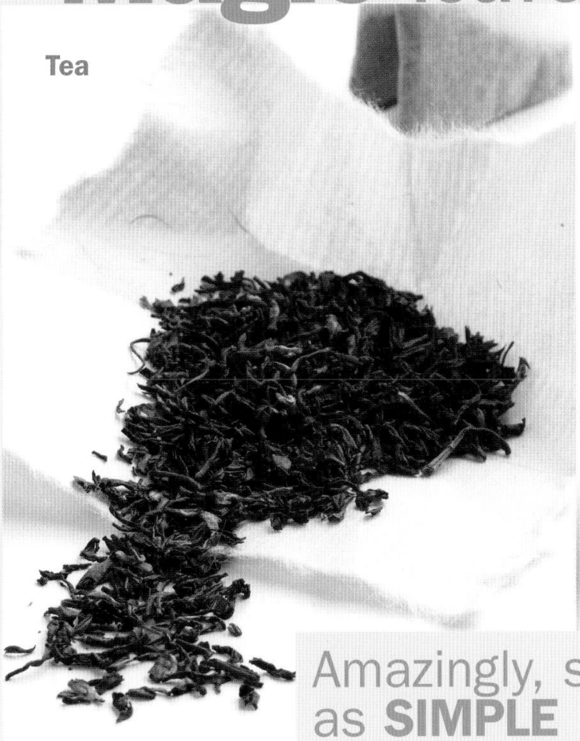

Tea

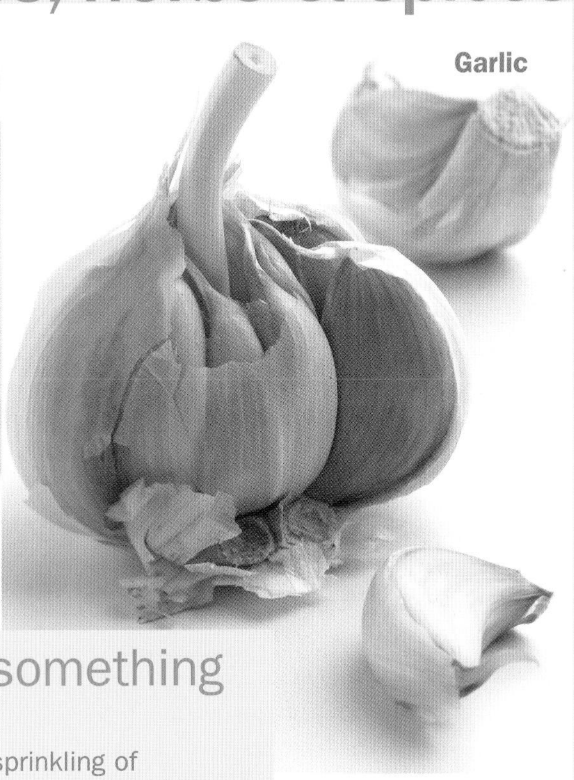

Garlic

Amazingly, something as **SIMPLE**

as a cup of tea or a sprinkling of cinnamon can help to keep your blood sugar in check.

- cinnamon
- coffee
- fenugreek
- garlic
- tea
- turmeric

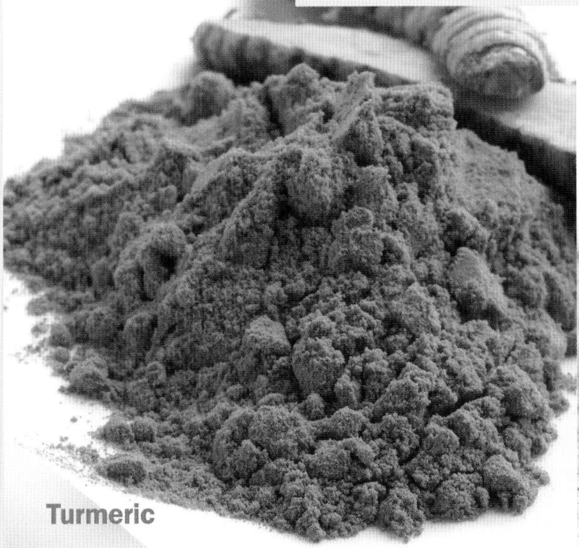

Turmeric

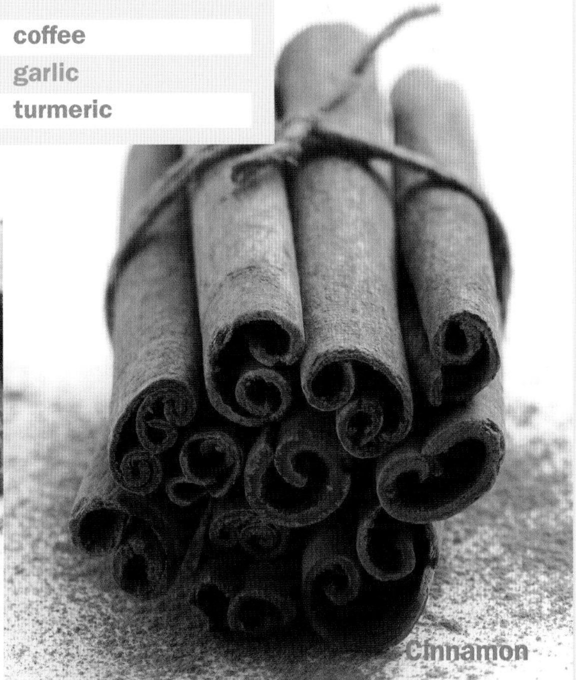

Cinnamon

tea a day for three weeks experienced an 11 per cent drop in 'bad' LDL cholesterol and a 6.5 per cent drop in total cholesterol. Again, that's a lot of tea, but it's likely that drinking even a cup or two a day offers some benefits. In another study, more moderate tea drinkers had a 28 per cent lower death rate after heart attacks than people who didn't drink tea.

Cooks' tips

You'll need to store tea properly if you want to keep the same subtle flavours that helped you to make it your choice in the first place. Always store tea, whether loose leaves or tea bags, in an airtight container away from light, moisture and strong odours, which the leaves may absorb.

Menu magic

While drinking a cup of hot tea is the obvious way to consume this Magic food, tea is actually a more versatile plant than you might imagine.

■ **Grind oolong** tea leaves in a pepper mill and blend them with freshly ground white pepper to sprinkle on chicken or pork.

■ **Tea also works** wonders in a marinade; just add ground leaves to the mixture.

■ **Add tea leaves** to chicken broth or stock for a dish with an Asian nuance.

Related recipes

Blueberry and melon compote with
  green tea and lime 288
Chai 210
Peachy iced tea 213

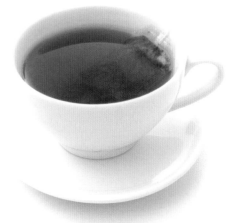

TEA glossary

True tea comes from the *Camellia sinensis* plant. Varieties are listed below. Herbal teas don't offer the same blood-sugar benefits.

■ **White tea:** it's picked and harvested before the leaf buds, which are covered with white fuzz, have opened. It's the least processed of the teas and has about half the amount of caffeine of black tea (about 15mg per cup).

■ **Green tea:** the leaves are picked, then dried, steamed or pan fried to keep enzymes in the tea from changing some of the antioxidant compounds and turning the tea dark.

■ **Oolong tea:** the leaves are dried for a longer time than for green tea, allowing the enzymes to work longer. Oolong is half-way between green and black tea in terms of processing.

■ **Black tea:** the leaves are processed longer to oxidise more of the compounds and produce a darker tea. Black tea contains the most caffeine (about 40mg per cup).

■ **Chai:** this isn't a result of processing but rather is tea (usually black) that's combined with spices such as cardamom, cinnamon, cloves and pepper.

tomatoes

GL very low This is a food that comes highly recommended. Tomatoes are terrific for your blood sugar. These juicy fruits are incredibly low in calories (a medium tomato has just 17kcal) and carbs (3g). What's more, they're rich in vitamin C, which helps to protect the body from blood sugar damage, and lycopene, a member of the carotenoid family along with beta-carotene.

Lycopene may be especially effective against diabetes. Researchers from the Centers for Disease Control and Prevention looked at 1,665 men and women with and without diabetes and found that those with impaired glucose tolerance (essentially, prediabetes) had blood levels of lycopene that were 6 per cent lower than those of healthy people. Levels averaged 17 per cent lower in people with newly diagnosed diabetes. Two other studies found similar connections.

Health bonus

A Harvard study found that men who ate tomatoes and tomato products such as tomato sauce and tomato paste at least twice a week lowered their risk of prostate cancer by 24 to 36 per cent. Studies also suggest that eating tomatoes may reduce your risk of osteoporosis and asthma and may improve circulation and reduce inflammation.

Cooks' tips

Store tomatoes on the counter; never keep them in the fridge. It ruins the texture and flavour.

Menu magic

The possibilities are virtually endless. Serve tomatoes raw, and you get the full vitamin C content (heat destroys the vitamin); serve them cooked with a little oil, and you get the maximum lycopene dose (the oil helps the body to absorb lycopene). Canned tomatoes, tomato sauce and tomato paste all count, too. Ketchup isn't such a good choice since it contains sugar, and while tomato juice is rich in lycopene, it's often loaded with salt.

■ **Include tomato wedges** or cherry tomatoes in green and pasta salads.
■ **Add tomato slices** to your sandwiches.
■ **Whip up fresh** tomato salsa.
■ **Marinate peeled tomatoes** in a mixture of olive oil, lemon juice, crushed garlic, salt, pepper and oregano and serve as a starter or side dish.
■ **Serve sliced tomatoes** with reduced-fat mozzarella, balsamic vinegar and olive oil as a snack or starter.
■ **Make a tomato** pizza on a wholemeal pitta. Brush the pitta with olive oil and top with sliced tomatoes and onions. Sprinkle with basil and grated Parmesan cheese and bake.

Related recipes

Caponata 201
Cherry tomatoes filled with creamy pesto
  cheese 203
Dahl with spinach 272
Garden pasta salad 223
Greek pasta and beef casserole 240
Lentil and bean chilli 273
Mediterranean salad with edamame 224
Penne with tomato and aubergine sauce 262
Prawn and orzo casserole 260
Seared fish steaks with tomato and
  olive sauce 256
Slow-cooker beef and red wine stew 238
Spiced cauliflower with peas 284
Turkey and bean chilli with avocado salsa 252

PERFECT PORTION: 1 medium

One juicy sliced tomato is a satisfying serving, but because tomatoes are so low in calories and carbs, feel free to have as many as you like.

turmeric

GL very low

Turmeric, the spice that gives mustard its bright yellow colour and curried dishes their warm glow, may help to tame wild blood sugar. That's because turmeric root, a relative of ginger, is one of Earth's most concentrated sources of curcumin, an antioxidant compound that's been shown to help to prevent blood sugar surges, at least in diabetic animals. (Cumin is another source of curcumin.) While turmeric the spice has not been well studied, researchers have set their sights on extracts containing curcumin, the active ingredient. One animal study, for example, found that 10mg of a turmeric extract lowered blood sugar levels by 37 per cent within 3 hours and by 55 per cent after 6 hours.

Exactly how curcumin works isn't known, but researchers point to a number of different possibilities. The main theory is that it acts on the pancreas to stimulate the release of insulin.

Curcumin also has very powerful antioxidant effects that could help to stave off heart disease as well as damage related to high blood sugar, including kidney disease, nerve damage and retinopathy (eye damage).

Health bonus

Turmeric has a long history as a folk medicine in India and other countries for treating stomach ailments, inflammation, arthritis and sprains. It's also being studied as an anti-cancer spice. Population studies find dramatically reduced rates of colon cancer in people whose diets are rich in curcumin. And in test-tube studies, curcumin has killed off cervical cancer cells and blocked harmful cell changes.

Most recently, researchers have begun to look at whether curcumin may help to prevent Alzheimer's disease. In India, where turmeric is widely used in cooking, there is a very low incidence of the disorder. In animal studies, curcumin decreased the formation of amyloid, the stuff that makes up the brain deposits characteristic of people with Alzheimer's. While the findings are promising, curcumin has not yet been studied for the treatment or prevention of Alzheimer's in humans.

Cooks' tips

Be careful to keep turmeric contained when you use it, because it will stain almost anything – your fingernails, plastic cups and utensils and even some kitchen worktops.

Menu magic

- **Purchase bright yellow** curry powder; it's likely to contain the most turmeric. Or you can add extra turmeric to your favourite brand of curry powder.
- **Use yellow mustard** on burgers and when cooking. Its colour comes from turmeric.
- **Add turmeric to** rice instead of saffron in paella and Spanish rice.
- **Include up to** a teaspoon of turmeric in your favourite pea soup recipe.
- **Add turmeric to** stews and casseroles.
- **A touch of turmeric** generally works very well in lentil dishes.

Related recipes

Crushed curried butternut squash 282
Spiced cauliflower with peas 284

PERFECT PORTION: 1/8 to 1/4 teaspoon

Most of the studies with turmeric have used curcumin extracts derived from turmeric, so it's hard to know exactly how much is beneficial. The best advice? Use turmeric **whenever you can.** *It adds deep colour and richness to dishes you won't get from anything else.*

vinegar

Fans of folk medicine swear by vinegar to treat just about anything that could ail a person, from sunburn to stomachache to dull hair. But there's one truly effective use for vinegar that most people don't know about. It turns out that simply adding a high-acid food like vinegar to your meals can reduce the blood sugar effect of the entire meal – by 19 to 55 per cent!

In one small Italian study, when five people consumed 1g of acetic acid (the equivalent of 1⅓ tablespoons of vinegar) and olive oil (sounds suspiciously like a vinaigrette salad dressing), followed by 50g of carbohydrates from white bread (the amount in about four small slices), their blood sugar went up 31 per cent less than when they ate just the bread.

In another study, from Arizona State University, healthy people consumed about 4 teaspoons of cider vinegar before eating a high-GI meal (a bagel, butter and orange juice), then repeated the exercise drinking water sweetened with saccharin before the meal. Their blood sugar was measured an hour after eating both meals and rose an average of 55 per cent less after the meal preceded by cider vinegar. In another study by the same researchers, people with insulin resistance who consumed vinegar before a bagel meal had a 34 per cent increase, on average, in insulin sensitivity, which of course translates to better blood sugar control.

Yet another study, this one from Japan, found that when vinegar was part of a meal, it reduced the glycaemic index of white rice by an impressive 20 to 40 per cent.

One reason for the dramatic findings: the acid in vinegar slows the rate at which food leaves your stomach, also slowing the transformation of a meal's carbohydrates into blood sugar. Animal studies also suggest the acid may help to increase the storage of glycogen (the form in which blood sugar is stored for future energy needs) in the liver and skeletal muscles, getting it out of the bloodstream.

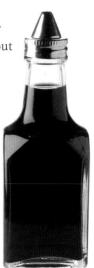

Health bonus

Some of the research showing that vinegar can lower blood sugar also shows that it can make you feel more satisfied after a meal – a boon to anyone trying to lose weight.

Cooks' tips

Don't limit yourself to plain old distilled vinegar. Try red or white wine vinegar, rice vinegar or apple cider vinegar. You can also buy flavour-infused vinegars such as tarragon, raspberry, strawberry and so on. See 'Enhance the flavour' on page 160 to learn how to make your own flavoured vinegar.

Menu magic

- **Start dinner with** a spinach salad dressed with balsamic vinegar and oil.
- **Add red wine** vinegar to lentil soup.
- **Mix up Asian** coleslaw with shredded red cabbage and carrots, mung bean sprouts, chopped bok choy, olive oil, rice vinegar, sesame seed oil, chopped coriander leaves and some toasted sesame seeds.
- **Make a balsamic** vinegar glaze for grilled salmon. In a saucepan, boil balsamic vinegar, red wine and a bit of honey until thick.

PERFECT PORTION: 3 to 4 teaspoons

Research suggests that making this much vinegar part of a meal can **significantly lower** *your blood sugar response to the meal.*

---

vinegar continued

- **Marinate chicken** in cider vinegar and rapeseed oil before baking or grilling.
- **Marinate sliced beetroot** in balsamic vinegar, rosemary, crushed garlic and herbes de Provence for about 20 minutes. Place the beetroot and marinade in a foil packet, seal tightly and grill until tender.
- **Serve soya-glazed** chicken. Sauté some chopped garlic and shallots in olive oil, then add chopped tomato, distilled vinegar, soya sauce, honey, salt and pepper. Stir well. Add cooked chicken breast and cook over medium-high heat, turning occasionally, until the vinegar mixture has thickened into a glaze.
- **Pickle some carrots.** In a medium saucepan mix 225ml distilled white vinegar, 2 tablespoons sugar, 1 teaspoon salt, pepper to taste and 150ml water. Bring to a boil, then remove from the heat and let cool slightly. Dice eight large carrots, place in sterile containers, and cover with the vinegar solution. Seal and refrigerate for 12 hours or overnight.
- **For dessert, serve** sliced strawberries splashed with balsamic vinegar and sprinkled with a few pinches of sugar.

Related recipes

Enhance the FLAVOUR

Here are basic instructions for making your own flavour-infused vinegar.

1 Use clean glass jars or bottles that are free of cracks or nicks and can be sealed.

2 Choose your flavouring and vinegar. White vinegar has a sharp, acidic taste and is good for delicately flavoured herbs. Wine and champagne vinegars work well with delicate herbs and lighter-flavoured fruits. Red wine vinegar has a bolder flavour and complements spices and strong herbs like rosemary.

3 In a saucepan, heat the vinegar to just below the boiling point (at least 88° to 90°C).

4 Place three or four sprigs of fresh herbs, 3 tablespoons of dried herbs, or the peel of one lemon or orange per 300ml of vinegar to be flavoured into the jar. For some herbs, you may want to 'bruise' the leaves or sprigs to release the flavours.

5 Pour the hot vinegar over the flavouring ingredient in the jar. Seal the jar and let stand undisturbed in a cool, dark place for three to four weeks.

6 Strain the vinegar through damp cheesecloth or a coffee filter until it's no longer cloudy, then pour it into a clean, dry glass jar.

Store all flavoured vinegars in a cool, dark place in an airtight glass jar. Flavoured vinegars will keep for three months in cool storage and for six to eight months in the fridge.

wheat berries

GL medium

Whole-grain foods are a cornerstone of this book. You may remember secret number 2 of Magic eating: 'Make three of your carb servings whole grains'. Well, you can't get any more 'whole grain' than wheat berries (also known as wheat kernels), which are the entire grain (or 'fruit') of the wheat plant, minus the hull. If you've read the bran and wheat-germ entries, you know how good those are for your blood sugar and your health in general. Wheat berries offer both in one package.

As mentioned earlier, people who eat at least three daily servings of whole-grain foods, like wheat berries, are much less likely to develop Type 2 diabetes.

It's no wonder. According to a British study, eating wheat berries resulted in significantly lower levels of blood sugar and insulin than eating the same amount of carbs from flour. A Swedish study had similar results when healthy volunteers ate either white bread or coarse wheat bread made with wheat berries.

If you've shopped for prepared salads lately, you may have noticed some made with wheat berries. They sometimes turn up in yoghurts, too. The berries have a nice, firm texture that requires some chewing, so they keep you from wolfing down your food. They're also more filling than other wheat products containing the same amount of carbohydrates, according to findings from Australia.

Health bonus

Large-scale studies have shown that eating whole-grain foods lowers the risk not only of diabetes but also of heart disease, stroke and several types of cancer.

Wheat berries supply minerals and other compounds that are lost when the grains are milled into white flour. Their germ portion is a rich source of cholesterol-lowering sterols.

Cooks' tips

As wheat berries take so long to cook (an hour or more, depending on whether you soak them first), you may want to cook extra, then store the surplus in a covered container in the refrigerator for up to two days or in the freezer for up to six months. If you have them to hand, it's easy to add them to salads, soups, pilafs and breads.

Menu magic

Wheat berries are most often enjoyed in salads featuring anything from cranberries and nuts to avocados and tomatoes. They can be served as side dishes or main dishes, warm or chilled. Here are a few other ideas for cooked wheat berries.

■ **Combine wheat berries** with avocado cubes and cherry tomatoes and toss with a vinaigrette.

■ **Mix them with** grilled peppers, place on a bed of lettuce and top with a vinaigrette.

■ **For a tasty** side dish, combine wheat berries with raisins, sliced almonds, chopped spring onions and curry powder.

■ **Use as a hot or** cold breakfast cereal, plain or with milk or soya milk and topped with a bit of brown sugar and a dash of cinnamon.

■ **Fold wheat berries** into bread dough or pancake batter.

■ **Combine them with** cooked lentils and season to taste.

■ **Use them in** Italian soups along with beans. They offer a nice textural contrast to the soft, creamy beans.

Related recipe

Wheat berry salad with dried apricots
    and mint 277

PERFECT PORTION: 60g cooked

There's no better way to get a whole grain into your diet.

wheat germ

GL very low

This food is another great example of good things that come in small packages. The germ (think of it as the grain's embryo) is the nutritional heart of the wheat kernel. Besides complex carbohydrates, it's packed with protein and sugar-stabilising, hunger-fighting 'good-for-you' fats as well as fibre, vitamins and minerals, including zinc, selenium and magnesium, which help the body to manage blood sugar.

Magnesium is a potential diabetes fighter. Harvard researchers studied the magnesium intakes of more than 127,000 men and women with no initial history of diabetes. After 18 years of follow-up research in women and 12 years in men, they found that people whose diets provided the most magnesium were about 34 per cent less likely to develop Type 2 diabetes than those whose diets provided the least.

Health bonus

Wheat germ is particularly rich in vitamin E – a powerful antioxidant that thwarts cell damage from free radicals, the rogue molecules that are suspected of playing a role in various chronic conditions such as heart disease, cataracts and Alzheimer's disease.

Like magnesium, diets rich in E may help to stave off diabetes. As part of the Insulin Resistance and Atherosclerosis Study, University of South Carolina researchers measured the levels of E in the blood of nearly 900 people without diabetes for five years. They found that among people who didn't take vitamin E

supplements, those with the highest blood levels of E were 88 per cent less likely to develop Type 2 diabetes than those with the lowest levels.

The 'good' fat in wheat germ, along with its cholesterol-lowering plant sterols, can also help to lower harmful (LDL) cholesterol.

Cooks' tips

Buy plain toasted wheat germ and steer clear of sweetened varieties. Once the packet has been opened, store it in the refrigerator to prevent the wheat germ from going rancid.

Menu magic

Wheat germ's crunchy texture and nutty flavour make it perfect for a variety of uses.

- **Add nutty crunch** to steamed vegetables and green salads with a sprinkling of wheat germ.
- **Sprinkle it on** porridge or cold cereal.
- **Top low-fat** yoghurt with a sprinkling of berries and wheat germ.
- **When coating chicken** or fish, skip the bread crumbs in favour of a mixture of wheat germ, grated Parmesan cheese and dried parsley.
- **Add wheat germ** to smoothies made with low-fat plain yoghurt and fruit.
- **Substitute wheat germ** for some of the meat in your favourite meat loaf or meatball recipe.
- **Add wheat germ** to muffins, pancakes, casseroles, pizza dough and savoury pastry.

Related recipes

Macaroni cheese with spinach 264
Multi-grain griddle cakes or waffles 192

PERFECT PORTION: 2 tablespoons

Wheat germ has a very low GL thanks to its fat and protein, but it does have calories (36kcal in 2 tablespoons), so portion size is important.

---

wholemeal bread and flour

GL medium

Some types of bread

– particularly refined white breads – are not particularly good for levelling your blood sugar. But if the bread is made with whole grains, there's every reason to eat it, as whole grains in your diet help you to reduce your risk of diabetes.

Whole grains also help to improve the body's sensitivity to insulin, the hormone that manages blood sugar. In one study of 978 men and women, the higher their intake of whole grains, the greater their insulin sensitivity, which translates into better blood-sugar control.

There's another reason to eat whole grains – your heart. Countless studies have confirmed that people who eat a lot of whole-grain foods cut their heart disease risk by anywhere from 15 to 30 per cent compared with people who eat only white bread (or avoid grains altogether). Chalk up wholemeal bread's heart benefits to its abundance of antioxidants, fibre and cholesterol-reducing plant sterols.

Want to lose weight? Switch to wholemeal. The Nurses' Health Study from the Harvard School of Public Health looked at more than 74,000 women and found that those who ate the most whole grains were a whopping 49 per cent less likely to gain weight over a 12-year period than those who ate the least. Why? Whole grains are filling, in large part because of their hefty fibre content (remember, fibre contains no calories, because it can't be digested). And, of course, they're gentler on your blood sugar than their refined-grain counterparts. Steadier blood sugar means steadier weight.

Blood sugar aside, wholemeal bread is better than white bread in other ways. It contains the germ of the wheat, where most of the nutrients are located (you may not know that wholemeal bread is a terrific source of antioxidants). The germ is stripped out to make white bread, as is the bran, where most of the fibre is found. To make sure the good stuff is still in your bread, read the label. See 'The whole truth about wholemeal' on page 164 to learn exactly what to look for.

Health bonus

Whole grains have surprising power to prevent certain cancers, including breast cancer and other hormone-related cancers, such as uterine and ovarian cancers. They are also thought to ward off gastrointestinal cancers, such as stomach and colorectal cancers. In fact, according to various studies, you can cut your overall risk of cancer by as much as 40 per cent by eating plenty of whole grains.

According to the American Institute for Cancer Research, for instance, when data from 40 recent studies on whole grains and cancer risk were combined and analysed, the risk of cancer was reduced by 34 per cent on average in people who ate a lot of whole grains compared to those who ate very little.

How can whole-grain bread help to prevent cancer? That depends on the cancer, but the ingredients at work probably include fibre, flavonoids (special types of antioxidants) and lignans, oestrogen-like compounds found in the bran and germ layers of the grain.

Probably thanks to their fibre, whole grains also help to prevent constipation as well as an intestinal disorder called diverticulitis.

PERFECT PORTION: 1 slice

One small slice of wholemeal bread provides about 70kcal. But be careful: some heftier slices have as many as 110kcal each.

wholemeal bread and flour continued

Cooks' tips

Since wholemeal flour contains more fat (it's the beneficial type) than white flour does, it's more perishable. Store it in an airtight container in the refrigerator or freezer.

You can usually replace up to half the white flour called for in recipes with wholemeal flour. But when making delicate baked goods like biscuits, opt for wholemeal pastry flour. It contains less gluten-forming protein than regular wholemeal flour and helps to ensure your biscuits do not end up dried out and crumbly.

Menu magic

■ **Use wholemeal** bread instead of refined white bread for sandwiches (when you're not using rye, pumpernickel or sourdough, which are all Magic foods, too).

■ **Make your pizza** with wholemeal dough.

■ **If you're using** croutons for soups or salads, make them wholemeal. The same goes for breadcrumbs in cooking and baking. To make croutons, cube two slices of wholemeal bread and toss with 2 teaspoons olive oil, then spread in a small baking pan and bake at 180°C/gas mark 4 for 15 to 25 minutes until crisp.

■ **Use wholemeal** pittas as the base for quick, healthy lunches. Stuff with grated carrots and tuna or other good-for-you fillings, or top with grilled vegetables, tomato sauce and a little grated cheese for a fast pizza.

Related recipes

Apple bran muffins 198
Chicken pot pie with a wholemeal crust 248
Chocolate fudge brownies 294
Honey-mustard turkey burgers 252
Lemony blueberry cheesecake bars 291
Oven-fried chicken 249
Quick wholemeal pizza dough 268
Wholemeal flaxseed bread 196

The whole truth about **WHOLEMEAL**

Buying wholemeal bread is not as simple as picking up a brown loaf from the shelf. Brown bread is often made with a mixture of wholemeal and white flour. To get your hands on a Magic foods type of loaf, you need to look for the words wholemeal on the label. Ideally it should be the first item on the ingredients list. That also goes for any bread labelled as multigrain.

You may have seen new breads on the market called 'wholegrain white breads.' Even though they're wholemeal, they look like white bread because they're made from a special variety of wheat (albino wheat) that's lighter in colour, plus a host of 'dough conditioners' that keep the bread soft like white bread. These breads are more processed than regular wholemeal breads because the whole grains are pulverised into tiny bits by special machinery to make the bread smooth. We don't know what effect this has on the bread's GL, but it certainly doesn't help it.

yoghurt

Like milk, yoghurt has a naturally low GL (after all, yoghurt is nothing more than fermented milk). The unidentified natural component in milk that experts think may help to prevent insulin resistance is there in yoghurt, too. Since it's fermented by bacteria, yoghurt also contains acids, and you've already read that acids can help to lower blood sugar.

You can drink your yoghurt in a smoothie or eat it with fresh fruit. Another reason we like yoghurt: it's a perfectly acceptable lower-fat substitute for some or all of the mayonnaise in creamy salads and the sour cream in baked goods, soups and dips.

Compared to milk, yoghurt is usually more easily digested by people who are lactose intolerant. Even though yoghurt contains lactose, or milk sugar, the bacterial cultures used to make it produce the lactase enzyme required for proper digestion.

When it comes to yoghurt types, low fat and fat free are, of course, your best choices. Skip 'fruit on the bottom' brands, which are usually loaded with added sugar. You can always add your own fresh fruit.

Health bonus

A 150ml portion of yoghurt counts as one of the three servings of dairy produce that we're recommended to eat each day. And it is one of the dairy foods in a special US diet that has been shown to control high blood pressure.

Yoghurt contains 'good' bacteria, the kind that offer numerous health benefits, including boosting the immune system and alleviating diarrhoea caused by some infections or treatment with antibiotics. It relieves constipation and even reduces the risk of developing colon cancer. Some people like to eat yoghurt whenever they're taking antibiotics to replace the beneficial bacteria in the gut that the drugs obliterate. As far as yoghurt's immune benefits go, more than 70 per cent of the body's natural immune defences are located in the digestive tract. Building up the population of good bacteria there may boost production of important immune system compounds, making you more resistant to viruses.

There's also evidence that women who regularly eat yoghurt with live *Lactobacillus acidophilus* cultures get fewer yeast infections.

Only yoghurts labelled 'contains live, active cultures' have bacteria that are still active (unless they were pasteurised after the bacterial cultures were added, which destroys the bacteria; these yoghurts should be labelled 'heat-treated after culturing').

DON'T fall for it ...

Frozen yoghurt may seem like the next best thing to regular yoghurt, but it's not. First, almost all frozen yoghurt is sweetened and flavoured. While there are several low-fat and fat-free options, they're typically high in sugar. In addition, levels of beneficial bacteria vary greatly. Some brands are heat treated after the bacterial cultures are added, rendering the bacteria useless to your health. In others, the bacteria are added to an ice cream–like mixture after the heat treatment.

PERFECT PORTION: 150ml

*This amount will give you a **low glycaemic load** and a good deal of **calcium** at the same time.*

yoghurt continued

Cooks' tips

To get the most bacterial benefit from yoghurt, use it by the expiration date on the carton. The 'friendly' bacteria begin dying when the yoghurt is no longer fresh. Cooking destroys the beneficial bacteria, but the cooked yoghurt will remain a low-GL food.

Cooking with yoghurt on top of the stove can be tricky since it usually curdles when boiled. When adding it to hot dishes, it's best to stabilise it first by mixing in 1 teaspoon of corn starch for every 150ml of yoghurt. Add it towards the end of the cooking time.

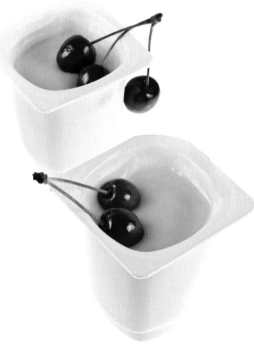

Menu magic

■ **Substitute yoghurt for** sour cream for use in baked goods.

■ **Make your favourite** dip using low-fat plain yoghurt instead of sour cream.

■ **Replace half the** mayonnaise in creamy salad dressings with yoghurt.

■ **Use yoghurt as a** restaurant-worthy garnish for puréed vegetable soups, such as a squash or carrot soup. Thin the yoghurt with low-fat milk until it is the same consistency as the soup. Drop spoonfuls of the mixture into the soup, then draw the tip of a knife through it to create swirls.

■ **Use a spoonful** on chilli instead of sour cream.

■ **Make cool, creamy** fruit 'soup' with low-fat plain yoghurt, sliced peaches, strawberries, orange juice and honey. Process in the blender, then garnish with fresh mint leaves.

■ **Serve a cucumber** salad made with grated cucumbers and carrots, diced onion, chopped dill and low-fat plain yoghurt.

■ **Top sliced fruit** with yoghurt or create a beautiful breakfast parfait. In a tall, chilled parfait glass, layer low-fat plain yoghurt with fresh blueberries and oat and nut muesli.

■ **Dip silces of Granny Smith apples** into yoghurt for a refreshing snack.

■ **Make a refreshing** yoghurt cooler (ayran, a traditional Turkish beverage) by combining equal parts yoghurt and cold water and a pinch of salt in a blender. Serve over crushed ice.

■ **To make yoghurt** creamier and richer tasting, make yoghurt 'cheese'. Spoon yoghurt into a cheesecloth-lined sieve, set over a bowl, and refrigerate for at least 6 hours or overnight. Discard the liquid (whey) that has accumulated in the bowl. Use the 'cheese' as a substitute for cream cheese or sour cream. Stir in chopped fresh herbs, spring onions, and garlic to make a delicious low-fat herby cheese spread.

Related recipes

Berry and flaxseed smoothie 212
Creamy coleslaw without mayonnaise 220
Dahl with spinach 272
Garden pasta salad 223
Instant strawberry frozen yoghurt 289
Nectarine, plum and mixed berry soup 289
Orange-glazed roasted plums 296
Porridge with apples and flaxseeds 192

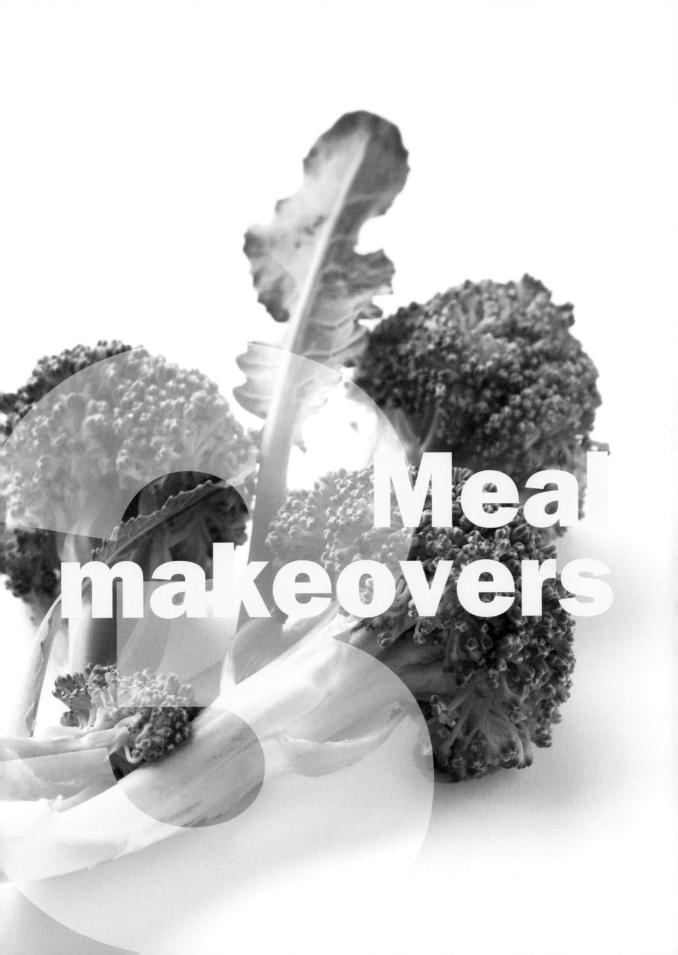

Meal makeovers

Breakfast makeovers

If your idea of breakfast is a Danish pastry, a bowl of cornflakes or a piece of toast and jam, help is here. Nothing sabotages your daily efforts to follow the Magic eating plan like a high-GL breakfast – the kind most of us eat. Breakfast is usually the most carbohydrate-filled meal of the day and therefore the one that raises your blood sugar the most dramatically. But you don't have to cut out all the carbohydrate. Just switching to 'slower-acting' carbs, and eating less of them, will do the trick. You should also try to find ways to add some protein to your plate.

Our top five breakfast guidelines:

1 **Limit carbohydrates to one serving** Have one slice of wholemeal bread instead of two of white and allow yourself 30g cereal (dry weight) instead of a huge bowlful.

2 **Choose lower-GL cereals** These usually include whole-grain cereals with at least 5g of fibre per serving (*see* 'How cereals rate' in the bran entry on page 85). Bran cereals such as All Bran and Bran Buds are good choices, along with high-fibre, high-protein cereals, such as Special K Sustain, and oat cereals, such as porridge or muesli.

3 **Cut out 'white' carbs** This means no Danish pastries or croissants, white toast with jam, or muffins made with white flour.

4 **Replace some carbohydrate calories** with fruit and a high-protein food. Sprinkle nuts and berries on your cereal, enjoy grapefruit along with a piece of toast, spread with peanut butter, or have a piece of fruit after your breakfast eggs. This will not only make the meal more filling, it will also lower its effect on your blood sugar.

5 **Use small glasses for juice** Fruit juice is fine for you – in moderation. Drink too much, and it quickly becomes a high-GL (and high-calorie) food.

In many ways breakfast really is the most important meal of the day. If you start the day with a Magic breakfast, you're more likely to stay off the blood sugar rollercoaster – and eat less – all day long.

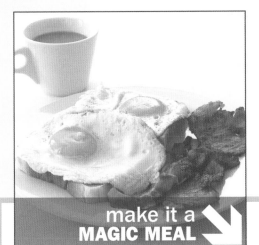

Typical weekend breakfast

2 slices of toasted white bread
   with 2 teaspoons of butter
2 fried rashers of streaky bacon
2 fried eggs cooked in 2 teaspoons of butter
1 cup white coffee (with whole milk)

TOTAL GL **HIGH**
TOTAL CALORIES **790kcal**

make it a
MAGIC MEAL

MAGIC brunch **1**

2 small slices toasted wholemeal bread
   with 1 teaspoon of polyunsaturated
   margarine
2 large eggs, scrambled
2 grilled rashers of lean back bacon
2 halves grilled tomatoes
30g cooked mushrooms
1 cup white coffee or tea (with low-fat milk)

The fixes

■ Substituted wholemeal bread for white
   bread to lower the GL.
■ Scrambled the eggs, instead of frying
   them, to decrease the fat.
■ Added Magic tomatoes and mushrooms
   to increase the bulk of the meal.
■ Substituted lean bacon for streaky bacon
   to reduce the saturated fat (which
   contributes to insulin resistance) and
   grilled, rather than fried it.
■ Replaced butter with polyunsaturated
   margarine and reduced the amount spread
   on the toast.

TOTAL GL: **MEDIUM**
TOTAL CALORIES: **500kcal**

Better still Swap wholemeal bread
   for rye bread.

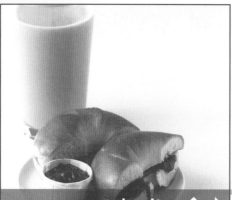

Typical breakfast

1 toasted large plain bagel with
  2 tablespoons jam
Large vanilla latte (350ml)

TOTAL GL **HIGH**
TOTAL CALORIES **500kcal**

**make it a
MAGIC MEAL**

MAGIC breakfast 2

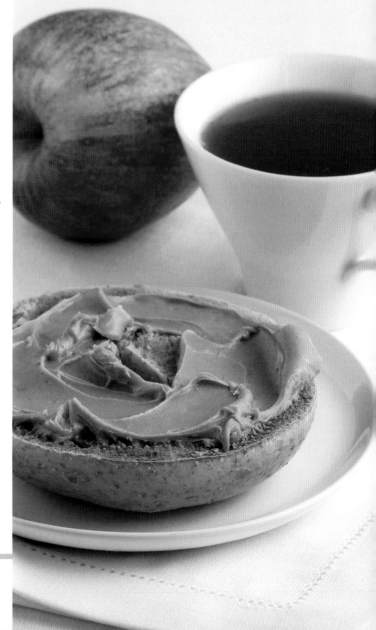

½ toasted large wholemeal bagel with
  1 tablespoon peanut butter
1 medium apple
1 cup coffee or tea

The fixes

- Substituted a wholemeal bagel for the white flour bagel for more fibre and a lower GL.
- Cut the bagel portion in half to limit carbs.
- Added peanut butter as a filling source of protein and 'good' fat to add back calories without increasing the GL.
- Replaced the high-calorie, high-GL coffee beverage with plain coffee or tea.

TOTAL GL: **MEDIUM**
TOTAL CALORIES: **256kcal**

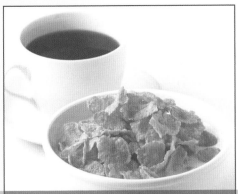

Typical breakfast

Large bowl (60g) cornflakes with
250ml semi-skimmed milk
1 cup coffee or tea

TOTAL GL **HIGH**
TOTAL CALORIES **340kcal**

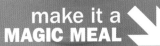

**make it a
MAGIC MEAL**

MAGIC breakfast 3

30g Bran Flakes with 80g strawberries,
2 teaspoons (14g) flaked almonds and
125ml skimmed milk
1 cup coffee or tea

The fixes
- Switched the high-GL cereal for a lower-GL
  cereal.
- Decreased the cereal serving to further
  cut the GL.
- Cut calories and fat by switching
  from semi-skimmed milk to skimmed milk.
- Added fruit and nuts to the cereal to make
  up for the smaller portion. The
  strawberries count as one of your 5-a-day
  servings and provide extra vitamins and
  phytochemicals. The nuts, with their
  healthy fats, slow the digestion of the
  meal for a slower rise in blood sugar.

TOTAL GL: **MEDIUM**
TOTAL CALORIES: **250kcal**

Better still *Go for All Bran cereal
instead of Bran Flakes.*

Lunch makeovers

Lunch can be a difficult meal because we often eat on the move, and healthy food can be harder to find when you're not at home. Regardless of where you eat lunch, though, you can make choices that will be gentler on your blood sugar.

Our top six lunch guidelines:

1 Make your lunch at home You'll have all the control you need over what you eat. If you do have to grab something from a fast-food restaurant or sandwich bar, we give some examples of smarter ordering.

2 Change your sandwich bread to whole-grain Choose rye or pumpernickel for the lowest possible GL. Wholemeal is also a good choice. If you do choose white bread, make it sourdough; its acids make its GL lower than that of other white breads.

3 Ask for mustard instead of mayonnaise Mustard might as well be a Magic food because of its vinegar and turmeric content. But mayonnaise ... well, it isn't.

4 Opt for fruit for dessert Try to eat one or more of your fruit servings for the day during the lunch hour (eat others between meals).

5 Select a nutritious salad Make sure it contains plenty of protein in the form of eggs, chicken, tuna, beans, tofu or low-fat cheese. And choose a Magic vinegar-based dressing, rather than a creamy one.

6 Skip the fizzy drink It has a sky-high GL unless you order a diet type or stick to 250ml – less than one can. Drink mineral water instead. If you prefer juice, look for one that's 100 per cent juice and unsweetened (too many have a lot of added sugar), and either stick to 180ml or less, or dilute the drink with sugar-free tonic or mineral water.

Finally, don't forget to have a snack between lunch and dinner to keep your blood sugar on an even keel. See our snack makeovers starting on page 178.

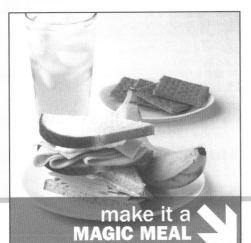

Typical lunch

2 slices white bread with 2 slices roast turkey,
  2 slices cheese, 1 tablespoon mayonnaise
1 medium banana
3 or 4 crackers
495ml apple juice

TOTAL GL HIGH
TOTAL CALORIES 891kcal

make it a MAGIC MEAL

MAGIC lunch 1

2 slices wholemeal bread with:
  2 slices roast turkey
  1 slice processed cheese
  Lettuce
  2 slices tomato
  1 tablespoon mustard
12 sweet cherries
30g dark chocolate-covered almonds
180ml unsweetened grapefruit juice

The fixes

- Swapped white bread for wholemeal to boost fibre and lower the GL.
- Cut approximately 60kcal by switching from mayonnaise to mustard.
- Exchanged the apple juice for grapefruit juice, which has a lower GL, and cut the quantity to reduce calories and further lower the GL.
- Swopped the banana for cherries. All stone fruits have lower GLs than bananas.
- Included dark chocolate-covered almonds instead of crackers. The almonds offer protein, 'good' fats, vitamins and fibre, while the crackers don't provide much in the way of nutrition and add significantly to the meal's GL.

TOTAL GL: MEDIUM
TOTAL CALORIES: 500kcal

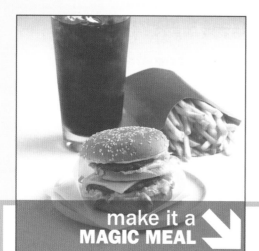

Typical lunch

Large cheeseburger
Large order of French fries
Large fizzy drink (525ml)

TOTAL GL **HIGH**
TOTAL CALORIES **1,175kcal**

make it a MAGIC MEAL ↘

MAGIC lunch 2

Medium hamburger
Yoghurt and fruit purée
Bottled water

The fixes

- Switched to the quarter pounder, which has less bread and more meat than the large cheeseburger. Ordered it without cheese to reduce the calories.
- Avoided chips and ordered yoghurt and fruit purée instead for fewer calories, less fat and more healthy nutrients.

TOTAL GL: **MEDIUM**
TOTAL CALORIES: **400kcal**

Better still: A small hamburger and a side salad with vinaigrette dressing.

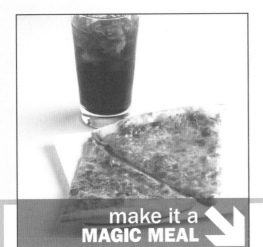

Typical lunch

2 slices cheese and tomato pizza (200g)
330ml fizzy drink

TOTAL GL HIGH
TOTAL CALORIES 690kcal

make it a
MAGIC MEAL ⬊

MAGIC lunch **3**

1 slice wholemeal pizza with cheese
and vegetables
1 portion of side salad with:
    lettuce, tomato and cucumber
    1 tablespoon oil-and-vinegar dressing
1 medium peach
1 can diet drink

The fixes

■ Cut carbohydrate, fat and calories by
limiting pizza to one slice.
■ Boosted fibre by switching to a wholemeal
base and adding vegetables.
■ Made up for the slice you're not eating by
adding a salad and a piece of fruit – both
nutritious, low-GL foods.

TOTAL GL: MEDIUM
TOTAL CALORIES: 366kcal

*Better still: Make your own pizza
at home by topping a wholemeal
pitta with 2 tablespoons tomato
sauce, 60g reduced-fat mozzarella,
and plenty of veggies.*

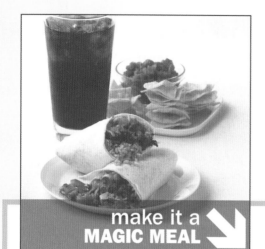

Typical lunch

1 large soft-flour tortilla or wrap, with
   60g minced beef filling
   30g Cheddar cheese,
   2 tablespoons salsa
45g tortilla chips
330ml cola
TOTAL GL HIGH
TOTAL CALORIES 800kcal

make it a MAGIC MEAL ⬊

MAGIC lunch 4

1 wholemeal tortilla with 42g roast chicken,
   2 tablespoons red kidney beans,
   15g Cheddar cheese and plenty of
   lettuce, tomato and salsa
½ mango
Bottled water

The fixes

- Cut carbs and lowered the GL by switching from a large white flour tortilla to a more reasonably sized wholemeal tortilla.
- Increased the fibre and lowered the GL by teaming lean chicken with red kidney beans.
- Added fruit instead of tortilla chips. These are an 'empty-calorie' food, whereas fruit is packed with fibre and vitamins, not to mention having a low GL.

TOTAL GL: MEDIUM
TOTAL CALORIES: 400kcal

Better still: *Replace the chicken with reduced-fat hummus and replace the full-fat Cheddar with reduced-fat cheese.*

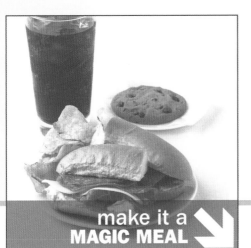

Typical lunch

1 large white roll filled with 4 slices salami,
   1 slice of processed cheese
   1 tablespoon mayonnaise
50g packet of potato crisps
1 large chocolate chip cookie
330ml cola

TOTAL GL HIGH
TOTAL CALORIES 980kcal

make it a MAGIC MEAL ⬊

MAGIC lunch 5

1 large wholemeal roll with:
   2 slices lean roast beef
   2 slices of processed cheese
   Green salad dressed with 1 tablespoon
   oil and vinegar dressing
1 medium apple
Mineral water with lemon

The fixes

- Switched to a large wholemeal roll,
  which has more fibre and is more filling.
- Substituted leaner meat for salami which
  is high in saturated fat, reduced the
  quantity of meat and 'beefed up'
  the sandwich with a generous helping
  of green salad.
- Replaced the crisps and chocolate chip
  cookie with fruit, for much less fat, fewer
  calories and more healthy nutrients.

TOTAL GL: MEDIUM
TOTAL CALORIES: 428kcal

Better still Enjoy a chef's salad
with lean cold cuts, cheese and
veggies.

Snack makeovers

It's 3pm and your energy is dipping. You want to raid the biscuit tin or grab a chocolate bar. The good news: snacking is allowed because it keeps your blood sugar steady. The bad news: biscuits and confectionery are the worst snack choices.

Our top three snacking guidelines:

1 **Pack your snack if you take a packed lunch** It's easy enough to grab some carrot or celery sticks, some grapes or grape tomatoes, a container of yoghurt, or some nuts, and put them in your lunchbox.

2 **Stay away from crisps and go easy on biscuits** which are usually packed with unhealthy starch, bad fats and sugar.

3 **Seek out protein** Nuts, seeds and yoghurt or a slice of lower-fat cheese are good snack sources.

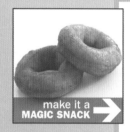

make it a
MAGIC SNACK ➡

2 cinnamon doughnuts

TOTAL GL: **HIGH**
TOTAL CALORIES: **484kcal**

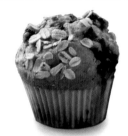

1 medium blueberry oat muffin
(*recipe on page 199*)

TOTAL GL: **MEDIUM**
TOTAL CALORIES: **170kcal**

The fixes
- Fat and saturated fat are decreased because this snack is baked, rather than fried.
- The fibre is increased and GL decreased by using ingredients such as oats and dried fruit.

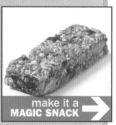

make it a
MAGIC SNACK ➡

1 fruit & nut cereal bar

TOTAL GL: **MEDIUM**
TOTAL CALORIES: **200kcal**

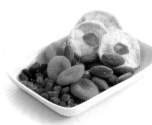

Dried fruit
10 almonds, 4 dried apricots,
3 dried apple rings, 15 sultanas

TOTAL GL: **LOW**
TOTAL CALORIES: **150kcal**

The fixes
- Reduced the saturated fat by including Magic almonds and no other fat source.
- Increased the fibre and minerals by adding more dried fruit than is in the cereal bar.

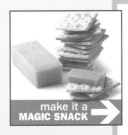

make it a
MAGIC SNACK →

15 plain salted crackers
85g Cheddar cheese

TOTAL GL: **HIGH**
TOTAL CALORIES: **527kcal**

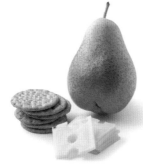

6 wholemeal crackers
30g Swiss cheese,
1 small pear

The fixes

- Switched to wholemeal crackers and cut the portion by more than half to decrease the GL.
- Limited the cheese to decrease saturated fat. Cheese is indeed a Magic food, but you need to eat it in moderation.
- Added a piece of fruit to replace some calories. Because of its fibre and water, the pear will fill you up more than the crackers.

TOTAL GL: **MEDIUM**
TOTAL CALORIES: **300kcal**

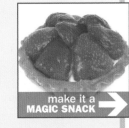

make it a
MAGIC SNACK →

1 rich strawberry tart
TOTAL GL: **MEDIUM**
TOTAL CALORIES:
175kcal

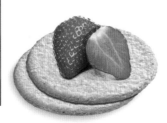

2 oatcakes topped with slices of strawberry

The fixes

- Swapped rich, custard-filled strawberry tart, packed with added sugar and 'bad' fats, for 2 high-fibre oatcakes to help you feel full, while lowering the GL and reducing the fat content.
- Added slices of Magic fresh strawberries to satisfy your sweet tooth without sending your blood sugar soaring.

TOTAL GL: **LOW**
TOTAL CALORIES: **130kcal**

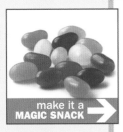

make it a
MAGIC SNACK →

14 jelly beans
TOTAL GL: **MEDIUM**
TOTAL CALORIES:
150kcal

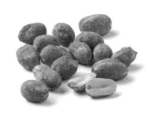

15 dry-roasted peanuts

The fix

- Slashed the GL to almost nothing by substituting peanuts, which are satisfying and full of protein, fibre and healthy fat. Jelly beans contain nothing but blood sugar-raising sugar.

TOTAL GL: **LOW**
TOTAL CALORIES: **90kcal**

Dinner makeovers

In many households, dinner time can be quite chaotic. You're tired, people are hungry and you just want to get something onto the table fast. The good news is that you can make your dinner more Magic without spending any extra time making the meal.

Our top five dinner guidelines:

1 **Limit yourself to one or two servings of carbohydrates** The sort of carbohydrates we mean here are pasta, potatoes, rice or stuffing.

2 **Fill the space on your plate with vegetables** This is your best opportunity for meeting your vegetable quota for the day. Even if you're having a salad on the side, put at least two types of veggies, such as sautéed carrots or green beans, on your plate. Use frozen vegetables and prewashed, bagged salad leaves if you're short of time.

3 **Cut out the bread** Bread isn't bad for you, but if you had a sandwich for lunch, that's probably all the bread you need for the day. Adding bread to dinner means you may not eat other, healthier foods. It almost always adds butter to your meal and certainly increases the GL.

4 **Keep your protein lean** Eat lean minced beef and lean cuts of meat, and chicken without the skin instead of fried chicken. Tofu, beans, fish and prawns are also good protein sources.

5 **Drink water rather than soft drinks** A glass of wine is also fine unless your doctor forbids it, but fizzy drinks and juice add calories and GL without adding much (or any) nutrition. Most of us don't drink enough water throughout the day and come home feeling wilted. Make it a habit to drink a cold glassful at dinner to rehydrate.

Dish the food up onto plates instead of placing a serving dish on the table for everyone to help themselves. You're likely to eat less. A final tip: after dinner (or dessert, if you have it), shut the kitchen door – firmly. For many people, late-night eating is a prime reason for consuming too many calories in a day.

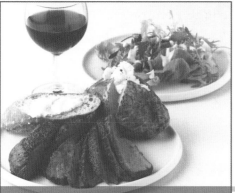

Typical dinner

200g grilled prime sirloin steak
1 medium baked potato with 1 tablespoon butter
Side salad with 1 tablespoon mayonnaise
1 slice French bread with 1 tablespoon butter
125ml red wine

TOTAL GL **HIGH**
TOTAL CALORIES **1,052kcal**

**make it a
MAGIC MEAL**

MAGIC dinner 1

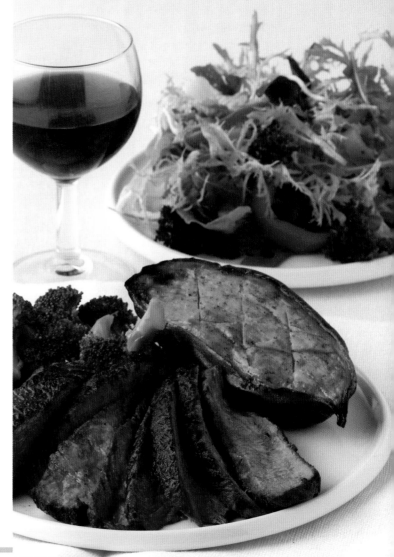

150g grilled prime sirloin steak
½ baked medium sweet potato with:
  1 teaspoon polyunsaturated margarine,
  cinnamon and nutmeg
80g steamed broccoli
Large salad with:
  roasted red and yellow peppers and
  1 tablespoon oil-and-vinegar dressing
125ml red wine

The fixes

- Replaced the white potato with half a
  sweet potato to dramatically decrease the
  GL. Eat the skin for added fibre.
- Doubled the salad size. Salad is filling and
  full of low-GL nutrition.
- Changed the mayonnaise dressing to oil
  and vinegar to decrease unhealthy
  saturated fat and provide extra acidity,
  which lowers the meal's GL.
- Replaced the bread with broccoli to add
  vitamins and fibre and lower the GL.

TOTAL GL: **LOW**
TOTAL CALORIES: **600kcal**

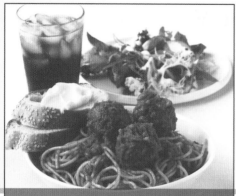

Typical dinner

Large serving spaghetti (270g) with
    200ml tomato sauce, 4 (100g) meatballs
1 bowl of salad with cucumber, tomato and
    1 tablespoon mayonnaise
2 slices of ciabatta
250ml fizzy drink
TOTAL GL HIGH
TOTAL CALORIES 1,000kcal

make it a
MAGIC MEAL

MAGIC dinner 2

Medium serving wholemeal spaghetti (150g)
    with 100ml tomato sauce
    4 (100g) meatballs, made with extra lean
    mince
Large bowl of salad with:
    tomato, cucumber, olives and red onion
    and 1 tablespoon oil-and-vinegar dressing
250ml sugar-free fizzy drink

The fixes

- Reduced the spaghetti portion and
  switched to wholemeal spaghetti to
  add fibre and lower the GL.
- Eliminated the bread and doubled the size
  of the salad (just as filling as bread), thus
  swapping empty calories for fibre and
  vitamins and lowering the GL.
- Topped the salad with oil-and-vinegar
  dressing instead of mayonnaise to reduce
  the saturated fat and add a dose of sugar-
  lowering acid from the vinegar.

TOTAL GL: MEDIUM
TOTAL CALORIES: 590kcal

Better still *To reduce the fat*
further, use minced turkey or
chicken instead of minced beef

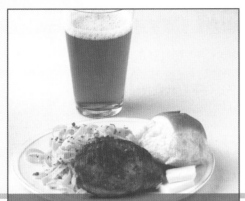

Typical dinner

125g pork chop
250g cooked fettucine with 1 tablespoon butter,
   1 tablespoon Parmesan cheese plus
   1 tablespoon chopped parsley
1 white roll with 1 tablespoon butter
340ml beer
TOTAL GL **HIGH**
TOTAL CALORIES **938kcal**

make it a
MAGIC MEAL ⬇

MAGIC dinner 3

125g pork chop
250g Bulghur wheat with ginger and orange
   (recipe on page 275)
Sautéed spinach with ginger and soy sauce
   (recipe on page 287)
340ml alcohol-free/low alcohol beer

The fixes

■ Swapped the fettucine for a better
carbohydrate choice, bulghur wheat.
Pasta's not bad for you, but bulghur has
more fibre and a lower GL.

■ Eliminated the white roll, which adds
nothing but GL to the meal.

■ Added sautéed spinach to replace the roll.
Spinach is loaded with fibre and nutrients
and has a very low GL (and far fewer
calories than a bread roll).

■ Changed the regular beer to alcohol-
free/low alcohol beer to reduce
carbohydrates and calories.

TOTAL GL: **MEDIUM**
TOTAL CALORIES: **571kcal**

Better still Substitute mineral
water for the beer.

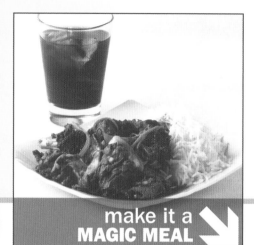

Typical dinner

300g beef and broccoli stir-fry (either take away
   or ready meal)
Large portion (180g) white rice
250ml fizzy drink

TOTAL GL HIGH
TOTAL CALORIES 633kcal

make it a
MAGIC MEAL

MAGIC dinner 4

100g unshelled edamame
1 serving Orange beef stir-fry with broccoli
   and red pepper (*recipe on page 234*)
Small portion (100g) brown rice
Black or green tea

The fixes

- Made the stir-fry at home using leaner
  beef, less oil and more vegetables. The
  result: fewer calories and less saturated
  fat, which clogs arteries and hampers
  insulin sensitivity.
- Substituted brown rice for white and
  cut the portion in half to dramatically
  decrease the meal's GL.
- Started the meal with edamame (steamed
  green soybeans) to fill you up on a low-GL,
  high-fibre, protein-rich food so you won't
  miss the rest of the rice. Edamame also
  slows eating because it takes time to get
  the beans out of their shells.
- Replaced high-GL fizzy drink with no-GL
  black or green tea.

TOTAL GL: MEDIUM
TOTAL CALORIES: 371kcal

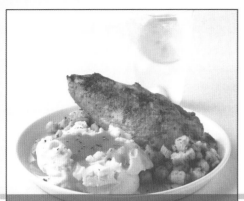

make it a
MAGIC MEAL

Typical dinner

1 roasted chicken breast with skin
Large serving (220g) mashed potatoes
100g stuffing
125ml gravy
Mineral water with lemon

TOTAL GL **HIGH**
TOTAL CALORIES **700kcal**

MAGIC dinner **5**

1 roasted chicken breast without skin
100ml gravy
50g apple and walnut stuffing
1 serving Moroccan spiced carrots
   (recipe on page 274)
Mineral water with lemon

The fixes

■ Took off the chicken skin, a significant
   source of saturated fat (which hampers
   insulin sensitivity) and calories.
■ Cut out the un-Magic mashed potatoes
   and replaced them with carrots to
   increase fibre and vitamins and
   substantially lower the GL of the meal.
■ Added apples and walnuts to the stuffing
   to decrease the GL (more apples and
   walnuts mean less bread) while adding
   some 'good' fat from the nuts to further
   lower the GL.

TOTAL GL: **MEDIUM**
TOTAL CALORIES: **414kcal**

Dessert makeovers

Everyone likes dessert – but nowhere else do the evils of white flour, sugar and saturated fat converge in such a perfect storm, making your blood sugar surge. In terms of glycaemic load and extra calories, most desserts are the last thing you need. But that doesn't mean dessert in general is off-limits. When the cake trolley comes around, don't say no; instead, say: 'I'll take half a slice please, with lots of berries on top.'

Our top four dessert guidelines:

1 **Think fruit, fruit, fruit** It's sweet and refreshing and easily transformed into an almost endless variety of attractive, easy-to-make desserts (for proof, look at the dessert recipes in Part 4).

2 **Watch portion sizes** The truth is, you can eat whatever you like if the portion is small enough. Use a small plate, such as a saucer, or a child-size cereal bowl, for ice cream to make smaller portions look more substantial. Or, to make your dessert fill up a big plate or bowl, add fruit such as pineapple, blueberries or banana.

3 **Hunt for whole grains** Most baked goods are made with white flour, but they don't have to be. In fact, many of our dessert recipes in Part 4 cut down the amount of white flour in favour of blood sugar-friendly oats, wholemeal flour and so on.

4 **Opt for low fat** Whether it's the ice cream you buy or the cream cheese you put in your cheesecake, make sure it's a low–fat type to avoid the nasty saturated fats that hamper your body's ability to handle blood sugar.

Finally, think of dessert as a treat – not a daily habit. Indulge twice a week to keep your sweet tooth happy. The rest of the week, why not top off dinner with an evening stroll instead?

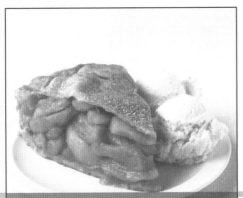

Typical dessert

1 slice apple pie plus
2 scoops (120g) ice cream

TOTAL GL **HIGH**
TOTAL CALORIES **480kcal**

**make it a
MAGIC MEAL**

MAGIC dessert **1**

1 serving Maple-walnut baked apples with
ice cream *(recipe on page 296)*

The fixes

- Kept the apple but got rid of the pastry
  and the extra sugar used for the filling.
  Both of these ingredients are responsible
  for increasing the GL of this dessert
  (plus, the pastry is high in calories and
  full of saturated fat).
- Added walnuts for protein and 'good' fat
  to fill you up and further lower the
  dessert's GL.
- Cut the ice cream down to one small
  scoop and switched to low-fat ice cream
  to reduce the saturated fat.

TOTAL GL: **MEDIUM**
TOTAL CALORIES: **214kcal**

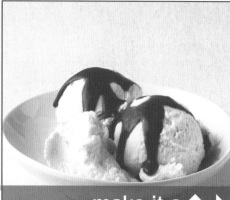

Typical dessert

2 scoops (120g) vanilla ice cream topped with
5 tablespoons hot fudge sauce

TOTAL GL **HIGH**
TOTAL CALORIES **500kcal**

make it a
MAGIC MEAL ↘

MAGIC dessert **2**

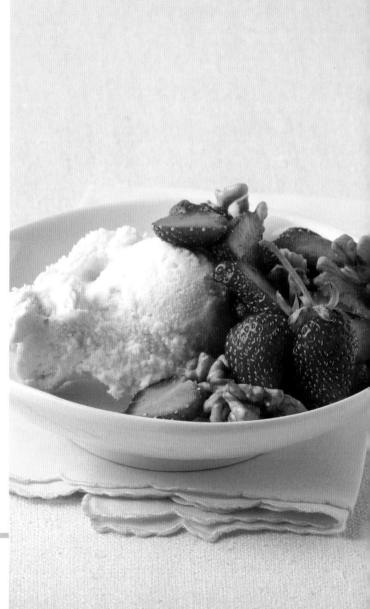

1 scoop (60g) vanilla ice cream with
80g strawberries
5 walnut halves

The fixes
■ Decreased the portion of ice cream as it
has a lot of sugar and a high GL, not to
mention saturated fat, which hampers
insulin sensitivity.
■ Scrapped the sugar-laden hot fudge, along
with its glycaemic load.
■ Added walnuts and strawberries to fill up
the bowl and provide fibre, nutrients and
healthy fats (from the walnuts) to help
improve insulin sensitivity.

TOTAL GL: **MEDIUM**
TOTAL CALORIES: **265kcal**

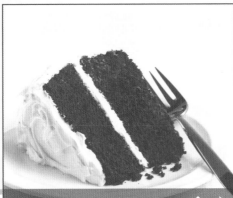

Typical dessert

1 large piece of chocolate cake (100g)
  with butter cream

TOTAL GL **HIGH**
TOTAL CALORIES **481kcal**

make it a
MAGIC MEAL

MAGIC dessert **3**

1 small piece chocolate cake (50g) dusted
  with confectioner's sugar
80g mixed blueberries and raspberries

The fixes
■ Decreased the portion size of the cake to
  cut refined carbohydrates and therefore
  the GL.
■ Eliminated the icing, which has a high GL.
■ Added berries to increase the nutritional
  value of the dessert and make the
  smaller portion of cake more satisfying.

TOTAL GL: **MEDIUM**
TOTAL CALORIES: **250kcal**

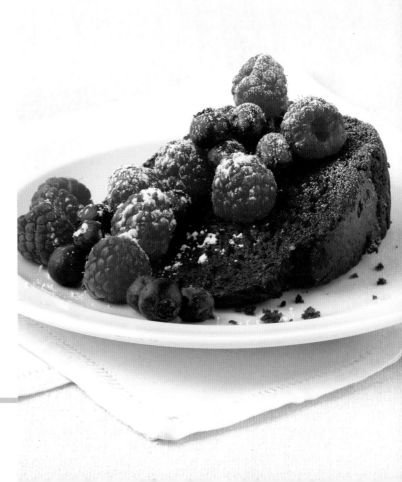

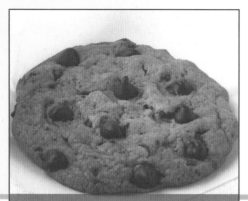

Typical dessert

1 large chocolate chip cookie (40g)

TOTAL GL **HIGH-MEDIUM**
TOTAL CALORIES **190kcal**

make it a MAGIC MEAL

MAGIC dessert 4

1 Oat and peanut butter bar *(recipe on page 210)*

The fix
- Swapped the cookie, made with the triple evils of sugar, butter and white flour, for an even more delicious bar made with whole grains (full of fibre) and peanut butter (full of protein and 'good' fat) to lower the GL a little and to keep you fuller longer. The bar also provides extra nutrition from dried fruit.

TOTAL GL: **LOW-MEDIUM**
TOTAL CALORIES: **175kcal**

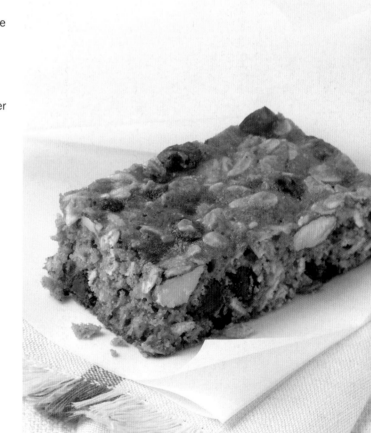

4

Magic recipes
and meal plans

Breakfasts

Porridge with apple and flaxseeds

serves 4

PREPARATION TIME: **5 MINUTES**

COOKING TIME: **10 MINUTES**

What better way to start your day than with a comforting bowl of steaming porridge? This simple breakfast packs not one or two but *six* Magic foods to steady your blood sugar and keep you feeling full until lunchtime.

500ml semi-skimmed **milk** or vanilla **soya milk**
60g rolled **oats**
1 medium **apple**, peeled, cored and chopped
50g dried cranberries or raisins
$1/2$ teaspoon ground **cinnamon**
40g whole **flaxseeds (linseeds)**, ground to a meal (*see* Tip, page 197)
4 tablespoons fat-free plain or vanilla **yoghurt**
4 tablespoons maple syrup, warmed, or
   2 tablespoons soft brown sugar

1 **Combine the milk,** rolled oats, apple, dried cranberries (or raisins) and cinnamon in a heavy medium saucepan. Bring to a simmer over a medium-high heat, stirring almost constantly.

2 **Reduce the heat** to medium-low and cook, stirring often, for 3–5 minutes or until creamy and thickened.

3 **Stir in the flaxseeds** Spoon the porridge into four individual bowls and top each serving with a dollop of yoghurt and a drizzle of maple syrup (or sprinkle of sugar). Any left-over porridge will keep, covered, in the refrigerator for up to 2 days. Reheat in the microwave.

PER SERVING: **282**kcal, **9g** protein, **19g** carbohydrate, **3g** fibre, **8g** total fat (**0.5g** saturated fat), **8mg** cholesterol, **0.15g** salt.

Multigrain griddle cakes or waffles

serves 8

PREPARATION TIME: **20 MINUTES**

COOKING TIME: **15–20 MINUTES**

Most griddle cakes, or Scotch pancakes, are anything but Magic, but here they have been entirely re-imagined. We've slashed the white flour and added wholemeal flour and oats, plus an unexpected dash of sugar-lowering cinnamon. Wheat germ provides healthy fats, extra fibre and deliciously nutty flavour.

500ml buttermilk (*see* Tip, page 199)
40g rolled **oats**
80g **wholemeal flour**
100g plain white flour
25g toasted **wheat germ**
$1^{1}/2$ teaspoons baking powder
$1/2$ teaspoon bicarbonate of soda
$1/4$ teaspoon salt
1 teaspoon ground **cinnamon**
2 medium **eggs**
50g soft brown sugar
1 tablespoon canola (rapeseed) oil
2 teaspoons pure vanilla extract
250ml maple syrup, warmed
225g mixed sliced **strawberries** and **blueberries**

1 **Mix the buttermilk** and oats in a small bowl. Leave to soak for 15 minutes.

2 **Whisk the wholemeal flour,** plain flour, wheat germ, baking powder, bicarbonate of soda, salt and cinnamon in a large bowl.

3 **Whisk the eggs** with the sugar, oil and vanilla extract in a medium bowl. Add the buttermilk mixture. Add this mixture to the flour mixture and combine with a rubber spatula just until the flour mixture is moistened.

4 **To cook the pancakes:** coat a large non-stick griddle or frying pan with cooking spray and heat over a medium heat. Spoon the batter into the pan (about 4 tablespoons for each pancake) and cook for 3 minutes or until the bases are golden and small bubbles start to form on top. Flip the pancakes and cook for a further 1–2 minutes or until they are browned on the other side and cooked through. (Adjust the heat as necessary for even browning.) Keep the pancakes warm in a very low oven while you finish cooking the remainder in the same way.

To cook the waffles: coat an electric or stovetop waffle iron with cooking spray and heat the iron. Spoon in enough of the batter to cover about three-quarters of the surface, then close the iron and cook for 4–5 minutes or until the waffle is crisp and golden brown. Keep the waffles warm in a very low oven while you finish cooking the remainder in the same way.

5 **Top with warm maple syrup** and mixed berries. One serving is two pancakes or waffles (depending on size). Wrap any left-over pancakes or waffles individually in cling film and refrigerate for up to 2 days, or freeze for up to a month. Reheat in a toaster or toaster oven.

PER SERVING: **274**kcal, **8g** protein, **50g** carbohydrate, **2.5g** fibre, **4.5g** total fat (**1g** saturated fat), **61mg** cholesterol, **0.7g** salt.

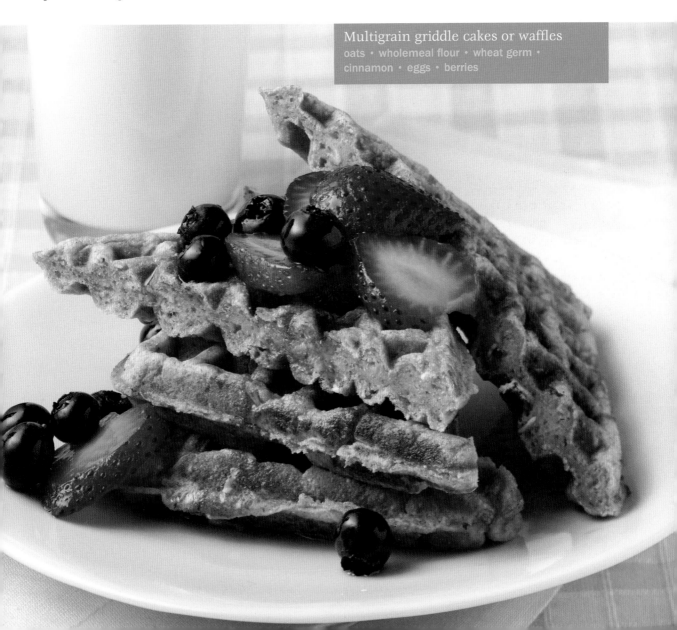

Multigrain griddle cakes or waffles
oats • wholemeal flour • wheat germ • cinnamon • eggs • berries

Spinach and goat's cheese omelette

serves	PREPARATION TIME: **10 MINUTES**
1	COOKING TIME: **2 MINUTES**

A French-style folded omelette is one of the easiest and fastest protein-rich meals you can make. It is also an excellent strategy for healthy solo dining. Omelette filling options are limitless. Try the variations given here or improvise with any cooked vegetables or other filling ingredients you have to hand.

200g baby **spinach** leaves, rinsed
2 tablespoons crumbled goat's **cheese**
    or feta cheese
1 tablespoon chopped **spring onion**
1 medium **egg**
2 medium **egg** whites
¼ teaspoon Tabasco sauce
Pinch of salt
Pinch of freshly ground black pepper
1 teaspoon **olive oil**

1 **Bring about 2.5cm** of water to the boil in a large saucepan. Drop in the spinach and cook for about 30 seconds or just until wilted. Drain,

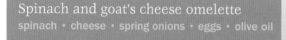

Spinach and goat's cheese omelette
spinach · cheese · spring onions · eggs · olive oil

pressing out the excess liquid, and chop coarsely. (Alternatively, if the spinach is ready-washed, microwave it, in its pierced plastic bag, for 1–2 minutes.) Place the spinach in a small bowl. Stir in the cheese and spring onion.

2 **Stir the egg,** egg whites, Tabasco, salt and pepper briskly with a fork in a medium bowl. Heat the oil in an 18–25cm non-stick omelette pan or frying pan over a medium-high heat. When hot, tilt the pan to swirl the oil over the surface. Pour in the egg mixture and stir with a heat-resistant rubber spatula or fork for a few seconds. Then use the spatula to push the cooked egg at the edges in towards the centre, tilting the pan to allow the uncooked egg mixture to fill the areas around the edges. Sprinkle the spinach mixture over the omelette and cook until almost set and the underside is golden. The entire cooking process should take about 1 minute.

3 **Use the spatula** to fold one-third of the omelette over the filling. Tip the pan and slide the omelette on to a plate so that it lands, folded in thirds, seam-side down. Serve hot.

PER SERVING: **285**kcal, **26g** protein, **4g** carbohydrate, **4.5g** fibre, **19g** total fat (**8g** saturated fat), **265mg** cholesterol, **2g** salt.

VARIATIONS
Mushroom omelette
Omit the spinach, goat's cheese and spring onion. In Step 1, heat 1 teaspoon olive oil in a medium non-stick pan over a medium-high heat. Add 35g sliced mushrooms. Cook for 3–4 minutes or until browned, stirring often. Stir in 1 tablespoon chopped parsley, a pinch of salt and pepper to taste. In Step 2, sprinkle the mushroom mixture over the omelette.

Broccoli and cheese omelette
Substitute 2 tablespoons chopped cooked broccoli and 2 tablespoons shredded Gruyère or Cheddar cheese for the spinach, goat's cheese and spring onion in the filling.

Courgette frittata

serves 2 PREPARATION TIME: **15 MINUTES**
COOKING TIME: **8–12 MINUTES**

Eggs are one of our favourite Magic foods because they're an inexpensive and remarkably complete source of protein that doesn't budge blood sugar a bit.

1 tablespoon **olive oil**
1 small **onion**, thinly sliced
1 small **courgette**, shredded
2 **garlic** cloves, finely chopped
4 medium **eggs**
½ teaspoon Tabasco sauce
Good pinch of salt, or to taste
Freshly ground black pepper to taste
50g Parmesan **cheese**, freshly grated
15g fresh basil leaves, chopped

1 **Heat 2 teaspoons oil** in a 25cm non-stick ovenproof frying pan over a medium heat. Add the onion and cook for 1½–2 minutes or until softened. Add the courgette and garlic and cook, stirring often, for 2–3 minutes or until the courgette is tender and most of the moisture has evaporated. Transfer to a plate and leave to cool slightly. Wash and dry the pan.

2 **Stir the eggs,** Tabasco, salt and pepper briskly with a fork in a medium bowl. Stir in the courgette mixture, Parmesan and basil.

3 **Preheat the grill.** Brush the remaining 1 teaspoon oil over the pan and heat over a medium-low heat. Pour in the egg mixture. Cook, lifting the edges with a heat-resistant rubber spatula and tilting the pan from time to time to allow the uncooked egg to flow underneath, for 3–4 minutes or until the underside is golden.

4 **Place the pan** under the grill and cook the frittata for 2–4 minutes or until the top is firm to the touch and set. Slide the frittata on to a plate and cut into wedges for serving.

PER SERVING: **355**kcal, **26g** protein, **5g** carbohydrate, **1g** fibre, **26g** total fat (**9g** saturated fat), **500mg** cholesterol, **1.1g** salt.

Wholemeal flaxseed bread

1 loaf

PREPARATION TIME: **20 MINUTES**
RISING/BAKING TIME (FOR FOOD PROCESSOR METHOD): **ABOUT 3 HOURS**

Many of the healthy-sounding multigrain and wholemeal breads on the supermarket shelves actually contain only a tiny proportion of whole grain. An enjoyable way to make sure you're getting at least 50 per cent wholegrain wholemeal flour in a loaf is to make your own. Flaxseed (linseed) is a Magic addition to this bread; it increases the amount of blood sugar-lowering soluble fibre and also contributes a delightful nutty taste. Note: Since bread machines can make loaves of different sizes, proportions are given here for both a small and a medium loaf.

FOR A 450–500G LOAF (8 SLICES):

160g **wholemeal bread flour**
80g white bread flour
3 tablespoons whole **flaxseeds**, ground to a meal (*see* Tip, opposite page)
2 tablespoons skimmed **milk** powder
1½ teaspoons easy-blend dried yeast
¾ teaspoon salt
180ml water, at room temperature
1 tablespoon molasses or clear honey
1 tablespoon **olive oil**

FOR A 675–750G LOAF (12 SLICES):

240g **wholemeal bread flour**
120g white bread flour
4 tablespoons whole **flaxseeds**, ground to a meal (*see* Tip, opposite page)
3 tablespoons skimmed **milk** powder
2 teaspoons easy-blend dried yeast
1 teaspoon salt
250ml water, at room temperature
2 tablespoons molasses or clear honey
1 tablespoon **olive oil**

TOPPING FOR FOOD PROCESSOR/OVEN METHOD

1 **egg** white, lightly beaten with 1 tablespoon water
1 tablespoon whole **flaxseeds**

To mix the dough and bake the bread in a bread machine:

Place all of the ingredients in a bread machine container in the order recommended by the manufacturer (do not place the yeast in direct contact with the liquids and salt). Select the wholemeal or basic cycle and medium crust, then press start. Once the dough is mixed, check the consistency; it should be smooth yet soft to the touch. Adjust if necessary by adding flour 1 tablespoon at a time or water 1 teaspoon at a time. When the bread has finished the baking cycle, transfer it to a rack to cool.

To mix the dough in a food processor and bake the bread in the oven:

1 **In a food processor** fitted with a metal chopping blade, combine the wholemeal flour, white bread flour, ground flaxseeds, milk powder, yeast and salt, and pulse several times to blend. In a measuring jug, stir together the water, molasses (or honey) and oil until the molasses is fully dissolved; set aside. With the motor running, slowly pour enough of the liquid through the hole in the lid to make a smooth dough that pulls away from the sides of the bowl. The consistency should be smooth yet soft to the touch; adjust if necessary by adding flour 1 tablespoon at a time or water 1 teaspoon at a time. Process for 1 minute to knead. Transfer the dough to a bowl coated with cooking spray and turn to coat. Cover with cling film and leave to rise at room temperature for 1½–1¾ hours or until doubled in bulk.

2 **Coat a baking tray** with cooking spray. When the dough has doubled, turn it out on to a lightly floured surface. Knock it back and shape into a round or oval loaf (or make two small loaves). Place the loaf on the baking tray. Coat a sheet of cling film with cooking spray and cover the loaf with it. Leave to rise for about 1 hour or until almost doubled in bulk.

3 **Meanwhile, place** a small metal baking tin on the bottom rack in the oven. Preheat the oven to 200°C/gas 6.

4 **When the loaf has risen,** brush it with the egg white mixture and sprinkle with the whole flaxseeds. Pour 250ml water into the baking tin in the oven to create steam. Use a serrated knife to score four 5mm deep slashes across the top of the loaf. Bake for 20–30 minutes or until the bread is golden and sounds hollow when tapped on the base. Transfer to a wire rack to cool. One serving is one slice.

PER SERVING: **152**kcal, **6g** protein, **22g** carbohydrate, **3g** fibre, **5g** total fat (**0.5g** saturated fat), **0mg** cholesterol, **0.5g** salt.

*Tip: **Grind flaxseeds to a coarse meal** using an electric spice mill, a clean coffee grinder or a blender. Flaxseeds need to be ground in order for your body to reap the full nutritional benefits.*

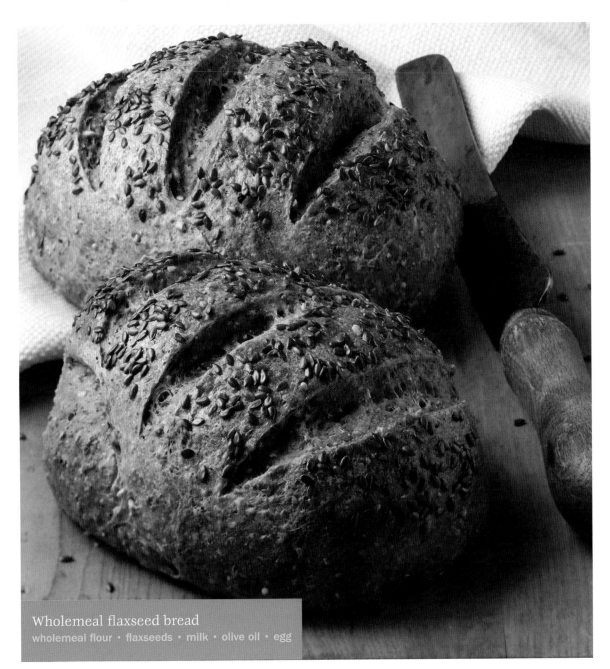

Wholemeal flaxseed bread
wholemeal flour · flaxseeds · milk · olive oil · egg

Apple bran muffins

12 muffins

PREPARATION TIME: **20 MINUTES**

BAKING TIME: **20 MINUTES**

Apple purée makes these low-fat, fibre-rich treats moist and tender. Bake a batch at the weekend, then wrap individually in cling film and freeze, to enjoy on busy weekday mornings.

2 medium **eggs**
100g soft light brown sugar
250ml unsweetened **apple** purée
180ml buttermilk (see Tip, next page)
60g natural **wheat bran**
3 tablespoons canola (rapeseed) oil
1 teaspoon pure vanilla extract
120g **wholemeal flour**
115g plain white flour
1½ teaspoons baking powder
½ teaspoon bicarbonate of soda
¼ teaspoon salt
2 teaspoons ground **cinnamon**
¼ teaspoon grated nutmeg
1 medium **apple**, peeled, cored and chopped
40g chopped **walnuts**

1 **Preheat the oven** to 200°C/gas 6. Coat a 12-hole muffin tray with cooking spray.

2 **In a medium bowl,** whisk together the eggs and brown sugar until smooth. Add the apple purée, buttermilk, bran, oil and vanilla extract, and whisk until blended.

3 **In a large bowl,** whisk the wholemeal flour and plain flour with the baking powder, bicarbonate of soda, salt, cinnamon and nutmeg. Add the egg and apple mixture and mix with a rubber spatula just until the dry ingredients are moistened. Fold in the chopped apple. Spoon the mixture into the muffin tray and sprinkle over the chopped walnuts.

4 **Bake for 18–22 minutes** or until the tops of the muffins spring back when touched lightly. Cool in the tray on a rack for 5 minutes, then loosen the edges of the muffins and turn out on to the rack. Allow to cool slightly before serving. One serving is one muffin.

PER SERVING: **185**kcal, **5**g protein, **28**g carbohydrate, **3.5**g fibre, **7**g total fat (**1**g saturated fat), **40**mg cholesterol, **0.4**g salt.

Tip: **To thaw a frozen muffin,** *remove the cling film, wrap in kitchen paper and microwave on defrost (20 per cent power) for 1–2 minutes. To thaw in the oven, wrap in foil and bake at 150°C/gas 2 for 25–35 minutes.*

Blueberry and oat muffins

12 muffins

PREPARATION TIME: **25 MINUTES**

BAKING TIME: **20 MINUTES**

Pairing rolled oats, which are filled with blood sugar-lowering soluble fibre, with antioxidant-rich blueberries makes for a Magic breakfast, especially when you add cinnamon, as we have. Maple syrup provides a subtle sweetness that complements the blueberries and lets their fruity flavour shine through – and it has a lower GL than table sugar.

105g **wholemeal flour**
115g plain white flour
1½ teaspoons baking powder
½ teaspoon bicarbonate of soda
¼ teaspoon salt
1 teaspoon ground **cinnamon**
90g rolled **oats**
1 medium **egg**
2 medium **egg** whites
125ml maple syrup
180ml buttermilk (see Tip)
3 tablespoons canola (rapeseed) oil
2 teaspoons grated orange zest
1 tablespoon orange juice
1 teaspoon pure vanilla extract
225g fresh **blueberries**, rinsed and patted dry

1 **Preheat the oven** to 200°C/gas 6. Coat a 12-hole muffin tray with cooking spray or insert paper cups.

2 **In a large bowl,** whisk together the wholemeal flour, plain flour, baking powder, bicarbonate of soda, salt and cinnamon. Reserve 2 tablespoons of the rolled oats and stir the rest of the oats into the flour mixture.

3 **In a medium bowl,** whisk the egg and egg whites with the maple syrup until smooth. Add the buttermilk, oil, orange zest and juice and vanilla extract, and whisk until blended. Add to the flour mixture and mix with a rubber spatula just until the dry ingredients are moistened. Fold in the blueberries. Spoon the mixture into the muffin tray, filling the cups almost to the top. Sprinkle the reserved 2 tablespoons rolled oats over the tops of the muffins.

4 **Bake for 18–22 minutes** or until lightly browned and the tops spring back when touched lightly. Loosen the edges of the muffins, turn out on to a wire rack and cool slightly before serving. One serving is one muffin.

PER SERVING: **170**kcal, **5g** protein, **21g** carbohydrate, **1.8g** fibre, **4g** total fat (**0.7g** saturated fat), **20mg** cholesterol, **0.4g** salt.

Tip: **If you can't get buttermilk,** *make your own 'sour milk' by mixing 1 tablespoon lemon juice or vinegar with 225ml semi-skimmed milk or plain soya milk. Or, blend equal proportions of fat-free plain yoghurt and semi-skimmed milk.*

Blueberry and oat muffins
wholemeal flour · cinnamon · oats · eggs · blueberries

Upside-down nectarine muffins

12 muffins

PREPARATION TIME: **25 MINUTES**

BAKING TIME: **20 MINUTES**

There is nothing ordinary about these muffins. A bit like individual upside-down cakes, they boast an irresistible caramelised fruit topping. They're tasty treats indeed – with the Magic benefits of wholegrains, stone fruit, nuts and cinnamon.

TOPPING

2 tablespoons soft light brown sugar

30g chopped **walnuts**

3 medium **nectarines** (about 350g total weight), stoned and cut into 5mm thick wedges

MUFFINS

120g **wholemeal flour**

150g plain white flour

1½ teaspoons baking powder

½ teaspoon bicarbonate of soda

¼ teaspoon salt

1½ teaspoons ground **cinnamon**

½ teaspoon grated nutmeg

2 medium **eggs**

100g soft light brown sugar

250ml buttermilk (see Tip, page 199)

3 tablespoons canola (rapeseed) oil

1 teaspoon pure vanilla extract

1 **Preheat the oven** to 200°C/gas 6. Coat a 12-hole muffin tray with cooking spray.

2 **To make the topping:** sprinkle about ½ teaspoon brown sugar into each muffin cup and pat into an even layer on the bottom, then sprinkle about 1 teaspoon walnuts into each cup. Arrange 3 or 4 nectarine slices, slightly overlapping, over the walnuts and brown sugar. Cover and set aside. Coarsely chop the remaining nectarines; set aside.

3 **To make the muffins:** in a large bowl, whisk together the wholemeal flour, plain flour, baking powder, bicarbonate of soda, salt, cinnamon and nutmeg.

4 **In a medium bowl,** whisk the eggs with the brown sugar until smooth. Whisk in the buttermilk, oil and vanilla extract. Add to the flour mixture and mix with a rubber spatula just until the dry ingredients are moistened, then fold in the chopped nectarines. Spoon the mixture into the muffin cups (they will seem quite full, but the nectarine slices on the bottom will collapse during baking).

5 **Bake for 18–22 minutes** or until the muffins are lightly browned and the tops spring back when touched lightly. Immediately loosen the edges and carefully turn the muffins out on to a wire rack. Replace any stray nectarine slices and spoon on any walnut pieces left in the muffin tray. Allow to cool slightly before serving. One serving is one muffin.

PER SERVING: **193**kcal, **5g** protein, **31g** carbohydrate, **1.7g** fibre, **6g** total fat (**1g** saturated fat), **40mg** cholesterol, **0.4g** salt.

VARIATION

Substitute 350g plums or apricots for the nectarines.

Snacks and drinks

Caponata

serves 12

PREPARATION TIME: 25 MINUTES

COOKING TIME: 30–35 MINUTES

Caponata is terrific for entertaining because you can make it ahead of time. In fact, it gets better as it sits. Serve it in an attractive bowl, surrounded by wholegrain crackers or toasted slices of wholemeal baguette. You can also use it to perk up a sandwich filling or enliven a tomato-based pasta sauce. Made with plenty of vegetables and well flavoured with olives and olive oil – a 'good fat' that may help reverse insulin resistance – this is a Magic way to begin a meal.

3 tablespoons **olive oil**

450g **aubergine**, cut into 1cm cubes

1 small **onion**, chopped

4 celery sticks, finely diced

4 **garlic** cloves, finely chopped

Good pinch of crushed dried chillies

400g can chopped **tomatoes** (undrained)

4 tablespoons finely chopped sun-dried **tomatoes** (not oil-packed)

3 tablespoons red wine **vinegar**

8 green **olives**, pitted and chopped

2 tablespoons drained capers, rinsed

1 tablespoon caster sugar

3 tablespoons currants

35g pine **nuts**, toasted (see Tip, page 262)

3 tablespoons chopped fresh parsley

1 **Heat 1 tablespoon of the oil** in a large non-stick frying pan or sauté pan over a medium-high heat. Add half of the aubergine cubes and cook, stirring and turning, for 4–6 minutes or until they are browned and tender. Transfer to a plate and set aside. Add another tablespoon of oil to the pan and repeat with the remaining aubergine. Set aside.

2 **Add the remaining 1 tablespoon** oil to the pan. When hot, add the onion and celery. Cook, stirring often, for 3–5 minutes or until softened. Add the garlic and crushed chillies and cook, stirring, for 30 seconds. Add the canned tomatoes, sun-dried tomatoes, vinegar, olives, capers, sugar and browned aubergine cubes. Bring to a simmer. Reduce the heat to medium-low, cover and cook for about 15 minutes or until the mixture has a chunky jam-like consistency, stirring occasionally.

3 **Add the currants** and cook, covered, for a further 1 minute. Remove from the heat. Stir in the pine nuts and parsley. Leave to cool before serving. One serving is $2\frac{1}{2}$ tablespoons.

PER SERVING: **94**kcal, **1.5g** protein,
7g carbohydrate, **1.4g** fibre, **6.5g** total fat
(**0.5g** saturated fat), **0mg** cholesterol, **0.3g** salt.

Marinated olives

serves 8

PREPARATION TIME: 5 MINUTES

COOKING TIME: 2 MINUTES

Full of 'good fats', these highly savoury nibbles are a perfect pre-dinner appetiser that will promote better blood sugar levels.

2 teaspoons **olive oil**
2 **garlic** cloves, peeled
4 strips orange peel (about 5 x 1cm)
1½ teaspoons fennel seeds
350g rinsed Kalamata **olives**
2 tablespoons orange juice

1 **Heat the olive oil** in a medium frying pan over a low heat until warm. Add the garlic, orange peel and fennel seeds. Cook, stirring, for 30–60 seconds or until fragrant. Add the olives and cook, stirring, for about 1 minute or until they are warmed through but not hot. Remove from the heat.

2 **Stir in the orange juice.** Transfer to a bowl, cover tightly and leave to marinate at room temperature for about 1 hour. Serve at room temperature. One serving is 2 tablespoons. Keep any leftovers, tightly covered, in the refrigerator.

PER SERVING: **70**kcal, **0.6g** protein,
0.3g carbohydrate, **1g** fibre, **7g** total fat
(**1g** saturated fat), **0mg** cholesterol, **1g** salt.

Cherry tomatoes filled with creamy pesto cheese

serves 16

PREPARATION TIME: 35 MINUTES

COOKING TIME: 0 MINUTES

This delicious and attractive appetiser is simple to prepare. You can make the creamy pesto filling ahead of time (keep it, covered, in the refrigerator for up to 2 days), but wait until shortly before serving to stuff the tomatoes.

135g fresh basil leaves, washed and dried
2 medium **garlic** cloves, finely chopped
½ teaspoon salt, or to taste
Freshly ground black pepper to taste
60g pine **nuts**, toasted (see Tip, page 262)
1 tablespoon extra virgin **olive oil**
250g low-fat soft **cheese**, cut into chunks
700g cherry **tomatoes**, washed and dried

1 **Combine the basil,** garlic, salt and pepper in a food processor. Reserve 2 tablespoons of the pine nuts and add the rest to the basil. Process until the pine nuts are ground. With the motor running, drizzle in the olive oil. Add the soft cheese and pulse until smooth and creamy.

2 **Shortly before serving,** make an X on the bottom side (opposite the stalk) of each cherry tomato with a serrated or sharp paring knife. Scoop out the seeds with a grapefruit spoon or your fingertips, taking care to keep the tomatoes intact.

3 **Scrape the pesto cheese** filling into a piping bag fitted with a star nozzle, or small plastic food bag with a 1cm hole snipped in one corner. Pipe a rosette of filling into each cherry tomato cavity. Garnish the cherry tomatoes with the remaining pine nuts. One serving is about three filled cherry tomatoes.

PER SERVING: **64**kcal, **2g** protein, **2g** carbohydrate,
0.6g fibre, **5g** total fat (**1.5g** saturated fat),
8mg cholesterol, **0.14g** salt.

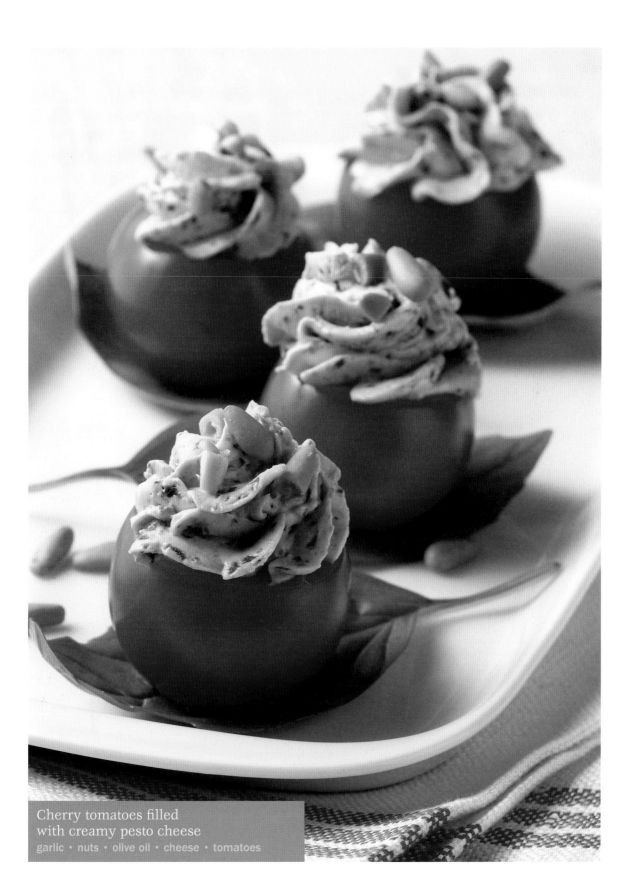

Cherry tomatoes filled
with creamy pesto cheese
garlic · nuts · olive oil · cheese · tomatoes

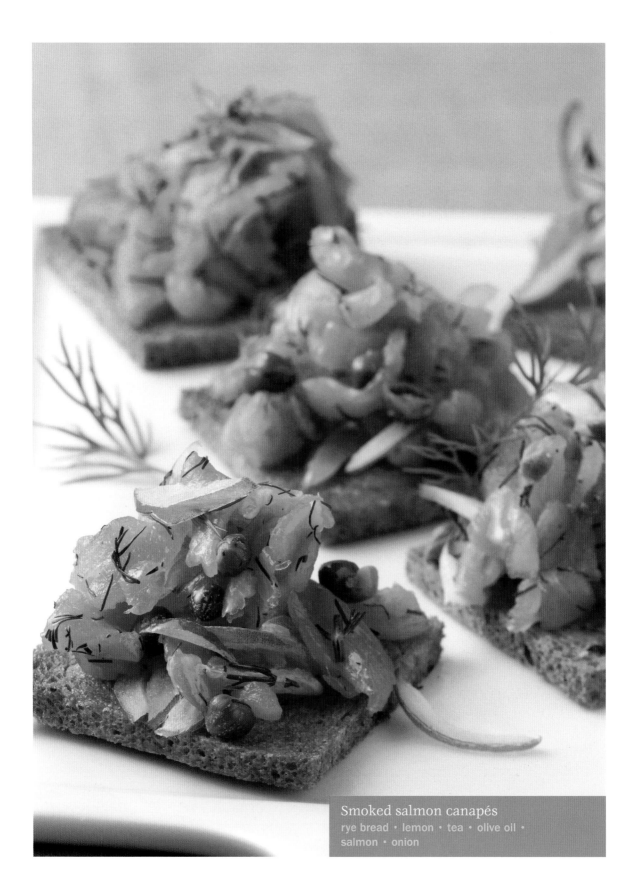

Smoked salmon canapés
rye bread • lemon • tea • olive oil • salmon • onion

Smoked salmon canapés

serves 12

PREPARATION TIME: 15 MINUTES

BAKING TIME: 15 MINUTES

These elegant party canapés offer a delectable bite of smoked salmon (a good source of protein and omega-3s), moistened with a light, lemony vinaigrette on a low-GL rye bread.

24 small slices **rye bread**
2 tablespoons **lemon** juice
2 tablespoons strong black **tea** or vodka
1 tablespoon extra virgin **olive oil**
2 teaspoons Dijon mustard
Freshly ground black pepper to taste
250g sliced smoked **salmon** or smoked salmon
    trimmings, finely chopped
60g finely diced red **onion**
3 tablespoons chopped fresh dill, plus
    sprigs to garnish
2 tablespoons drained capers, rinsed and
    coarsely chopped

1 Preheat the oven to 160°C/gas 3. Coat a baking tray with cooking spray. Arrange the slices of rye bread in a single layer on the baking tray. Spray the tops of the slices lightly with cooking spray. Bake for 12–15 minutes or just until the slices are crisp.

2 Whisk the lemon juice, tea (or vodka), oil, mustard and pepper in a medium bowl. Add the smoked salmon, red onion, dill and capers. Toss to mix well.

3 Shortly before serving, mound about 1 tablespoon of the smoked salmon topping on each slice of toast. Garnish each with a dill sprig. One serving is two canapés.

PER SERVING: **160**kcal, **9g** protein,
    24g carbohydrate, **2.5g** fibre, **4g** total fat
    (**0.5g** saturated fat), **0mg** cholesterol, **0.9g** salt.

Spiced almonds

serves 8

PREPARATION TIME: 5 MINUTES

COOKING TIME: 25–30 MINUTES

Warm spices turn plain almonds into irresistible nibbles. And thanks to the protein and 'good fat' in almonds, these are blood sugar–smart.

150g unpeeled whole **almonds**
1 teaspoon **olive oil**
³⁄₄ teaspoon ground cumin
¹⁄₄ teaspoon salt
Good pinch of cayenne pepper

1 Preheat the oven to 180°C/gas 4. Toss the almonds with the olive oil, cumin, salt and cayenne in a small baking tray or a shallow baking tin.

2 Bake for 25–30 minutes or until fragrant, stirring the almonds occasionally. Allow to cool. One serving is 2 tablespoons. The spiced almonds can be kept, in an airtight container, for up to a week.

PER SERVING: **118**kcal, **4g** protein,
    1g carbohydrate, **1.5g** fibre, **11g** total fat
    (**1g** saturated fat), **0mg** cholesterol, **0.2g** salt.

Warm artichoke and bean dip

serves 8

PREPARATION TIME: **10 MINUTES**

BAKING TIME: **20–25 MINUTES**

Beans are the Magic ingredient in this lower-fat, higher-fibre version of a classic hot artichoke dip. It makes a very tempting and savoury appetiser with pre-dinner drinks. Try serving it with Wholemeal pitta crisps (page 210) or low-fat wholegrain crispbread or crackers.

400g can cannellini **beans**, drained and rinsed
400g can artichoke hearts in water or brine, drained and rinsed
3 **garlic** cloves, finely chopped
1 tablespoon reduced-fat mayonnaise
Pinch of cayenne pepper
Freshly ground black pepper to taste
100g Parmesan **cheese**, freshly grated
4 tablespoons chopped fresh parsley
1 teaspoon grated lemon zest

1 Preheat the oven to 200°C/gas 6. Coat a 500–750ml capacity ovenproof dish with cooking spray.

2 Place the beans, artichoke hearts, garlic, mayonnaise, cayenne pepper and black pepper in a food processor. Process until almost smooth, stopping to scrape down the sides of the processor bowl once or twice. Transfer to a medium bowl.

3 Reserve 2 tablespoons of the Parmesan. Add the rest of the Parmesan to the artichoke mixture together with the parsley and lemon zest and stir to mix. Scrape into the ovenproof dish and smooth the top with a spatula. Sprinkle with the reserved Parmesan.

4 Bake the dip, uncovered, for 20–25 minutes or until it is heated through. Serve warm. One serving is 4 tablespoons.

PER SERVING: **115**kcal, **9g** protein,
9.5g carbohydrate, **3g** fibre, **4.5g** total fat
(**2.5g** saturated fat), **12mg** cholesterol, **0.3g** salt.

Oriental peanut dip

serves 8

PREPARATION TIME: **10 MINUTES**

COOKING TIME: **0 MINUTES**

Silken tofu stretches the peanut butter in this spicy dip, reducing calories and giving it a velvety consistency. Serve with crudités, or use as a spread to fill sandwiches made with wholemeal bread, grated carrot, sliced cucumber and shredded lettuce. The dip also can be used as a dressing for an Asian noodle salad.

130g smooth, unsweetened **peanut butter**
75g silken **tofu**
3 tablespoons soft light brown sugar
2 tablespoons reduced-salt soy sauce
2 tablespoons **lime** juice
½–¾ teaspoon crushed dried chillies
2 **garlic** cloves, crushed

Place all of the ingredients in a food processor and process until smooth and creamy, stopping once or twice to scrape down the sides of the processor bowl. One serving is 2 tablespoons. The dip can be kept, covered, in the refrigerator for up to 2 days.

PER SERVING: **130**kcal, **5g** protein,
9g carbohydrate, **1g** fibre, **9g** total fat
(**2g** saturated fat), **0mg** cholesterol, **0.6g** salt.

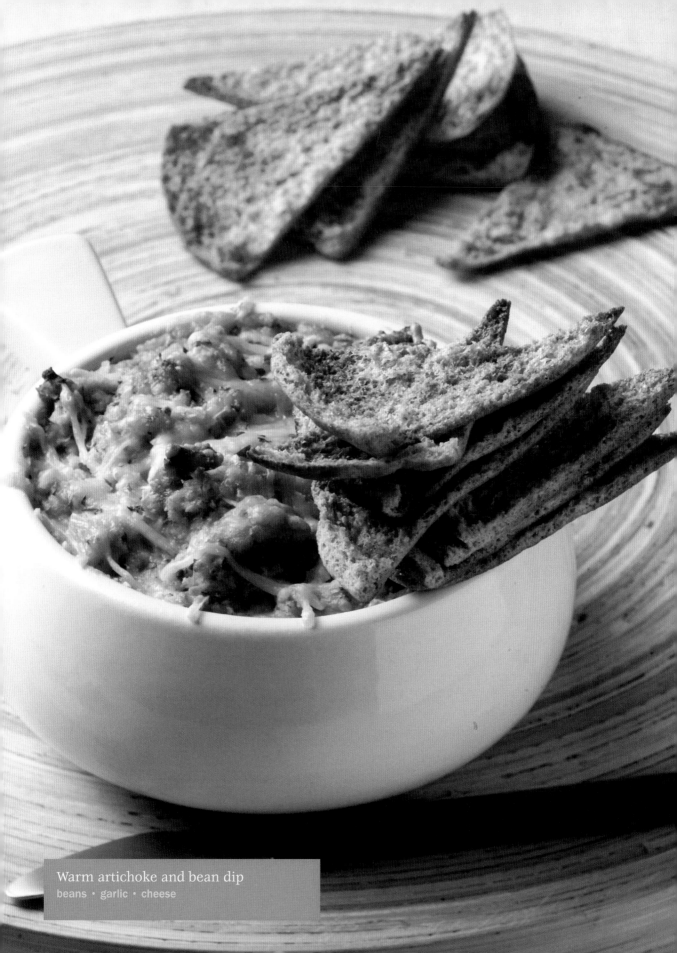

Warm artichoke and bean dip
beans · garlic · cheese

Mediterranean split pea spread

serves 16

PREPARATION TIME: 10 MINUTES

COOKING TIME: 50 MINUTES

This Greek appetiser illustrates how the traditional Mediterranean diet can be healthy and at the same time delicious. The base of the spread is humble yellow split peas – which boast slow-acting complex carbohydrates. When seasoned with cumin, garlic, lemon juice and fruity olive oil, they are transformed. Enjoy this spread as a starter for a casual meal with friends, accompanied by Wholemeal Pitta Crisps (*see* page 210) or wholegrain crackers, olives and cubes of feta cheese. It also makes a delicious sandwich filling.

150g dried yellow **split peas** (or chana dhal),
   picked over and rinsed
550ml water
6 **garlic** cloves, crushed
Good pinch of crushed dried chillies
3 tablespoons **lemon** juice
3 tablespoons extra virgin **olive oil**
1½ teaspoons ground cumin
¾ teaspoon salt, or to taste
2 tablespoons finely diced red **onion**
2 tablespoons coarsely chopped fresh dill

1 **Put the split peas** (or chana dhal), water, garlic and crushed chillies in a heavy medium saucepan. Bring to the boil. Reduce the heat to low, partly cover the pan and simmer, stirring occasionally, for 40–50 minutes or until the split peas are tender and most of the liquid has been absorbed. (Add more water during cooking, if necessary.) If the mixture seems too soupy at the end of cooking, simmer, uncovered and stirring constantly, for a few minutes or until the mixture has the consistency of very thick split pea soup. Remove from the heat.

2 **Allow the split pea mixture** to cool slightly, then transfer to a food processor. Add the lemon juice, 2 tablespoons of the olive oil, the cumin and salt. Process until smooth, stopping once or twice to scrape down the sides of the processor bowl. Spoon the purée into a shallow serving dish and smooth the top.

3 **Drizzle the remaining 1 tablespoon** oil over the spread, then sprinkle with the red onion and dill. One serving is 2 tablespoons. The spread can be kept, covered, in the refrigerator for up to 4 days.

PER SERVING: **50**kcal, **2g** protein,
   6g carbohydrate, **0.6g** fibre, **2.3g** total fat
   (**0.3g** saturated fat), **0mg** cholesterol, **0.2g** salt.

White bean spread with Italian flavours

serves 12

PREPARATION TIME: 10 MINUTES

COOKING TIME: 0 MINUTES

So quick to make and simply delicious, this could be the perfect spread.

400g can cannellini **beans**, drained
   and rinsed
2 tablespoons extra virgin **olive oil**
2 tablespoons **lemon** juice
1 **garlic** clove, finely chopped
Pinch of cayenne pepper
Pinch of salt
Freshly ground black pepper to taste
1½ teaspoons chopped fresh rosemary

Combine the cannellini beans, olive oil, lemon juice, garlic, cayenne pepper, salt and black pepper to taste in a food processor. Pulse to a chunky purée, stopping once or twice to scrape down the sides of the processor bowl. Transfer to a medium bowl and stir in the rosemary. One serving is 2 tablespoons.

PER SERVING: **50**kcal, **2g** protein,
   4.5g carbohydrate, **1.5g** fibre, **2g** total fat
   (**0.3g** saturated fat), **0mg** cholesterol, **0.08g** salt.

Chickpea spread with Indian flavours

serves 12

PREPARATION TIME: **10 MINUTES**

COOKING TIME: **1 MINUTE**

This has a bit of a chilli kick, balanced nicely by the cool yoghurt.

2 tablespoons canola (rapeseed) oil
2 fresh green chillies, deseeded and finely chopped
1 tablespoon finely chopped fresh root ginger
2 **garlic** cloves, finely chopped
2 teaspoons ground cumin
1 teaspoon ground coriander
400g can **chickpeas**, drained and rinsed
85g fat-free plain **yoghurt**
2 tablespoons **lime** juice
Good pinch of salt
Freshly ground black pepper to taste
2 tablespoons chopped fresh coriander (or parsley)

1 **Heat the oil** in a small frying pan over a medium-high heat. Add the chillies, fresh ginger and garlic, and cook, stirring, for about 30 seconds or until fragrant. Stir in the cumin and ground coriander. Transfer the spice mixture to a food processor.

2 **Add the chickpeas,** yoghurt, lime juice, salt and pepper to taste. Process until smooth, stopping once or twice to scrape down the sides of the processor bowl. Spoon into a medium bowl and stir in the fresh coriander (or parsley). One serving is 2 rounded tablespoons.

PER SERVING: **51**kcal, **2.3g** protein, **5g** carbohydrate, **1g** fibre, **2.5g** total fat (**0.3g** saturated fat), **0mg** cholesterol, **0.3g** salt.

Black bean spread with Mexican flavours

serves 12

PREPARATION TIME: **10 MINUTES**

COOKING TIME: **0 MINUTES**

Fibre-rich canned beans provide the base for an easy spread that makes a satisfying snack served with Baked Tortilla Chips (*see* page 210) or with crudités. It can also be used as a sandwich filling – spread it on sourdough or wholemeal bread and top with grated carrot, avocado and tomato slices, and lettuce leaves.

400g can black **beans**, drained and rinsed
2 tablespoons **lime** juice
1 tablespoon extra virgin **olive oil**
1 **garlic** clove, finely chopped
1 teaspoon ground cumin
$\frac{1}{4}$ teaspoon Tabasco sauce
Pinch of salt
Freshly ground black pepper to taste
2 tablespoons chopped fresh coriander (or parsley)

1 **Combine the black beans,** lime juice, olive oil, garlic, cumin, Tabasco sauce, salt and pepper in a food processor. Process until smooth, stopping once or twice to scrape down the sides of the processor bowl.

2 **Transfer to a medium bowl** and stir in the fresh coriander (or parsley). One serving is 2 tablespoons. The spread will keep, covered, in the refrigerator for up to 4 days.

PER SERVING: **40**kcal, **2g** protein, **4g** carbohydrate, **1g** fibre, **1.7g** total fat (**0g** saturated fat), **0mg** cholesterol, **0.4g** salt

Baked tortilla chips

serves 8

PREPARATION TIME: **2 MINUTES**

COOKING TIME: **10–15 MINUTES**

These are a smart, and tasty, alternative to store-bought tortilla chips, which are much higher in fat and salt.

300g pack corn tortillas (8–12 tortillas)
¼ teaspoon salt

Preheat the oven to 200°C/gas 6. Stack the tortillas and cut into four wedges. Spread the wedges in a single layer on two baking trays. Spray lightly with cooking spray and sprinkle with salt. Bake for 10–15 minutes or until light golden and crisp. One serving is six chips.

PER SERVING: **98**kcal, **2.7g** protein, **22g** carbohydrate, **1g** fibre, **0.4g** total fat (**0g** saturated fat), **0mg** cholesterol, **0.4g** salt.

Wholemeal pitta crisps

serves 8

PREPARATION TIME: **3 MINUTES**

COOKING TIME: **8–10 MINUTES**

Here's a healthy wholegrain partner for any of the dips and spreads on pages 206–209.

4 **wholemeal pitta** breads

Preheat the oven to 220°C/gas 7. Cut each pitta bread into four triangles. Separate each triangle into two halves at the fold. Arrange, rough side up, on a baking tray. Spray lightly with olive oil cooking spray. Bake for 8–10 minutes or until crisp. One serving is four crisps.

PER SERVING: **96**kcal, **3.5g** protein, **12.5g** carbohydrate, **1.5g** fibre, **7.5g** total fat (**1.5g** saturated fat), **10mg** cholesterol, **0.2g** salt.

Chai

serves 2

PREPARATION TIME: **2 MINUTES**

COOKING TIME: **10 MINUTES**

Chai is a sweet, milky, spiced tea drink that originated in India. It's easy to make your own blend of this warming tea, and it's a good way to get some milk into your diet. This homemade version has a fraction of the calories and fat grams of ready-made chai – and it's much easier on your pocket.

¼ teaspoon ground **cinnamon**
¼ teaspoon ground cloves
¼ teaspoon ground ginger
375ml water
150ml semi-skimmed **milk** (or vanilla **soya milk**)
3 black **tea** bags
2 teaspoons clear honey, or to taste

1 **Combine the cinnamon,** cloves and ginger with the water in a small saucepan. Bring to a simmer. Reduce the heat to low, then cover and simmer for 5 minutes. Add the milk (or soya milk) and heat until steaming but not boiling. Remove from the heat.

2 **Add the tea bags,** cover the pan again and leave to steep for 3–4 minutes. Pour the chai into two mugs and sweeten with honey to taste.

PER SERVING: **50**kcal, **2.5g** protein, **7g** carbohydrate, **0g** fibre, **1.3g** total fat (**0.8g** saturated fat), **4mg** cholesterol, **0.08g** salt.

Oat and peanut butter bars

24 bars

PREPARATION TIME: 25 MINUTES
BAKING TIME: 20–25 MINUTES

When you bake your own snack bars, you can be sure that they include wholegrains like rolled oats and wholemeal flour, and healthy fats such as those from canola (rapeseed) oil and nuts. Peanut butter stands in for butter, reducing the saturated fat and boosting protein. The bars make ideal snacks – tuck one into your pocket when you head out the door.

60g **wholemeal flour**
1 teaspoon ground **cinnamon**
½ teaspoon bicarbonate of soda
Good pinch of salt
130g smooth, unsweetened **peanut butter**
   (see Ingredient note, next page)
100g soft brown sugar
115g clear honey
1 medium **egg**
2 medium **egg** whites (see Tip, next page)
2 tablespoons canola (rapeseed) oil
2 teaspoons pure vanilla extract
160g rolled **oats**
140g dried cranberries (or raisins)
60g **walnuts** or **almonds**, coarsely chopped
85g plain dark chocolate chips

1 **Preheat the oven** to 180°C/gas 4. Coat a 23 x 33cm baking tin with cooking spray.

2 **Whisk together the flour,** cinnamon, bicarbonate of soda and salt in a medium bowl. Set aside.

3 **In a large bowl,** beat the peanut butter with the sugar and honey using an electric mixer until blended. Stir the egg and egg whites with a fork in a small bowl. Add to the peanut butter mixture, together with the oil and vanilla extract and beat until smooth. Add the flour mixture and mix in with a rubber spatula. Mix in the oats, dried cranberries (or raisins), walnuts (or almonds) and chocolate chips.

4 **Scrape the mixture** into the prepared baking tin. Use a piece of cling film to spread the mixture into an even layer, then discard the cling film.

5 **Bake for 20–25 minutes** or until lightly browned and firm to the touch. Allow to cool completely in the tin on a wire rack before cutting into 24 bars. One serving is one bar.

PER SERVING: **161**kcal, **3.5g** protein, **12.5g** carbohydrate, **1.5g** fibre, **7.5g** total fat (**1.5g** saturated fat), **10mg** cholesterol, **0.2g** salt.

Ingredient note: **If you must avoid peanut butter** because of an allergy, you can substitute other nut or seed butters such as soya nut butter or pumpkin seed butter. You can replace the nuts with unsalted roasted pumpkin seeds and/or sunflower seeds (look for unsalted seeds in healthfood and whole foods shops).

Tip: **To avoid wasting egg yolks,** instead of fresh egg whites use reconstituted dried egg whites, which you can find in the cake decorating section of the supermarket.

Berry and flaxseed smoothie

serves 2

PREPARATION TIME: **5 MINUTES**

COOKING TIME: **0 MINUTES**

A smoothie is a smart way to start your day, especially when it includes this tasty mix of Magic foods. Flaxseeds (linseeds) may seem like an unusual addition, but they blend in seamlessly and make this breakfast drink an excellent source of fibre, too.

2 tablespoons whole **flaxseeds**
125ml orange juice
125g fat-free vanilla **yoghurt**
250g unsweetened frozen mixed **berries**
    or **blueberries**
1 small banana, sliced

Place the flaxseeds in a blender and blend until ground into a fine powder. Add the orange juice, yoghurt, mixed berries (or blueberries) and banana. Blend until smooth and creamy. Pour into two glasses and serve immediately.

PER SERVING: **200**kcal, **9g** protein, **27g** carbohydrate, **4g** fibre, **6.5g** total fat (**0.7g** saturated fat), **0mg** cholesterol, **0.1g** salt.

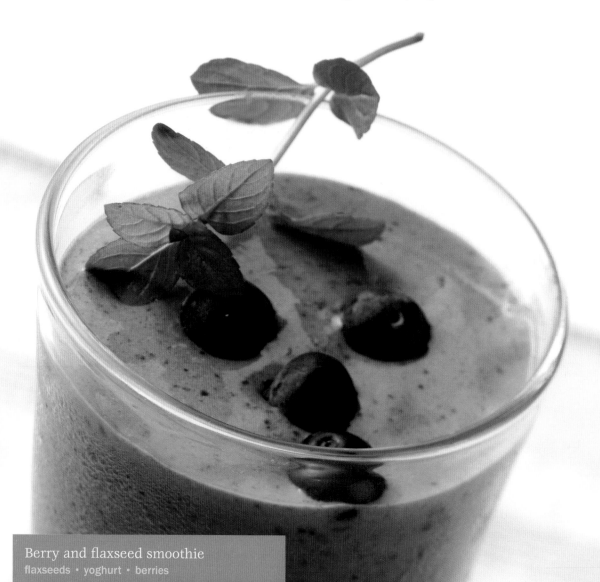

Berry and flaxseed smoothie
flaxseeds · yoghurt · berries

Peachy iced tea

serves 8

PREPARATION TIME: **5 MINUTES**

COOKING TIME: **2 MINUTES**

CHILLING TIME: **3 HOURS**

Here's a great alternative to sugary fizzy drinks and juice drinks – a delightfully refreshing iced tea enhanced with the sweet perfume of peach. When buying the peach juice, be sure it is pure juice, and contains no added sugar.

7 black or green **tea** bags
1.5 litres boiling water
500ml unsweetened peach juice
2 medium **peaches**, stoned and sliced
Ice cubes
Mint sprigs (optional)

1 **Steep the tea bags** in the boiling water for 5 minutes. Remove the tea bags. Combine the brewed tea and peach juice in a large jug and stir in the peaches. Place in the refrigerator to chill for at least 3 hours, or overnight.

2 **Serve in tall glasses** over ice cubes and garnished with mint sprigs, if you like. One serving is 250ml.

PER SERVING: **30**kcal, **0.5g** protein,
   7g carbohydrate, **0.5g** fibre, **0g** total fat
   (**0g** saturated fat), **0mg** cholesterol, salt (trace).

VARIATION
Berry iced tea
Substitute blackberry or blueberry juice (or blueberry and apple) for the peach juice, and fresh berries for the peaches.

Iced coffee frappé

serves 1

PREPARATION TIME: **5 MINUTES**

COOKING TIME: **0 MINUTES**

Coffee bar drinks may seem innocent enough, but they are often outrageously high in calories, especially if you opt for the typical oversize portion. It is very easy to make your own frothy coffee-flavoured drink. Our recipe has less than half the calories of a Starbucks Frappuccino.

2 teaspoons instant **coffee**
1 teaspoon caster sugar, or to taste
2 ice cubes
60ml cold water
85ml chilled vanilla **soya milk** (or
   semi-skimmed **milk**)
Pinch of ground **cinnamon**

1 **Combine the instant coffee,** sugar, ice cubes and water in a cocktail shaker or a wide-mouth jar with a tight-fitting lid (about 700ml capacity). Put on the lid and shake vigorously for about 30 seconds or until frothy.

2 **Pour into a tall glass.** Add the soya milk (or semi-skimmed milk) and stir to mix. Sprinkle with cinnamon and serve with a straw.

PER SERVING: **60**kcal, **3g** protein,
   9g carbohydrate, **0g** fibre, **1.5g** total fat
   (**1g** saturated fat), **5mg** cholesterol, salt (trace).

Salads, sandwiches and soups

Grilled chicken salad with orange

serves 4

PREPARATION TIME: 25 MINUTES
MARINATING TIME: 20 MINUTES
COOKING TIME: 10–15 MINUTES

Slices of grilled chicken breast, sweet fresh oranges and crunchy pistachios transform a leafy green salad into a satisfying summer main dish that's packed with flavour – and Magic foods. When marinating poultry (as well as meat and fish), be sure to reserve a few tablespoons of the marinade for basting during cooking, rather than using the marinade that has been in contact with the raw chicken.

85ml orange juice

2 tablespoons **lemon** juice

3 tablespoons extra virgin **olive oil**

1 tablespoon Dijon mustard

2 **garlic** cloves, finely chopped

¼ teaspoon salt, or to taste

Freshly ground black pepper to taste

450g **chicken** breast fillets, trimmed

30g **pistachio nuts** (or slivered or coarsely chopped **almonds**)

140g mixed baby salad leaves, rinsed and dried

1 small red **onion**, thinly sliced

2 medium **oranges**, peeled, quartered and sliced (or segmented)

1 **Combine the orange juice,** lemon juice, oil, mustard, garlic, salt and pepper in a small bowl or a screw-top jar; whisk or shake to blend. Reserve 5 tablespoons of this dressing for the salad and 3 tablespoons for basting the chicken during cooking.

2 **Put the remaining dressing** in a shallow glass dish or a resealable plastic bag. Add the chicken and turn to coat. Cover or seal and leave to marinate in the refrigerator for at least 20 minutes or up to 2 hours.

3 **Preheat the grill to medium.** Lightly oil the grill rack by rubbing it with a piece of crumpled, oil-soaked kitchen paper. Remove the chicken from the dish or bag and discard the marinade. Grill the chicken for 4–6 minutes on each side, brushing it with the dressing reserved for basting when you turn it over, until no longer pink in the centre. Transfer to a chopping board and leave to rest for 5 minutes.

4 **Meanwhile, toast the pistachios** (or almonds) in a small dry frying pan over a medium-low heat for 2–3 minutes or until light golden. Stir constantly and be sure the nuts don't get too brown. Transfer to a bowl and cool.

5 **Place the salad leaves** and onion in a large bowl. Toss with the dressing reserved for the salad. Divide the salad among four plates. Slice the chicken and arrange on the salads. Scatter the orange slices over the top and sprinkle with the toasted nuts.

PER SERVING: **311**kcal, **27g** protein, **0g** carbohydrate, **2g** fibre, **18g** total fat (**3g** saturated fat), **96mg** cholesterol, **0.7g** salt.

Grilled chicken salad with orange
lemon • olive oil • garlic • chicken • nuts •
onion • oranges

Barley salad with mangetout and lemon dressing

serves 8

PREPARATION TIME: 30 MINUTES

COOKING TIME: 40–45 MINUTES

As this colourful salad attests, sugar-lowering barley isn't just for soups. Mangetout add even more sugar-busting, cholesterol-bashing soluble fibre, and the refreshing lemon dressing helps slow down your body's conversion of carbohydrates into blood sugar.

DRESSING

2 teaspoons grated lemon zest
4 tablespoons fresh **lemon** juice
4 tablespoons finely chopped **shallot**
1 **garlic** clove, finely chopped
1/2 teaspoon salt, or to taste
Freshly ground black pepper to taste
85ml extra virgin **olive oil**

SALAD

200g pearl **barley**, rinsed
600ml water
1/4 teaspoon salt, or to taste
170g **mangetout** (or sugarsnap peas)
1 medium red pepper, deseeded and diced
3 medium **carrots**, grated
4 tablespoons chopped fresh parsley
4 tablespoons snipped fresh chives

1 **To make the dressing:** whisk the lemon zest and juice with the shallot, garlic, salt and pepper in a medium bowl. Whisk in the oil.

2 **To make the salad:** put the barley, water and salt in a large saucepan and bring to a simmer over a medium-high heat. Reduce the heat to low, cover and cook for 40–45 minutes or until tender and most of the liquid has been absorbed. Tip into a large bowl and cool, fluffing with a fork occasionally to prevent sticking.

3 **Meanwhile, remove** the stem ends and strings from the mangetout. Cut in half on the diagonal. Cook in a large saucepan of lightly salted boiling water, or steam them, for about 2 minutes or until just tender. Drain and rinse with cold running water.

4 **Add the mangetout,** red pepper, carrots, parsley and chives to the barley. Drizzle the dressing over the salad and toss to coat well. (To make ahead, prepare the dressing and salad and refrigerate in separate covered containers for up to a day. Toss the salad with the dressing shortly before serving.)

PER SERVING: **180**kcal, **3g** protein, **27g** carbohydrate, **2g** fibre, **7.5g** total fat (**1g** saturated fat), **0mg** cholesterol, **0.5g** salt.

Black bean and barley salad

serves 6

PREPARATION TIME: 25 MINUTES

COOKING TIME: 40–45 MINUTES

With an all-star Magic foods line-up of barley, beans, vinegar and citrus, this hearty salad is a real winner. It's great for picnics and barbecues and is an excellent accompaniment for grilled chicken, pork or fish.

150g pearl **barley**
500ml chicken or vegetable stock, made without salt
4 tablespoons cider **vinegar**
4 tablespoons orange juice
4 tablespoons extra virgin **olive oil**
1 1/2 teaspoons ground cumin
1 teaspoon dried oregano
1 **garlic** clove, finely chopped
1/4 teaspoon salt, or to taste
Freshly ground black pepper to taste
400g can black **beans**, drained and rinsed
1 large red or yellow pepper, deseeded and diced
1 bunch **spring onions** (or salad onions), trimmed and chopped
25g fresh coriander, coarsely chopped
Lime wedges

1 **Combine the barley** and stock in a large saucepan and bring to a simmer over a medium-high heat. Reduce the heat to low, cover the pan and cook for 40–45 minutes or until the barley is tender and most of the liquid has been absorbed. Transfer the barley to a large bowl and leave to cool, fluffing with a fork occasionally to prevent sticking.

2 **Meanwhile,** combine the vinegar, orange juice, oil, cumin, oregano, garlic, salt and pepper in a screw-top jar, or in a small bowl. Shake or whisk to blend.

3 **Add the black beans,** red or yellow pepper, spring onions and coriander to the barley. Drizzle over the dressing and toss to coat well. Garnish with lime wedges. The salad will keep, covered, in the refrigerator for up to 1 day.

PER SERVING: **250**kcal, **10g** protein, **33g** carbohydrate, **3g** fibre, **10g** total fat (**1.5g** saturated fat), **0mg** cholesterol, **0.9g** salt.

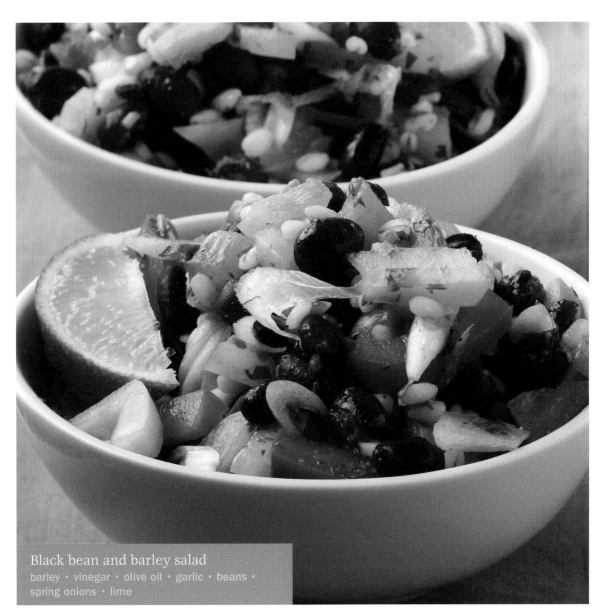

Black bean and barley salad
barley • vinegar • olive oil • garlic • beans •
spring onions • lime

Tuna and cannellini salad with lemon

serves 4

PREPARATION TIME: 25 MINUTES

COOKING TIME: 0 MINUTES

Tuna and beans are a classic combo as well as a practical and nutritious one. If you keep canned tuna and canned beans on hand, you can put this recipe together from your storecupboard staples – just add some fresh greens and cherry tomatoes. This version is distinguished by a seasoning of lemon zest and rosemary. It is perfect for an al fresco lunch or dinner when it's too hot to cook and eat indoors.

LEMON AND GARLIC DRESSING

3 tablespoons **lemon** juice

1 **garlic** clove, finely chopped

¼ teaspoon salt, or to taste

Good pinch of crushed dried chillies

4 tablespoons extra virgin **olive oil**

Freshly ground black pepper to taste

SALAD

400g can cannellini **beans**, drained
    and rinsed

200g can light **tuna** in water, drained
    and flaked

½ red **onion**, finely diced

2 teaspoons chopped fresh rosemary

1½ teaspoons grated lemon zest

6 handfuls of wild rocket, washed and dried

175g cherry **tomatoes**, quartered

1 **To make the dressing:** combine the lemon juice, garlic, salt and crushed chillies in a small bowl. Gradually whisk in the oil. Season with pepper.

2 **To make the salad:** combine the cannellini beans, tuna, onion, rosemary and lemon zest in a medium bowl. Add 4 tablespoons of the dressing and toss to coat well. (The salad can be kept, covered, in the refrigerator for up to 1 day.)

3 **Just before serving,** put the rocket in a large bowl. Add the remaining dressing and toss to coat well. Divide the rocket among four plates. Top each with one-quarter of the tuna and bean salad and garnish with a quarter of the cherry tomatoes.

PER SERVING: **300**kcal, **20g** protein, **17g** carbohydrate, **5g** fibre, **17g** total fat (**2.5g** saturated fat), **25mg** cholesterol, **0.6g** salt.

Tip: **Canned beans are high in salt,** *but you can reduce the salt by about 40 per cent just by draining them. A good rinse under the cold tap for about 30 seconds reduces salt content by another 3 per cent. In our nutrition analyses we've assumed you've drained and rinsed the canned beans.*

beans thanks to their soluble fibre, there's no better food for your blood sugar

tomato when raw, tomatoes retain their full complement of vitamin C

garlic great in dressings, garlic may boost insulin secretion

tuna fish no further for sugar-stabilising protein without saturated fat

lemon acidic lemon lowers a meal's GL

onions eat them raw for maximum antioxidant power

olive oil it slows the emptying of your stomach, curbing blood sugar spikes

Tuna and cannellini salad with lemon

Wholemeal noodles with peanut sauce and chicken

serves 8

PREPARATION TIME: 35 MINUTES

COOKING TIME: 8–10 MINUTES

This dish will be a big hit at your next supper party. Nutty-tasting wholemeal spaghetti complements the peanut sauce. Tofu stretches the peanut butter in the recipe, helping to keep calories in check and giving the sauce a velvety consistency. For a vegetarian version, replace the chicken with baked, diced seasoned tofu. If you are making the salad ahead, it is best to prepare all the components and toss the salad with the dressing shortly before serving.

DRESSING

130g smooth, unsweetened **peanut butter**

85g silken **tofu**

4 tablespoons reduced-salt soy sauce

3 tablespoons **lime** juice

3 **garlic** cloves, finely chopped

2 tablespoons soft light brown sugar

¾ teaspoon crushed dried chillies

SALAD

340g **wholemeal spaghetti**

2 teaspoons toasted sesame oil

350g cooked skinless **chicken** breast meat, shredded

3 medium **carrots**, grated

1 small red pepper, deseeded and finely diced

1 medium cucumber, grated

15g fresh coriander leaves, coarsely chopped

50g **spring onions** (or salad onions), chopped

3 tablespoons chopped unsalted dry-roasted **peanuts**

Lime wedges

1 **Bring a large pan** of lightly salted water to the boil for cooking the spaghetti.

2 **To make the dressing:** combine all of the dressing ingredients in a food processor. Process until smooth and creamy, stopping once or twice to scrape down the sides of the processor bowl. Set aside.

3 **To make the salad:** cook the spaghetti in the boiling water for 6–9 minutes, or according to packet instructions, until *al dente*. Drain and refresh under cold running water. Transfer to a large bowl. Drizzle with the oil and toss to coat.

4 **Add the chicken,** carrots and red pepper to the spaghetti. Add the peanut dressing and toss to coat. Sprinkle with the grated cucumber, chopped coriander, spring onions and peanuts. Serve with lime wedges.

PER SERVING: **385**kcal, **22g** protein, **42g** carbohydrate, **6g** fibre, **16g** total fat (**4g** saturated fat), **37mg** cholesterol, **1.3g** salt.

Creamy coleslaw without mayonnaise

serves 6

PREPARATION TIME: 20 MINUTES

COOKING TIME: 0 MINUTES

The traditional way to make coleslaw is to drown the cabbage and other vegetables in a rich mayonnaise-based dressing. Our version uses yoghurt enriched with olive oil (a 'good fat') instead of mayonnaise. If you have red cabbage on hand, use a mix of red and green cabbage for extra colour and to take advantage of the red variety's anthocyanins – pigments that may help boost insulin production and lower blood sugar.

85g fat-free plain **yoghurt**

4 teaspoons Dijon mustard

4 teaspoons cider **vinegar**

4 teaspoons extra virgin **olive oil**

1½ teaspoons caster sugar

½ teaspoon caraway **seeds** (or celery seeds)

¼ teaspoon salt

¼ teaspoon freshly ground black pepper

½ medium green **cabbage**, finely shredded

3 medium **carrots**, grated

1 **Whisk together the yoghurt,** mustard, vinegar, oil, sugar, caraway seeds, salt and pepper in a small bowl until smooth.

2 **Combine the cabbage** and carrots in a large bowl. Add the yoghurt dressing and toss to coat well. The coleslaw can be kept, covered, in the refrigerator for up to a day.

PER SERVING: **71**kcal, **3g** protein,
    9g carbohydrate, **3g** fibre, **3g** total fat
    (**0.4g** saturated fat), **0mg** cholesterol, **0.4g** salt.

Creamy coleslaw without mayonnaise
yoghurt · vinegar · olive oil · seeds ·
cabbage · carrots

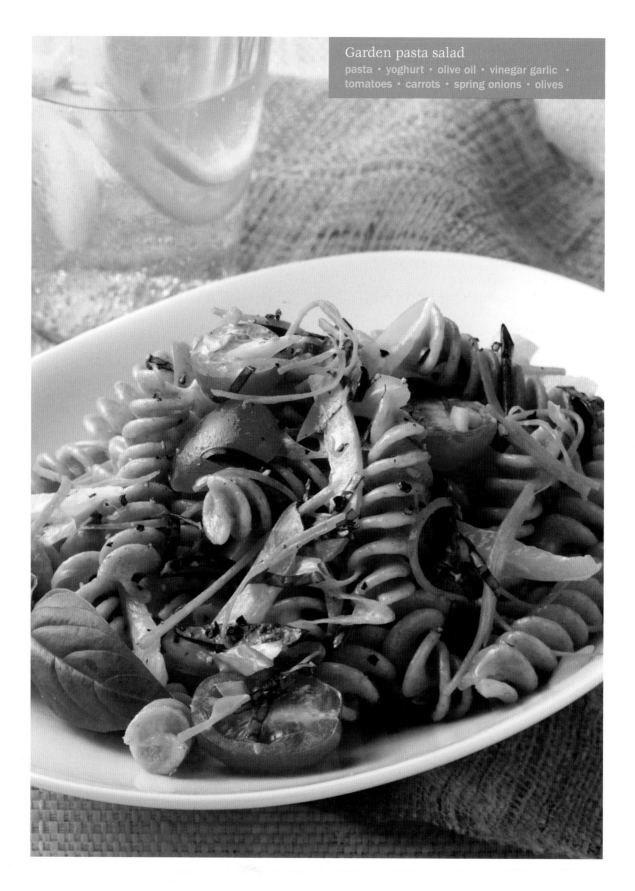

Garden pasta salad

pasta • yoghurt • olive oil • vinegar garlic •
tomatoes • carrots • spring onions • olives

Garden pasta salad

serves **6**

PREPARATION TIME: **30 MINUTES**
COOKING TIME: **8–10 MINUTES**

Pasta salads are perfect for al fresco lunches and barbecues. This version has been upgraded with wholemeal pasta and a generous quantity of colourful vegetables. Reduced-fat mayonnaise, blended with low-fat yoghurt, makes a creamy dressing that has a fraction of the saturated fat and calories of typical mayonnaise-based dressings. If you'd like to make this salad more substantial, toss in canned tuna or chickpeas, or cubes of cooked chicken.

170g wholemeal rotini or fusilli **pasta**
85ml reduced-fat mayonnaise
85g low-fat plain **yoghurt**
2 tablespoons extra virgin **olive oil**
1 tablespoon red wine **vinegar** or **lemon juice**
1 **garlic** clove, finely chopped
Good pinch of salt, or to taste
Freshly ground black pepper to taste
175g cherry or baby plum **tomatoes**, halved
1 small yellow or red pepper, deseeded and diced
3 medium **carrots**, grated
4 **spring onions**, chopped
70g Kalamata **olives**, chopped
5 tablespoons finely shredded fresh basil

1 **Bring a large pan** of lightly salted water to the boil. Add the pasta and cook for 8–10 minutes, or according to packet instructions, until *al dente*. Drain and refresh under cold running water.

2 **Whisk together the mayonnaise,** yoghurt, oil, vinegar (or lemon juice), garlic, salt and pepper in a large bowl until smooth. Add the pasta and toss to coat. Add the tomatoes, yellow or red pepper, carrots, spring onions, olives and basil. Toss to coat well. The salad can be kept, covered, in the refrigerator for up to 1 day.

PER SERVING: **222**kcal, **6g** protein, **27g** carbohydrate, **4.5g** fibre, **11g** total fat (**2g** saturated fat), **3mg** cholesterol, **0.9g** salt.

Greek lentil salad

serves **6**

PREPARATION TIME: **20 MINUTES**
COOKING TIME: **25–30 MINUTES**

Prized for their content of vegetable protein, soluble fibre and folate, lentils are an essential *Magic Foods* storecupboard staple. There is no need to wait for chilly weather to enjoy lentils – they are equally delicious in warming soups and in summer salads like this one. Feel free to substitute 2 x 425g cans of lentils (drained and rinsed) for the dried lentils.

200g dried Puy **lentils**, rinsed
1 teaspoon salt
3 tablespoons **lemon** juice
2 tablespoons extra virgin **olive oil**
1 **garlic** clove, finely chopped
Freshly ground black pepper to taste
1 bunch **spring onions** (or salad onions), chopped
350g roasted red peppers from a jar, rinsed
    and diced
60g feta **cheese**, crumbled
5 tablespoons chopped fresh dill
6 handfuls of wild rocket or watercress sprigs,
    washed and dried

1 **Place the lentils** in a large saucepan and cover with water. Bring to a simmer. Reduce the heat to medium-low, partly cover and simmer for 15–20 minutes or until tender but still keeping their shape. Drain. Add ½ teaspoon of salt and leave to cool slightly.

2 **Whisk together the lemon juice,** oil, garlic, the remaining ½ teaspoon salt and some pepper in a large bowl. Add the warm lentils and toss gently to mix. Add the spring onions, roasted red peppers, feta and dill. Toss again. To serve, mound the lentil salad on a bed of rocket or watercress sprigs.

PER SERVING: **210**kcal, **11g** protein, **28g** carbohydrate, **4g** fibre, **7g** total fat (**2g** saturated fat), **7mg** cholesterol, **1g** salt.

Spinach, grapefruit & avocado salad with poppy seed dressing

serves 4

PREPARATION TIME: 30 MINUTES

COOKING TIME: 0 MINUTES

Juicy, sharp grapefruit makes a delicious contrast to creamy avocado and crisp spinach. Serve as an impressive starter salad or add prawns and enjoy it as a refreshing summer main dish.

2 pink **grapefruit**
1 tablespoon white-wine **vinegar** or rice vinegar
1 large **shallot**, finely chopped
2 teaspoons poppy **seeds**
1 teaspoon clear honey
1 teaspoon Dijon mustard
3 tablespoons extra virgin **olive oil**
1/2 teaspoon salt, or to taste
Freshly ground pepper to taste
170g baby **spinach** leaves, rinsed and dried
1 bunch of radishes, sliced
2 Haas **avocados**, peeled, stoned and sliced

1 **Place a sieve** over a medium bowl. Using a sharp knife, remove the grapefruit's skin and white pith. Cut all the grapefruit segments from their surrounding membrane, letting the segments collect in the sieve and the juices collect in the bowl. Then, squeeze the membrane to extract as much juice as possible.

2 **Place 4 tablespoons** of the grapefruit juice (reserve the remainder for another use) in a small bowl or a screw-top jar. Add the vinegar, shallot, poppy seeds, honey, mustard, oil, salt and pepper. Whisk or shake to blend.

3 **Just before serving,** place the spinach and radishes in a large bowl. Toss with half of the dressing. Divide the salad among 4 plates. Strew the avocado slices and grapefruit segments over the salads and drizzle with the remaining dressing.

PER SERVING: **212**kcal, 3.5g protein, **9g** carbohydrate, **4g** fibre, **19g** total fat, (**3.5g** saturated fat), **8mg** cholesterol, **0.6g** salt.

Mediterranean salad with edamame

serves 8

PREPARATION TIME: 25 MINUTES

COOKING TIME: 4 MINUTES

This variation of a classic Greek salad features fragrant herbs and protein-rich edamame beans – baby soya beans, which are sold frozen – podded or in their pods – in many supermarkets as well as healthfood shops.

150g frozen podded **edamame** beans
85ml extra virgin **olive oil**
3 tablespoons **lemon** juice
2 **garlic** cloves, finely chopped
1/4 teaspoon salt, or to taste
1/4 teaspoon caster sugar
Freshly ground black pepper to taste
1/2 small romaine lettuce, shredded
350g cherry **tomatoes**, halved, or 2 medium tomatoes, cored and cut into 5 x 2.5cm wedges
150g cucumber, sliced
65g **spring onions**, chopped
70g Kalamata **olives**, halved
25g fresh mint leaves, torn into 1cm pieces
25g fresh flat-leaf parsley leaves, washed, dried and torn into 1cm pieces
135g feta **cheese**, crumbled

1 **Bring a large saucepan** of lightly salted water to the boil. Add the edamame beans, cover the pan and cook over a medium heat for 3–4 minutes or until tender. Drain and rinse under cold running water. Set aside.

2 **Combine the oil,** lemon juice, garlic, salt, sugar and some black pepper in a screw-top jar. Shake to blend.

3 **Mix the other salad** ingredients and cooked edamame beans in a large bowl. Just before serving, drizzle the lemon dressing over the salad and toss to coat well. Divide among plates and sprinkle each serving with feta.

PER SERVING: **151**kcal, **6g** protein, **4g** carbohydrate, **2g** fibre, **13g** total fat (**4g** saturated fat), **12mg** cholesterol, **1g** salt.

Mediterranean salad with edamame
edamame · olive oil · lemon · garlic · tomatoes
· spring onions · olives · cheese

Salmon sandwiches with wasabi mayonnaise

6 tablespoons reduced-fat mayonnaise
2 tablespoons rice **vinegar**
1 tablespoon grated fresh root ginger
1½ teaspoons wasabi powder
    (see Ingredient note)
1 teaspoon mirin (*see* Ingredient note)
200g can **salmon**, drained and flaked
2 tablespoons chopped **spring onions**
1 tablespoon sesame **seeds**, toasted (*see* Tip)
8 slices **pumpernickel bread**
⅓ cucumber, thinly sliced
100g trimmed watercress sprigs,
    rinsed and dried

serves	PREPARATION TIME: **20 MINUTES**
4	COOKING TIME: **0 MINUTES**

When you get tired of tuna sandwiches, try this recipe, which takes its inspiration from the sushi bar. Canned salmon is an essential storecupboard staple and a convenient way to get the omega-3 benefits of oily fish, as well as useful calcium (from the salmon bones).

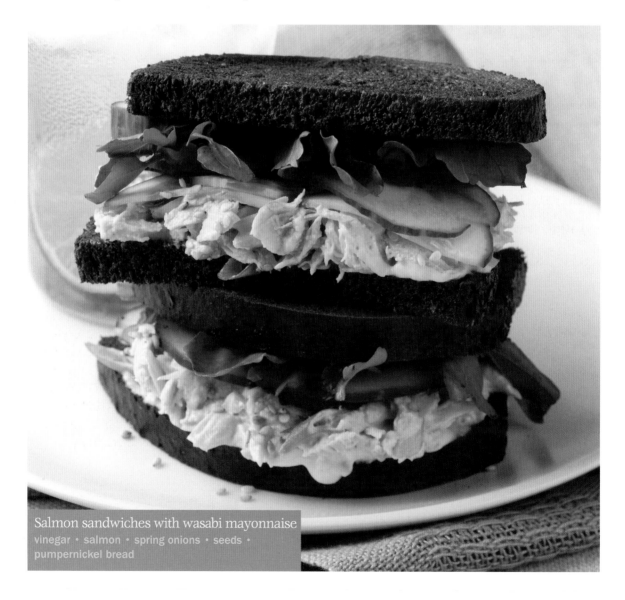

Salmon sandwiches with wasabi mayonnaise
vinegar • salmon • spring onions • seeds •
pumpernickel bread

1 **Whisk 3 tablespoons** of the mayonnaise with the rice vinegar, ginger, wasabi powder and mirin in a medium bowl. Add the salmon, spring onions and sesame seeds. Mix well.

2 **Spread the remaining** 3 tablespoons mayonnaise over one side of each slice of bread. Divide the salmon mixture among four of the slices, spreading evenly. Top with cucumber slices and watercress. Set the remaining bread slices on top. Cut the sandwiches in half to serve.

PER SERVING: **284**kcal, **18g** protein, **25g** carbohydrate, **3g** fibre, **13g** total fat (**2g** saturated fat), **19mg** cholesterol, **1.8g** salt.

Tip: Toast the sesame seeds in a small, dry frying pan, stirring constantly, for 2–3 minutes or until light golden and fragrant.

Ingredient notes:
■ *Wasabi, the pungent sushi condiment sometimes called Japanese horseradish, is made from the stalk of a semi-aquatic member of the cabbage family. You can find both wasabi paste and powder (mix with water) in the ethnic foods section of most supermarkets.*

■ *Mirin is a sweet wine made from glutinous rice. It has a low alcohol content. Look for it in the ethnic foods section of supermarkets.*

Grilled aubergine sandwiches with red pepper and walnut sauce

PREPARATION TIME: **30 MINUTES**

serves 4 COOKING TIME: **0 MINUTES**

This sophisticated and delicious sandwich uses low-GL sourdough bread. It is perfect for lunch or supper. To turn into panini, spritz the outside of the sandwiches with cooking spray and grill in a panini grill or on a griddle pan.

RED PEPPER AND WALNUT SAUCE
30g **walnuts**
1 tablespoon fine dried breadcrumbs
1 **garlic** clove, finely chopped
1 teaspoon ground cumin
Good pinch of crushed dried chillies
Good pinch of salt, or to taste
200g roasted red peppers from a jar, drained and rinsed
1 tablespoon **lemon** juice

SANDWICHES
2 medium-large baby **aubergines**, cut crossways into 1cm thick slices
1/4 teaspoon salt, or to taste
Freshly ground black pepper to taste
8 small slices **sourdough bread**, toasted if you like
125g creamy goat's **cheese**, cut into 1cm slices
50g wild rocket leaves, washed and dried

1 **Combine the walnuts,** breadcrumbs, garlic, cumin, chillies and salt in a food processor and process until the walnuts are ground. Add the peppers and lemon juice and process until smooth. Set aside. (The sauce can be kept, covered, in the refrigerator for up to 4 days.)

2 **Preheat the grill.** Lightly oil the grill rack. Spritz both sides of the aubergine slices with cooking spray and season with salt and pepper. Grill for 4–6 minutes on each side or until very tender and browned.

3 **Spread about** 1½ tablespoons of the sauce over one side of each slice of bread. Layer the slices of aubergine and goat's cheese on four slices of bread and top with the rocket. Set the remaining bread on top. Cut the sandwiches in half to serve. (If the bread is not toasted, the sandwiches can be kept, wrapped in cling film or foil, in the refrigerator for up to 2 days.)

PER SERVING: **351**kcal, **14g** protein, **35g** carbohydrate, **5g** fibre, **18g** total fat (**6g** saturated fat), **29mg** cholesterol, **1.7g** salt.

Tip: Instead of grilling the aubergine slices, you can cook them on a ridged griddle pan.

Tuna and carrot sandwich on rye

carrot • lemon • olive oil • spring onion •
tuna • rye bread

Tuna and carrot sandwich on rye

serves 2

PREPARATION TIME: 15 MINUTES

COOKING TIME: 0 MINUTES

Here's a great sandwich, with a lemony grated carrot salad to add vegetable crunch and rye bread to help lower your blood sugar.

1 medium **carrot**, grated
2 teaspoons **lemon** juice
2 teaspoons extra virgin **olive oil**
1 tablespoon chopped **spring onion**
1 tablespoon chopped fresh dill or parsley
Good pinch of salt, or to taste
100g can light **tuna** in water, drained and flaked
30g finely chopped celery
2 tablespoons reduced-fat mayonnaise
4 slices **rye** or **pumpernickel bread**
4 lettuce leaves, rinsed and dried

1 **Combine the carrot,** lemon juice, olive oil, spring onion, dill (or parsley) and salt in a small bowl. Toss with a fork to mix.

2 **Mix the tuna** and celery with 1 tablespoon of the mayonnaise in another bowl. Spread the remaining mayonnaise over the bread. Cover two of the slices with the tuna mixture, add the carrot salad and lettuce, and top with the remaining bread slices. Cut each sandwich in half to serve. The sandwiches will keep, well wrapped, in the refrigerator for up to a day.

PER SERVING: **215**kcal, **18g** protein, **27g** carbohydrate, **4g** fibre, **4.5g** total fat (**0.7g** saturated fat), **0mg** cholesterol, **1.4g** salt.

Barley-bean soup

serves 8

PREPARATION TIME: 30 MINUTES

COOKING TIME: 40 MINUTES

This nourishing, yet low-calorie soup focuses on low-GL beans and barley, and Magic vegetables such as carrots and spinach.

2 litres unsalted chicken or vegetable stock
6 **garlic** cloves, crushed
2 sprigs fresh rosemary
Good pinch of crushed dried chillies
400g can red kidney **beans**, drained and rinsed
2 teaspoons **olive oil**
1 medium **onion**, chopped
3 medium **carrots**, diced
1 celery stick, diced
400g can chopped **tomatoes** (undrained)
200g pearl **barley**
400g baby **spinach**, washed
Freshly ground black pepper to taste
50g Parmesan **cheese**, freshly grated

1 **Bring the stock** to the boil in a large pan. Add the garlic, rosemary and chillies. Partly cover the pan and simmer for 15 minutes to intensify the flavour. Strain the stock through a sieve into a large bowl. Discard the flavourings.

2 **Mash half** the kidney beans in a small bowl with a fork, then set aside. Heat the oil in a large saucepan over a medium heat. Add the onion, carrots and celery. Cook, stirring often, for 3–4 minutes or until softened. Pour in the infused stock. Add the tomatoes, barley and reserved mashed and whole beans. Bring to a simmer, stirring occasionally. Reduce the heat to medium-low, cover and cook for about 35 minutes or until the barley is almost tender.

3 **Stir in the spinach.** Cover and cook for a further 3–5 minutes or until the spinach has wilted and the barley is tender. Season with pepper. Serve hot, topped with Parmesan cheese.

PER SERVING: **200**kcal, **9g** protein, **34g** carbohydrate, **5g** fibre, **4g** total fat (**1.5g** saturated fat), **6mg** cholesterol, **0.7g** salt.

Hearty split pea soup with rye croutons

serves 4

PREPARATION TIME: 15 MINUTES
COOKING TIME: 1 HOUR

An old-fashioned split pea soup is back on the menu for Magic eating. Split peas, which are a good source of plant protein and fibre, are amazingly filling, making this soup wonderful for a midweek supper. It's also handy to take to the office for lunch – it will easily sustain you through the afternoon. The rye bread croutons are really easy to make and give the soup a final flourish. They're a far healthier alternative to ready-made croutons, which are typically made with white flour and often contain trans fats.

4 teaspoons **olive oil**
60g diced back bacon
1 medium **onion**, chopped
3 medium **carrots**, chopped
1.25 litres chicken stock made without salt
200g green **split peas**, picked over and rinsed
1 teaspoon dried summer savory or thyme
Good pinch of cayenne pepper
1 bay leaf
2 slices **rye bread**, cut into small cubes

1 **Heat 2 teaspoons** of the oil in a large saucepan over a medium heat. Add the bacon, onion and carrots. Cook, stirring often, for 3–5 minutes or until softened and lightly browned. Add the stock, split peas, savory (or thyme), cayenne and bay leaf. Bring to a simmer, then reduce the heat to medium-low, cover and cook for about 1 hour or until the split peas have broken down and thickened the soup.

2 **Meanwhile, preheat** the oven to 180°C/gas 4. Toss the bread cubes with the remaining 2 teaspoons oil in a medium bowl. Spread out in a small baking tray and bake for 15–20 minutes or until crisp.

3 **When the soup** is ready, discard the bay leaf. Ladle into bowls and garnish each serving with rye croutons. The soup can be kept, covered, in the refrigerator, for up to 2 days.

PER SERVING: **350**kcal, **27g** protein, **45g** carbohydrate, **6g** fibre, **10g** total fat (**2g** saturated fat), **8mg** cholesterol, **0.5g** salt.

Curried red lentil soup

serves 8

PREPARATION TIME: 15 MINUTES
COOKING TIME: 25 MINUTES

You may think of lentils as something to store in the back of your storecupboard until a day when you have lots of time to soak them and then wait for them to cook. But lentils, especially the red variety, are surprisingly convenient. They require no presoaking and cook up quickly – red lentils in just 20 minutes and brown lentils in about 30 minutes.

2 teaspoons canola (rapeseed) oil
2 medium **onions**, chopped
4 **garlic** cloves, finely chopped
4–5 teaspoons mild curry powder
285g red **lentils**, rinsed and picked over
1.5 litres chicken or vegetable stock made without salt
180ml water
2 tablespoons **tomato** purée
¼ teaspoon ground **cinnamon**
2 tablespoons **lemon** juice
¼ teaspoon salt, or to taste
Freshly ground black pepper to taste
125g fat-free plain **yoghurt**
4 tablespoons chopped **spring onion** greens

1 **Heat the oil** in a large saucepan over a medium heat. Add the onions and cook, stirring frequently, for 2–3 minutes or until softened. Add the garlic and curry powder, and cook, stirring, for 30 seconds.

2 **Add the lentils** and stir to coat. Add the stock, water, tomato purée and cinnamon. Bring to a simmer, then reduce the heat to low, cover and simmer for 20 minutes or until the lentils are very tender.

3 **In batches,** transfer the soup to a food processor or blender and process to a smooth purée. (Take care as the liquid will be very hot.) Return the purée to the pan and heat through.

4 **Season with the lemon juice,** salt and pepper. Ladle into bowls and garnish each serving with a dollop of yoghurt and a sprinkling of spring onion greens. The soup can be kept, covered, in the refrigerator for up to 2 days.

PER SERVING: **142**kcal, **11g** protein, **23g** carbohydrate, **2.3g** fibre, **1g** total fat (**0.2g** saturated fat), **0mg** cholesterol, **0.2g** salt.

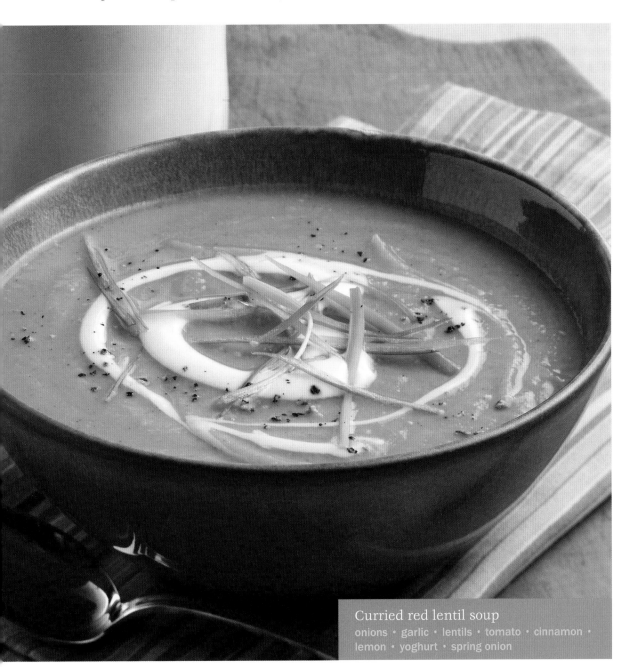

Curried red lentil soup

onions • garlic • lentils • tomato • cinnamon • lemon • yoghurt • spring onion

Peanut and chicken soup

serves
8

PREPARATION TIME: 20 MINUTES

COOKING TIME: 25 MINUTES

If you think peanut butter is just for toast, think again. The secret ingredient in this soup (based on a traditional African recipe), it contributes exceptionally rich flavour and body, but without the saturated fat. It also boosts the protein content of this simple but tasty recipe.

2 teaspoons canola (rapeseed) oil

1 medium **onion**, chopped

3 **garlic** cloves, finely chopped

1 tablespoon mild curry powder

750ml chicken stock made without salt

400g can chopped **tomatoes** (undrained)

1 small **sweet potato**, peeled and cut into 1cm pieces

450g **chicken** breast fillets, trimmed and cut into 1cm pieces

85g smooth, unsweetened **peanut butter**

20g fresh coriander leaves, chopped

2 tablespoons **lime** juice

Dash of Tabasco sauce

1 **Heat the oil** in a large saucepan over a medium-high heat. Add the onion and cook, stirring often, for 2–3 minutes or until softened. Add the garlic and curry powder and cook, stirring, for about 20 seconds or until fragrant.

2 **Add the stock,** tomatoes and sweet potato and stir to mix. Bring to a simmer, then reduce the heat to medium-low, cover and simmer for 10 minutes.

3 **Add the chicken.** Cover the pan again and simmer for a further 10 minutes or until the sweet potatoes are tender and the chicken is cooked through.

4 **Add the peanut butter** and stir until it has blended into the soup. Stir in the coriander, lime juice and Tabasco. Ladle into bowls and serve hot. The soup can be kept, covered, in the refrigerator for up to 2 days.

PER SERVING: **165**kcal, **17g** protein, **9g** carbohydrate, **1.7g** fibre, **7g** total fat (**1.7g** saturated fat), **39mg** cholesterol, **0.3g** salt.

*Ingredient note: **Unsweetened peanut butter,** which will say 'no added sugar' on the label, is made just with peanuts, oil (usually palm oil) and salt. The flavour of unsweetened peanut butter is richer and nuttier than peanut butters that contain sweeteners.*

Oriental noodle hotpot

serves 8

PREPARATION TIME: 15 MINUTES

COOKING TIME: 30 MINUTES

Serving noodles in a fragrant, spicy broth is a good way to ensure an appropriate portion size. The stock base for this soup is infused with ginger and garlic to give it a characteristic oriental flavour. Rounding out the broth and noodles are several key Magic foods: cabbage, carrots, tofu and vinegar. You can substitute diced cooked chicken for the tofu, if you prefer.

1.25 litres chicken or vegetable stock made without salt
3 slices (5mm thick) peeled fresh root ginger
2 **garlic** cloves, crushed
¼ teaspoon crushed dried chillies
2 teaspoons canola (rapeseed) oil
125g fresh shiitake mushrooms, stalks removed, wiped clean and sliced
½ medium head **Chinese leaves** or green cabbage, shredded
225g firm **tofu**, drained, patted dry and cut into 2.5cm cubes
3 medium **carrots**, grated
2 teaspoons reduced-salt soy sauce
2 teaspoons rice **vinegar**
1 teaspoon toasted sesame oil
125g **wholemeal linguine** or spaghetti
2 medium **spring onions**, chopped

1 **Bring a large saucepan** of lightly salted water to the boil.

2 **Bring the stock** to a simmer in another large saucepan. Add the ginger, garlic and chillies. Partly cover and simmer over a medium-low heat for 15 minutes to intensify the flavour. Strain the stock through a sieve into another large saucepan and discard the flavourings. Set the pan of stock aside.

3 **Heat the oil** in a large non-stick frying pan over a medium-high heat. Add the sliced mushrooms and cook, stirring often, for 3–5 minutes or until tender. Add the Chinese leaves (or cabbage) and cook, stirring often, for a further 2–3 minutes or until almost tender.

4 **Add the mushrooms** and Chinese leaves to the pan of infused stock. Simmer, partly covered, over a medium-low heat for about 5 minutes or until the Chinese leaves are tender. Add the tofu and carrots and heat through. Stir in the soy sauce, vinegar and sesame oil.

5 **Meanwhile, cook** the linguine (or spaghetti) in the boiling water for 6–9 minutes, or according to the packet instructions, until *al dente*. Drain the linguine and divide among four large soup bowls. Ladle the soup over the noodles and garnish each serving with the chopped spring onions.

PER SERVING: **110**kcal, **6g** protein, **15g** carbohydrate, **3g** fibre, **3.5g** total fat, (**0.5g** saturated fat), **0mg** cholesterol, **0.5g** salt.

Ingredient note: **Tofu, or bean curd,** *is a high-protein food made from soya beans. The two main types are firm tofu, which comes in a block packed in water (or vacuum-packed), and silken tofu. Firm tofu has a texture similar to feta cheese, while silken tofu is – as its name suggests – creamy in texture. Firm tofu is also available smoked.*

Beef, lamb and pork

Orange beef stir-fry with broccoli and red pepper

serves 4

PREPARATION TIME: **30 MINUTES**
COOKING TIME: **8 MINUTES**

Recipes for beef and broccoli stir-fries may be commonplace, but this one stands out, because stir-frying orange zest with fresh ginger gives the sauce extraordinary fragrance and flavour. The dish provides a generous quantity of vegetables balanced with lean protein, which means you get excellent nutritional value for the calories. For convenience, you can substitute frozen broccoli florets for fresh and frozen stir-fry vegetables for the fresh red pepper and onion.

125ml orange juice
2 tablespoons reduced-salt soy sauce
1 tablespoon oyster sauce
1 tablespoon rice **vinegar**
1½ teaspoons Thai chilli sauce or other
    hot chilli sauce
1½ teaspoons cornflour
1 tablespoon vegetable oil
340g rump **steak**, trimmed and cut into strips
    about 5cm long and 5mm thick
1 tablespoon very finely chopped fresh
    root ginger
2 teaspoons grated orange zest (see Tip)
3 **garlic** cloves, finely chopped
1 medium **onion**, sliced
450g **broccoli** crowns, cut into 2.5cm florets
1 red or yellow pepper, deseeded and cut into
    strips about 5cm long and 5mm thick

1 **In a small bowl,** whisk together the orange juice, soy sauce, oyster sauce, vinegar, chilli sauce and cornflour. Set aside.

2 **Heat 1 teaspoon oil** in a large wok or non-stick frying pan over a high heat. Add half of the steak and cook, without stirring or turning, for about 1 minute or until browned on the underside. Stir and turn the strips, then cook for about 30 seconds or just until browned on the other side. Transfer to a plate. Add another 1 teaspoon oil to the wok and brown the rest of the steak; transfer to the plate.

3 **Add the remaining** 1 teaspoon oil to the wok, then add the ginger, orange zest and garlic and stir-fry for 10–20 seconds or until fragrant. Add the onion and stir-fry for 1 minute. Add the broccoli and red pepper and stir-fry for 30 seconds. Add 4 tablespoons water. Cover the wok and cook for about 1½ minutes or until the vegetables are just tender but still crisp.

4 **Push the vegetables** to the outside of the wok. Stir the reserved sauce mixture, then pour it into the centre of the wok and cook, stirring, for 1 minute or until glossy and thickened. Stir the vegetables into the sauce. Return the steak to the wok and turn to coat with the sauce. Serve immediately.

PER SERVING: **200**kcal, **24g** protein, **11g** carbohydrate, **3.3g** fibre, **7g** total fat (**2g** saturated fat), **50mg** cholesterol, **1g** salt.

*Tip: **A citrus zester is the easiest way** to remove very fine shreds of zest from oranges and lemons. If you haven't got one, use a vegetable peeler to take a very thin layer of zest from the fruit, then finely chop the zest. Or cover a grater with cling film and use the fine holes to grate off the zest from the fruit.*

onions look here for chromium, a key mineral for blood sugar control

broccoli add this bulky vegetable to meat dishes to stretch the meat

beef when low-fat, it's a Magic source of protein

vinegar tart and tangy, it lowers a meal's GL

Orange beef stir-fry with broccoli and red pepper

garlic no stir-fry is complete without this heart-helper

Rump steak with balsamic sauce

vinegar · garlic · steak · shallot · olive oil

Rump steak with balsamic sauce

serves 6   PREPARATION TIME: 20 MINUTES

MARINATING TIME: 2 HOURS

COOKING TIME: 12–14 MINUTES

One of the leaner cuts of beef, rump steak is an excellent choice when you're craving steak for dinner. It has lots of flavour, and becomes really juicy and tender when marinated. Since you slice the steak before serving, it's easy to control portion sizes. In this recipe, the zesty marinade is transformed into a rich-tasting sauce. We use a ridged griddle pan, but you can also cook the steak on the barbecue or grill it.

85ml orange juice or port wine

4 tablespoons balsamic **vinegar**

1 teaspoon Worcestershire sauce

1 tablespoon chopped fresh thyme or 1 teaspoon
   dried thyme

2 **garlic** cloves, finely chopped

½ teaspoon salt, or to taste

Freshly ground black pepper to taste

700g rump **steak**, trimmed

2 tablespoons finely chopped **shallot**

1 teaspoon **olive oil**

Small knob of unsalted butter (about 10g)

1 **In a small bowl,** whisk together the orange juice (or port), vinegar, Worcestershire sauce, thyme, garlic, salt and pepper. Place the steak in a shallow glass dish, pour over the orange juice mixture and turn to coat. Cover and leave to marinate in the refrigerator for at least 2 hours or up to 8 hours, turning several times.

2 **Remove the steak** from the marinade and pour the marinade into a small saucepan. Add the shallot and set aside. Heat a ridged griddle pan (or a heavy frying pan). Brush with the oil, then add the steak and cook over a medium-high heat for 6–7 minutes on each side for medium-rare (depending on the thickness of the steak). If you prefer your meat well done, cook for longer. Transfer to a chopping board and allow to rest for 5 minutes.

3 **Meanwhile,** bring the marinade to the boil over a medium-high heat and cook for 3–5 minutes or until reduced to about 5 tablespoons. Remove from the heat, add the butter and whisk until melted.

4 **Slice the steak** thinly across the grain. Add any accumulated juices on the chopping board to the sauce and serve the sauce with the steak. Any leftover steak can be kept, covered, in the refrigerator for up to 2 days.

PER SERVING: **183**kcal, **26g** protein,
   4.5g carbohydrate, **0g** fibre, **7g** total fat
   (**3g** saturated fat), **7mg** cholesterol, **0.6g** salt.

Slow-cooker beef and red wine stew

8

PREPARATION TIME: 30 MINUTES
COOKING TIME: 15 MINUTES ON THE
STOVETOP, THEN 4–4½ HOURS IN THE
SLOW COOKER ON HIGH OR 7–8 HOURS ON LOW

The trick to making a healthful, hearty meat stew is to include lots of vegetables and a rich-tasting yet low-fat sauce. This stew keeps well and is even better the next day.

700g lean boneless **beef**, cut into 4cm cubes
¼ teaspoon salt, or to taste
½ teaspoon freshly ground black pepper
1 tablespoon **olive oil**
1 medium **onion**, chopped
2 tablespoons plain flour
4 **garlic** cloves, finely chopped
250ml dry red wine
400g can chopped **tomatoes** (undrained)
180ml chicken stock made without salt
1 teaspoon Worcestershire sauce
1½ teaspoons dried thyme
2 bay leaves
300g baby **carrots**, peeled
2 medium white turnips, peeled and cut into
    bite-size chunks
170g baby **onions**, blanched and peeled
20g fresh parsley, chopped

1 **Pat the beef dry** with kitchen paper and sprinkle with the salt and pepper. Heat 2 teaspoons oil in a large non-stick frying pan over a medium-high heat. Add half of the beef and cook, turning occasionally, for 3–5 minutes or until browned all over. Transfer to a plate. Repeat with the remaining beef and transfer to the plate.

2 **Add the remaining** 1 teaspoon oil to the pan, then add the chopped onion and cook, stirring frequently, for 1–2 minutes or until softened and lightly browned. Add the flour and garlic and cook, stirring, for 30–60 seconds. Add the wine and bring to the boil, stirring to scrape

up any browned bits from the pan. Add the tomatoes and mash in with a potato masher. Stir in the stock, Worcestershire sauce, thyme and bay leaves. Bring to a simmer.

3 **Place the browned beef** in a slow cooker (4 litre capacity) and spoon over half of the tomato and wine sauce. Place the carrots, turnips and baby onions on top of the sauce and spoon the remaining sauce over them evenly. Cover the slow cooker and cook for 4–4½ hours on high, or 7–8 hours on low, or until the beef and vegetables are very tender.

4 **When the stew is ready,** discard the bay leaves. Ladle on to warmed plates and sprinkle with the parsley before serving.

PER SERVING: **194** kcal, **21g** protein,
    11g carbohydrate, **2.3g** fibre, **5g** total fat
    (**1.7g** saturated fat), **52mg** cholesterol, **0.4g** salt.

VARIATIONS
Lamb stew with spring vegetables

In Step 1, instead of beef use boneless lean leg of lamb, trimmed and cut into cubes. In Step 2, substitute dry white wine for the red wine and 2 tablespoons chopped fresh rosemary for the thyme. In Step 3, omit the turnips. In Step 4, cook 225g frozen peas according to packet instructions, then add to the stew after discarding the bay leaves.

Pork stew with Mexican flavours

In Step 1, instead of beef use boneless lean pork (choose a leg cut rather than shoulder, which is higher in fat), trimmed and cut into cubes. In Step 2, substitute 1½ teaspoons ground cumin and ¾ teaspoon dried oregano for the dried thyme and bay leaves, and add a good pinch of crushed dried chillies (or more to taste). In Step 3, omit the carrots and turnips, and instead add 1 medium sweet

Savoury beef and vegetable loaf

serves

8

PREPARATION TIME: 20 MINUTES
BAKING TIME: 1 HOUR AND 5 MINUTES TO
1 HOUR AND 20 MINUTES

An old-fashioned favourite gets a new lease of life with this Magic meat loaf makeover. We stretched the minced beef with grated carrots and courgettes, thus reducing the saturated fat, boosting the vegetable quota and adding moisture. Wholegrain rolled oats play the role of filler and help keep the meat loaf tender. If you're running late and can't wait for the large meat loaf to bake, make individual loaves: divide the meat mixture among eight muffin cups coated with cooking spray and bake them for about 30 minutes.

450g extra-lean minced or ground **beef**
60g rolled **oats**
1 medium **onion**, chopped
3 medium **carrots**, grated
1 medium **courgette**, grated
1 medium **egg**, lightly beaten
2 medium **egg** whites, lightly beaten
2 tablespoons tomato ketchup
1 tablespoon Worcestershire sauce
2 teaspoons Dijon mustard
1 teaspoon dried thyme
¾ teaspoon salt
½ teaspoon freshly ground black pepper

1 **Preheat the oven** to 180°C/gas 4. Line a loaf tin (measuring about 20–23 x 10–12cm) with foil, leaving a 2.5cm overhang along the two long sides. Coat the foil with cooking spray.

2 **In a large bowl,** combine the mince, oats, onion, carrots, courgette, egg, egg whites, 1 tablespoon ketchup, the Worcestershire sauce, mustard, thyme, salt and pepper and mix together well. Transfer to the loaf tin and press down firmly into all the corners. Spread the remaining ketchup over the top of the loaf.

3 **Set the tin** on a baking tray and place in the oven. Bake for 1 hour. Drain off the fat from the tin, then continue baking for 5–20 minutes or until firm (timing depends on the depth of the tin). Drain off the fat again, then leave the meat loaf to rest for 5 minutes. Use the foil overhang to lift it out and transfer to a chopping board. Cut into slices to serve. Any leftover meat loaf will keep, covered, in the refrigerator for up to 2 days.

PER SERVING: **170**kcal, **16g** protein, **11g** carbohydrate, **1.7g** fibre, **7g** total fat (**2.5g** saturated fat), **61mg** cholesterol, **0.9g** salt.

Greek pasta and beef casserole

serves 8

PREPARATION TIME: 50 MINUTES

BAKING TIME: 40–50 MINUTES

Known as pastitsio, this hearty Greek casserole serves up layers of creamy macaroni cheese separated by cinnamon-scented meat sauce. Like its Italian cousin, lasagne, it's an ideal make-ahead meal (assemble it up to the end of Step 7, then cover and keep in the refrigerator for up to 2 days). While there are several parts to this lightened version, none is difficult to make, and you can break up the workload by preparing the meat sauce a day ahead (it's also delicious on its own, tossed with wholemeal pasta).

MEAT SAUCE

340g extra-lean minced or ground **beef**

2 teaspoons **olive oil**

1 large **onion**, chopped

3 **garlic** cloves, finely chopped

1½ teaspoons dried oregano

1 teaspoon ground **cinnamon**

½ teaspoon sugar

¼ teaspoon salt, or to taste

125ml dry white wine or chicken stock made without salt

400g can chopped **tomatoes** (undrained)

65g **tomato** purée

20g fresh parsley, chopped

Freshly ground black pepper to taste

MACARONI CHEESE

600ml semi-skimmed **milk**

50g plain flour

1 medium **egg**

2 medium **egg** whites

225g low-fat cottage **cheese**

85g Gruyère **cheese**, grated

¼ teaspoon grated nutmeg

¼ teaspoon salt, or to taste

Freshly ground black pepper to taste

250g **wholemeal macaroni** (see Ingredient note)

15g Parmesan **cheese**, freshly grated

1 **Preheat the oven** to 200°C/gas 6. Coat an ovenproof dish, measuring about 23 x 35cm, with cooking spray. Bring a large saucepan of water to the boil.

2 **To make the meat sauce:** cook the mince in a medium non-stick frying pan over a medium-high heat, breaking it up with a wooden spoon, for 3–4 minutes or until browned. Tip into a colander and leave to drain.

3 **Heat the oil** in a flameproof casserole or large saucepan over a medium heat. Add the onion and cook, stirring frequently, for 3–4 minutes or until softened. Add the garlic, oregano, cinnamon, sugar and salt and cook, stirring, for 30 seconds. Add the wine (or stock) and stir to mix, then bring to a simmer.

4 **Add the tomatoes** and mash them in with a potato masher. Bring back to a simmer and stir in the tomato purée and browned mince. Reduce the heat to medium-low, partly cover the pan and simmer, stirring occasionally, for 20 minutes. At the end of this time, stir in the parsley and black pepper.

5 **While the meat sauce is simmering,** make the macaroni cheese. In a small bowl, whisk 125ml of the milk with the flour until smooth. Heat the remaining milk in a medium saucepan over a medium heat until steaming. Add the flour mixture and cook, whisking constantly, for 3–4 minutes or until the sauce bubbles and thickens. Remove from the heat. In a small bowl, blend the egg and egg whites with a fork, then gradually whisk into the hot sauce. Stir in the cottage cheese, Gruyère cheese, nutmeg, salt and pepper. Set aside.

6 **Add the macaroni** to the pan of boiling water and cook for just 4½ minutes, then drain and rinse under cold running water (the macaroni is only blanched at this stage as it will continue to cook during baking). Transfer to a large bowl, add the cheese sauce and toss to coat.

7 **Spread half of the macaroni cheese** in the ovenproof dish, then spread the meat sauce on top. Cover with the remaining macaroni cheese and sprinkle over the Parmesan.

8 **Place the dish in the oven** and bake for 40–50 minutes or until the top is golden and the casserole is bubbling. Remove from the oven and leave to stand for 5 minutes before serving. Any leftovers can be kept, tightly covered, in the refrigerator for up to 2 days.

PER SERVING: **350**kcal, **27g** protein, **34g** carbohydrate, **3.6g** fibre, **12.5g** total fat (**6g** saturated fat), **72mg** cholesterol, **1.1g** salt.

Ingredient note: **Although macaroni** *is the traditional pasta to use for this casserole, you can substitute other pasta shapes such as penne and rigatoni.*

Mustard-crusted lamb chops

serves 4

PREPARATION TIME: **15 MINUTES**
MARINATING TIME: **30 MINUTES**
COOKING TIME: **10 MINUTES**

A full-flavoured marinade of grainy mustard, rosemary and garlic brings out the best in delicate lamb chops and forms an appealing crust during grilling or barbecuing. You can also use the marinade for grilled lamb kebabs, or increase the proportions to make a marinade for a leg of lamb to be roasted.

3 tablespoons coarse-grain mustard
2 tablespoons chopped fresh rosemary
2 tablespoons red wine **vinegar**
1 tablespoon extra virgin **olive oil**
½ teaspoon Worcestershire sauce
4 **garlic** cloves, finely chopped
¼ teaspoon salt
Freshly ground black pepper to taste
8 loin **lamb** chops (85g each), trimmed

1 **In a shallow glass dish,** whisk the mustard, rosemary, vinegar, oil, Worcestershire sauce, garlic, salt and pepper together until blended. Add the lamb chops and turn to coat well. Cover and leave to marinate in the refrigerator for at least 30 minutes or up to 4 hours.

2 **Preheat the grill** to high, or prepare a charcoal fire in the barbecue (when the flames die down and the coals are grey you are ready to cook).

3 **Lightly oil the grill** or barbecue rack by rubbing a piece of oil-soaked kitchen paper over the surface. Place the lamb chops on the rack and grill or barbecue for 4–5 minutes on each side for medium-rare (cook for longer if you prefer them medium). Serve hot.

PER SERVING: **340**kcal, **42g** protein, **1g** carbohydrate, **0g** fibre, **19g** total fat (**7g** saturated fat), **134mg** cholesterol, **1.4g** salt.

Pork chop and cabbage pan-fry

serves 4

PREPARATION TIME: 20 MINUTES

COOKING TIME: 20 MINUTES

Teamed with a low-calorie cabbage and carrot mix, pork chops make a hearty meal in minutes, especially when everything is cooked in the same pan (this saves on washing-up, too). If you use thin-cut boneless loin chops (about 1cm thick), you can ensure an appropriate portion size and still get all the protein benefits of lean meat. To trim the preparation time, use the food processor slicing disc to slice and shred the onion, carrots and cabbage.

1 teaspoon dried thyme

¼ teaspoon salt

¼ teaspoon freshly ground black pepper, or to taste

4 thin-cut boneless **pork** loin chops, about 450g, trimmed

1 tablespoon canola (rapeseed) oil

1 medium **onion**, sliced

½ medium green **cabbage**, shredded

2 medium **carrots**, sliced

350ml chicken stock made without salt

180ml water

2 teaspoons coarse-grain mustard

1 teaspoon cider **vinegar**

1 **In a small bowl,** combine the thyme, salt and pepper. Rub the mixture over the pork chops. Heat 2 teaspoons oil in a large non-stick frying pan over a medium heat. Add the chops

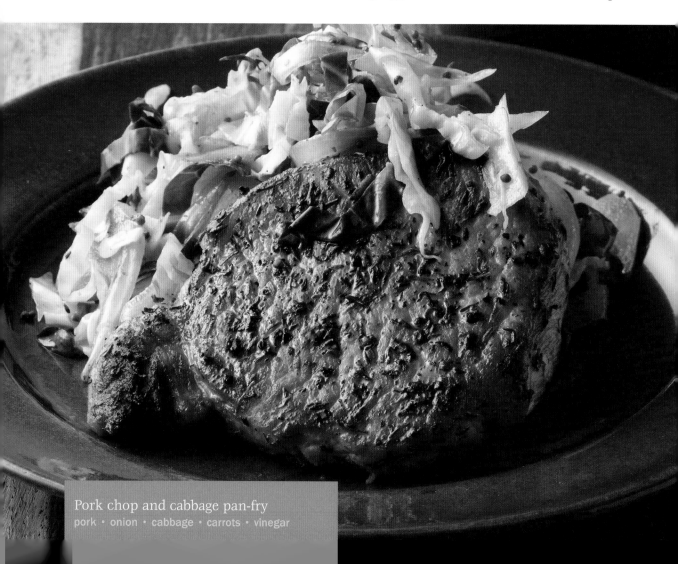

Pork chop and cabbage pan-fry

pork · onion · cabbage · carrots · vinegar

and cook for 2–3 minutes on each side or until browned and just cooked through. Transfer the chops to a plate, cover loosely with foil to keep them warm and set aside.

2 **Add the remaining** 1 teaspoon oil to the pan. Add the onion and cook over a medium heat, stirring frequently, for 1–2 minutes or until softened. Add the cabbage and carrots and cook, stirring, for about 2 minutes or until the cabbage is wilted. Add the stock and water and bring to a simmer. Cover and cook for 10–15 minutes or until the cabbage is tender. Stir in the mustard and vinegar and season with pepper.

3 **Place the chops** on individual warmed plates and spoon the cabbage alongside the chops. Serve immediately.

PER SERVING: **200**kcal, **26g** protein, **7g** carbohydrate, **2.5g** fibre, **8g** total fat (**2g** saturated fat), **71mg** cholesterol, **0.6g** salt.

Spice-crusted pork tenderloin with peach salsa

serves 4

PREPARATION TIME: **35 MINUTES**
COOKING TIME: **20–25 MINUTES**

Luscious peaches – one of the sweet Magic foods – are not just for desserts. Try them in this lively salsa, which sets off lean pork tenderloin beautifully. If you prefer to roast the pork, brown the tenderloin in 1 teaspoon vegetable oil in a frying pan for 2–4 minutes, then transfer to a roasting tin and roast in a 200°C/gas 6 oven for 15–20 minutes.

SALSA
1 large **peach**, peeled, stoned and diced (see Tip, page 244)
½ small red pepper, deseeded and diced
2 medium **spring onions**, chopped
1 fresh green chilli, deseeded and finely chopped
2 tablespoons **lime** juice
1 tablespoon chopped fresh coriander
Pinch of salt

PORK
2 teaspoons ground cumin
1 teaspoon soft brown sugar
1 teaspoon paprika
½ teaspoon ground **cinnamon**
½ teaspoon ground ginger
½ teaspoon salt, or to taste
¼ teaspoon freshly ground black pepper
1 teaspoon canola (rapeseed) oil
450g **pork** tenderloin (fillet), trimmed

1 **Preheat the grill** to medium. Lightly oil the grill rack by rubbing it with a piece of oil-soaked kitchen paper.

2 **To make the salsa:** in a medium bowl, combine the peach, red pepper, spring onions, chilli, lime juice, coriander and salt, and toss to mix well together. Set aside.

3 **To prepare the pork:** in a small bowl, combine the cumin, brown sugar, paprika, cinnamon, ginger, salt and pepper. Add the oil and mix well. Rub the spice paste over the pork.

4 **Grill the pork,** turning occasionally, for 20–25 minutes or until it is cooked through. Transfer to a carving board and allow to rest for 5 minutes. Cut into slices 1cm thick and serve with the salsa.

PER SERVING: **165**kcal, **25g** protein, **5g** carbohydrate, **0.8g** fibre, **5g** total fat (**2g** saturated fat), **71mg** cholesterol, **1g** salt.

Tip: **When working with chillies,** *wear rubber or latex gloves to protect your hands from the irritating oils, and be sure not to touch your eyes, lips and other sensitive areas.*

poultry

Chicken fillets with peaches and fresh ginger

serves 4

PREPARATION TIME: **25 MINUTES**
COOKING TIME: **10–12 MINUTES**

Squeezing more fruit into your diet has never been simpler or more delicious. Here, sweet peaches, accented with fresh root ginger, dress up a simple chicken sauté. The vinegar in the sauce balances the sweet flavours and helps lower your blood sugar response to the meal. You can substitute a nectarine or two plums for the peach (there's no need to peel these).

1 bunch **spring onions** (or salad onions), trimmed
450g **chicken** breast fillets, trimmed
¼ teaspoon salt, or to taste
Freshly ground black pepper to taste
2 teaspoons canola (rapeseed) oil
3 tablespoons cider **vinegar**
2 tablespoons sugar
125ml unsweetened peach juice (or apple juice)
2 tablespoons grated fresh root ginger
300ml chicken stock made without salt
1 large **peach**, peeled (see Tip), stoned and
    cut into 1cm wedges
2 teaspoons cornflour
2 teaspoons water

1 **Chop the spring onions,** reserving all of the white part and 4 tablespoons of the green part. Keep the white and green separate.

2 **If the chicken fillets** are large, cut them in half lengthways so that you have at least four pieces. Place each piece of chicken between two sheets of cling film and pound with a rolling pin or meat bat until about 1cm thick. Season the fillets with the salt and some pepper.

3 **Heat the oil** in a large non-stick frying pan over a medium-high heat. Add the chicken and cook for 3–3½ minutes on each side or until they are browned and no longer pink in the centre. Transfer the fillets to a plate.

4 **Add the vinegar** and sugar to the pan and stir to dissolve the sugar. Cook, swirling the syrup in the pan, for 30–60 seconds or until it turns dark amber. Add the white part of the spring onions, peach juice (or apple juice) and ginger. Bring to the boil, stirring to scrape up any caramelized bits in the pan. Cook for 1 minute.

5 **Add the stock** and peaches and bring back to the boil. Cook, turning the peaches from time to time, for 2–4 minutes or until tender. Mix the cornflour and water and add to the sauce. Cook, stirring, for about 30 seconds or until slightly thickened.

6 **Reduce the heat to low** and return the chicken and any accumulated juices to the pan. Simmer gently for about 1 minute or until the chicken is heated through. Serve hot, garnished with the spring onion greens.

PER SERVING: **200**kcal, **28g** protein,
    16g carbohydrate, **0.8g** fibre, **3g** total fat
    (**0.5g** saturated fat), **79mg** cholesterol, **0.4g** salt.

Tips:
■ *To peel peaches, immerse them in boiling water for 20–30 seconds to loosen the skins. Remove with a slotted spoon and cool slightly, then slip off the skins with a small, sharp knife.*
■ *Pounding the chicken fillets to make them thinner ensures that they will cook quickly and evenly.*

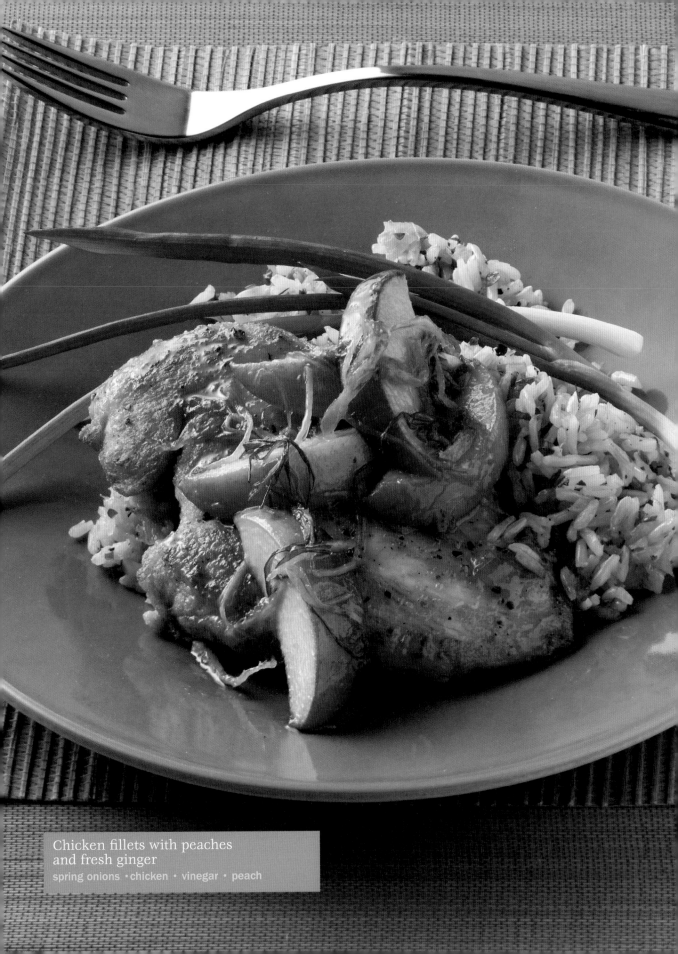

Chicken fillets with peaches
and fresh ginger
spring onions · chicken · vinegar · peach

Chicken sauté with apples

serves
4
PREPARATION TIME: 20 MINUTES
COOKING TIME: 15 MINUTES

This simple chicken sauté features delectable morsels of boneless chicken and a generous amount of a creamy sauce that tastes deceptively rich, thanks to fresh apples and a small amount of half-fat crème fraîche.

450g **chicken** breast fillets, trimmed and cut into 1cm thick slices
Good pinch of salt, or to taste
Freshly ground black pepper to taste
1 tablespoon **olive oil**
1 medium dessert **apple**, peeled, cored and sliced (prepare just before cooking)
1 large **shallot**, finely chopped
¾ teaspoon dried thyme
125ml apple juice
300ml chicken stock made without salt
1½ teaspoons cornflour
2 teaspoons water
4 tablespoons half-fat crème fraîche
2 teaspoons coarse-grain mustard
1 tablespoon chopped fresh parsley or chives

1 **Season the chicken** with salt and pepper. Heat 2 teaspoons of the olive oil in a large non-stick frying pan over a medium-high heat. Add the chicken and cook, turning from time to time, for 5–6 minutes or until the slices are browned all over and no longer pink in the centre. Transfer to a plate, cover loosely with foil to keep warm and set aside.

2 **Add the remaining** 1 teaspoon of oil to the pan. Add the apple, shallot and thyme, and cook, stirring often, for 2–3 minutes or until the apple is lightly browned. Add the apple juice and bring to the boil, stirring well to scrape up any browned bits from the pan. Cook for 1½ minutes. Add the stock and bring back to the boil. Cook for 3 minutes, stirring occasionally.

3 **Mix the cornflour** and water in a small bowl. Add to the sauce and cook, stirring, until slightly thickened. Reduce the heat to low. Whisk in the crème fraîche and mustard until smooth.

4 **Return the chicken** slices to the pan with any juices that have accumulated on the plate. Cook for about 1 minute or just until heated through; do not allow to boil. Garnish with parsley (or chives) to serve.

PER SERVING: **211**kcal, **28g** protein, **16g** carbohydrate, **0.6g** fibre, **4.5g** total fat (**2g** saturated fat), **79mg** cholesterol, **0.5g** salt.

All-new chicken cordon bleu

serves
4
PREPARATION TIME: 25 MINUTES
COOKING TIME: 22 MINUTES

Crisp-coated chicken breasts with a surprise cheese filling are a family favourite. This version trims fat and calories by avoiding deep-frying. Instead, the chicken is browned on one side in a frying pan and then finished in a hot oven, producing a crisp crust without all the fat and fuss. To get things ready ahead of time, prepare the recipe to the end of Step 3, then cover and refrigerate for up to 8 hours.

30g Gruyère or half-fat mozzarella **cheese**, grated
2 tablespoons chopped lean cooked ham
1 tablespoon reduced-fat mayonnaise
2 teaspoons Dijon mustard
Good pinch of freshly ground black pepper
4 **chicken** breast fillets (450–700g total weight), trimmed
50g dried breadcrumbs
1 medium **egg** white
2 teaspoons **olive oil**

1 **Preheat the oven** to 200°C/gas 6. Coat a baking tray with cooking spray. Mix together the cheese, ham, mayonnaise, mustard and pepper in a small bowl. Set aside.

2 **Using a small, sharp knife,** make a horizontal slit along the thinner, long edge of one of the chicken fillets, cutting nearly through to the opposite side. Open up the fillet and place about 1 tablespoon of the cheese mixture in the centre. Close the fillet over the filling and press the edges firmly together to seal. Repeat with the remaining fillets and cheese mixture.

3 **Place the breadcrumbs** in a shallow dish. Lightly beat the egg white with a fork in a medium bowl. Holding each stuffed chicken fillet together, dip it in the egg white, then coat it all over in the breadcrumbs.

4 **Heat the oil** in a large non-stick frying pan over a medium-high heat. Add the chicken fillets and cook for about 2 minutes or until browned on the underside. Using tongs, transfer the fillets to the baking tray, placing them browned side up.

5 **Place the tray in the oven** and bake the chicken for about 20 minutes or until no longer pink in the centre. Serve hot.

PER SERVING: **233**kcal, **32g** protein, **10g** carbohydrate, **0.5g** fibre, **7g** total fat (**2g** saturated fat), **91mg** cholesterol, **1g** salt.

Moroccan-style chicken thighs with butternut squash and baby onions

serves 4
PREPARATION TIME: **25 MINUTES**
COOKING TIME: **40–45 MINUTES**
Try this dish from a roasting tin for a special meal that's really easy to make and serve. Boneless skinless chicken thighs, which cook in the same time as the vegetables, are convenient for roasting. A flavourful spice rub gives them a fat-free 'skin' that seals in their juices.

450g peeled, seeded butternut squash, cut into 2cm cubes
250g baby **onions**, blanched and peeled
4 teaspoons **olive oil**
½ teaspoon salt
Freshly ground black pepper to taste
2 teaspoons clear honey
5 teaspoons **lemon** juice
2 teaspoons paprika
½ teaspoon ground cumin
450g boneless skinless **chicken** thighs, trimmed
12 fresh coriander sprigs, plus coarsely chopped coriander to garnish
250ml chicken stock made without salt

1 **Preheat the oven** to 230°C/gas 8. Coat a large roasting tin with cooking spray.

2 **Combine the butternut squash,** onions, 2 teaspoons oil, ¼ teaspoon salt and some pepper in a large bowl. Toss to coat. Set aside.

3 **Mix the remaining** 2 teaspoons oil with the honey and 2 teaspoons lemon juice in a small bowl until smooth. Add the paprika, cumin, remaining ¼ teaspoon salt and pepper. Rub this mixture over the chicken thighs.

4 **Place the coriander sprigs** in the centre of the roasting tin. Set the chicken thighs on the coriander sprigs and surround with the squash and onions. Place in the oven and roast for 40–45 minutes or until chicken is cooked through and the vegetables are tender, turning the vegetables twice. Transfer the chicken and vegetables to a platter or individual plates (leave the coriander sprigs in the roasting tin).

5 **Add the chicken stock** and remaining lemon juice to the roasting tin and place over a high heat. Bring to a simmer, stirring to scrape up any browned bits. Simmer for 1 minute. Strain the sauce through a sieve into a medium bowl. Spoon the sauce over the chicken and vegetables, sprinkle with chopped coriander and serve.

PER SERVING: **216**kcal, **29g** protein, **16g** carbohydrate, **2.7g** fibre, **4.5g** total fat (**0.8g** saturated fat), **79mg** cholesterol, **0.7g** salt.

Chicken pie with a wholemeal crust

serves
5

PREPARATION TIME: 1 HOUR

BAKING TIME: 30–40 MINUTES

Everyone loves chicken pie, but it can be a killer when it comes to calories. We've topped ours with a tender, low-fat scone pastry and included a generous serving of vegetables bathed in a light yet creamy sauce. Bake this whenever you have leftover cooked chicken, or buy a ready-roasted chicken from the deli counter.

FILLING

2 teaspoons canola (rapeseed) oil
250g button mushrooms, sliced
150g **carrots**, sliced
4 tablespoons plain white flour
550ml chicken or turkey stock made without salt
4 tablespoons half-fat crème fraîche
1½ teaspoons grated lemon zest
Good pinch of salt, or to taste
Good pinch of freshly ground black pepper
325g cooked skinless **chicken**, diced
180g frozen **peas**, rinsed under cold water to thaw

SCONE PASTRY

125g plain **wholemeal flour**
1 teaspoon caster sugar
¾ teaspoon baking powder
¼ teaspoon bicarbonate of soda
Good pinch of salt
60g cold low-fat soft **cheese**, cut into small pieces
15g cold unsalted butter, cut into small pieces
1 tablespoon canola (rapeseed) oil
About 85ml buttermilk
1 teaspoon semi-skimmed **milk** for brushing

1 **Preheat the oven** to 200°C/gas 6. Coat a 20cm square ovenproof dish (or a similar 2 litre capacity dish) with cooking spray.

2 **To make the filling:** heat the oil in a large non-stick frying pan over a medium-high heat. Add the mushrooms and cook, stirring from time to time, for 5–7 minutes or until they are browned and tender. Meanwhile, steam the carrots for 3–5 minutes or until just tender. Rinse them with cold running water to stop them cooking any further. Set the carrots aside with the mushrooms.

3 **Whisk the white flour** with 125ml of the cold stock in a small bowl until smooth. Bring the remaining stock to a simmer in a medium saucepan over a medium-high heat. Gradually whisk in the flour mixture. Cook, whisking, until the sauce boils and thickens. Reduce the heat to low and simmer for 1 minute. Remove from the heat and whisk in the crème fraîche, lemon zest, salt and pepper.

4 **Stir in the chicken,** peas, mushrooms and carrots. Pour the filling into the ovenproof dish, spreading evenly. (You can prepare the filling to this point up to 1 day ahead. Allow the sauce to cool completely before mixing with the vegetables and chicken, then cover and keep in the refrigerator.)

5 **To make the pastry:** whisk the flour, sugar, baking powder, bicarbonate of soda and salt together in a large bowl. Using two knives (or cool fingers), cut or rub in the soft cheese and butter until the mixture resembles coarse crumbs. Add the oil and toss with a fork to blend. With the fork, stir in just enough of the buttermilk to make a soft, slightly sticky dough. Turn out on to a lightly floured surface and knead briefly, just until smooth.

6 **Pat or roll out the dough** into a rough 23 x 18cm rectangle that is about 1cm thick. With a sharp knife, cut the dough in half lengthways, then cut each half into five triangles, trimming to make the sides straight as needed. Arrange the triangles over the filling and brush the top of the scones with milk.

7 **Place the dish** in the oven and bake the pie for 30–40 minutes or until the filling is bubbling and the scone topping is golden and firm. Serve hot.

Tips:

■ *Cutting the scone dough into triangles,* rather than the more traditional circles, allows you to cover a square baking dish efficiently, minimising waste.

■ *If you are cooking for a crowd,* double the recipe and use a 23 x 33cm ovenproof dish.

VARIATION

Turkey pie with a wholemeal crust

In Step 4, substitute diced cooked skinless turkey breast for the chicken. If you have any leftover turkey gravy (unthickened), add it to the sauce at the end of Step 3.

Oven-fried chicken

PREPARATION TIME: 20 MINUTES

serves 4 MARINATING TIME: 30 MINUTES
BAKING TIME: 40–50 MINUTES

This simple chicken recipe, with Magic extras like sesame seeds and mustard (which contains vinegar, a Magic food), makes a great family meal. Marinating the chicken in buttermilk keeps it moist and succulent. A light coating of wholemeal flour, sesame seeds and spices replaces the fatty chicken skin and forms an appealing crust during baking.

1.25–1.5kg **chicken** leg joints, skin removed and fat trimmed
125ml buttermilk
1 tablespoon Dijon mustard
2 **garlic** cloves, finely chopped
1 teaspoon Tabasco sauce
60g **wholemeal flour**
2 tablespoons sesame **seeds**
1½ teaspoons baking powder
1½ teaspoons paprika
1 teaspoon dried thyme
Pinch of salt
Freshly ground black pepper to taste

1 **Cut through the joint** in the chicken legs to separate the thighs and drumsticks. Whisk the buttermilk with the mustard, garlic and Tabasco sauce in a shallow glass dish until well blended. Add the chicken and turn to coat. Cover and leave to marinate in the refrigerator for at least 30 minutes or up to 8 hours.

2 **Preheat the oven** to 220°C/gas 7. Line a roasting tin with foil. Set a wire rack on the tin and coat it with cooking spray.

3 **Whisk the flour,** sesame seeds, baking powder, paprika, thyme, salt and pepper together in a small bowl. Tip the flour mixture into a large plastic food bag. One at a time, put the chicken pieces in the bag and shake to coat. Shake off excess flour and place the chicken on the rack in the roasting tin. (Discard any leftover flour mixture and marinade.) Spray the chicken pieces lightly with cooking spray.

4 **Bake the chicken** for 40–50 minutes or until golden brown and no longer pink in the centre. One serving is a drumstick and a thigh.

Turkey cottage pie with sweet potato topping

serves 6

PREPARATION TIME: 45 MINUTES

BAKING TIME: 35–40 MINUTES

A Magic version of a time-honoured favourite, this cottage pie uses lean minced turkey instead of beef mince, and sweet potatoes in place of white potatoes for the topping. The result is sure to please all the family. To make the pie ahead, prepare to the end of Step 5, then cover and keep in the refrigerator for up to 2 days.

FILLING

600g lean minced **turkey** breast (see Ingredient note)

2 teaspoons **olive oil** or canola (rapeseed) oil

1 medium **onion**, chopped

3 medium **carrots**, chopped

2 **garlic** cloves, finely chopped

1 teaspoon dried thyme

50g plain flour

550ml chicken stock made without salt

150g frozen **peas**, rinsed under cold water to thaw

1 teaspoon Worcestershire sauce

Freshly ground black pepper to taste

TOPPING

2 medium-large **sweet potatoes**, peeled and cut into chunks

125ml semi-skimmed **milk**

$^1/_2$ teaspoon grated lemon zest

$^3/_4$ teaspoon salt, or to taste

Freshly ground black pepper to taste

1 **Preheat the oven** to 200°C/gas 6. Coat a large ovenproof dish (measuring about 28 x 18cm or 23 x 33cm) with cooking spray.

2 **To make the filling:** cook the turkey in a large non-stick frying pan over a medium-high heat, breaking it up with a wooden spoon, for 4–5 minutes or until no longer pink. Transfer to a plate.

3 **Add the oil** to the pan. Add the onion and carrots and cook over a medium-high heat, stirring often, for 2–4 minutes or until softened. Add the garlic and thyme and cook, stirring, for 30 seconds. Sprinkle in the flour and stir to coat well. Gradually stir in the stock and bring to a simmer, stirring.

4 **Return the turkey** to the pan and reduce the heat to medium. Partly cover and simmer, stirring occasionally, for about 10 minutes or until the carrots are tender. Stir in the peas and Worcestershire sauce. Season with pepper. Transfer the turkey mixture to the prepared ovenproof dish.

5 **To prepare the topping:** put the sweet potatoes in a large saucepan. Add enough lightly salted water to cover and bring to a simmer. Reduce the heat. cover and simmer for 10–15 minutes or until the sweet potatoes are tender. Drain the sweet potatoes and return to the saucepan. Mash with a potato masher or electric mixer. Gradually stir or beat in the milk. Season with the lemon zest, salt and pepper. Spoon the sweet potato mixture over the turkey filling and use the back of the spoon to spread evenly and make decorative swirls.

6 **Place the dish in the oven** and bake the pie for 35–40 minutes or until the filling is bubbling up around the edge of the topping. Serve immediately.

PER SERVING: **262**kcal, **28g** protein, **32g** carbohydrate, **4.9g** fibre, **2.8g** total fat (**0.7g** saturated fat), **57mg** cholesterol, **0.8g** salt.

*Ingredient note: **When shopping** for minced turkey, check the pack labels. If made from breast and leg meat (and often skin), turkey mince is almost as high in calories and fat as extra-lean minced beef. Minced turkey breast, on the other hand, is truly lean.*

Turkey and pasta bake with spinach

serves 8

PREPARATION TIME: 40 MINUTES

COOKING/BAKING TIME: 50–60 MINUTES

Left-over turkey begs to be made into a creamy bake. Ours contains wholemeal pasta, a light lemony sauce and plenty of vegetables. This is an ideal dish to make ahead. Prepare it to the end of Step 5, then cover and keep in the refrigerator for up to 2 days. Or you can freeze it for up to 3 months (thaw before baking).

2 tablespoons plus 1 teaspoon **olive oil**

1 medium **onion**, chopped

75g plain flour

1 litre turkey or chicken stock made without salt, heated

125g half-fat crème fraîche

2 teaspoons grated lemon zest

1 tablespoon **lemon** juice

¼ teaspoon salt, or to taste

Freshly ground black pepper to taste

250g **wholemeal pasta** shapes, such as rotini or fusilli

4 medium **carrots**, sliced

300g baby **spinach** leaves, rinsed

340g cooked skinless **turkey** or **chicken**, diced

50g Parmesan **cheese**, freshly grated

30g fine dried breadcrumbs

1 **Bring a large saucepan** of lightly salted water to the boil. Preheat the oven to 200°C/gas 6. Coat a large ovenproof dish (about 23 x 33cm) with cooking spray.

2 **Heat 2 tablespoons** of the oil in a large saucepan over a medium heat. Add the onion and cook, stirring often, for 2–3 minutes or until softened. Add the flour and cook, stirring, for 30–60 seconds. Remove from the heat. Add the hot stock and whisk to blend.

3 **Place the saucepan** back over a medium-high heat and bring the sauce to a simmer, whisking constantly. Reduce the heat to low and simmer the sauce, whisking occasionally, for about 5 minutes or until it is slightly thickened. Remove from the heat and whisk in the crème fraîche, lemon zest and juice, salt and pepper. Keep the sauce warm.

4 **Add the pasta** and carrots to the pan of boiling water and cook for 5 minutes. Add the spinach and stir for 30–60 seconds or until wilted. Drain the pasta and vegetables in a colander and refresh under cold running water. (The pasta will seem quite firm but it will continue to cook during baking.)

5 **Transfer the pasta** and vegetables to a large bowl and add the warm sauce and turkey (or chicken). Toss to coat everything with the sauce. Turn into the prepared ovenproof dish, spreading evenly. Sprinkle with the Parmesan. Mix the breadcrumbs and remaining 1 teaspoon oil in a small bowl and sprinkle over the top.

6 **Place the dish in the oven** and bake for 35–45 minutes or until the sauce is bubbling around the edge and the topping is lightly browned. Serve hot.

PER SERVING: **322**kcal, **24g** protein, **37g** carbohydrate, **5g** fibre, **10g** total fat (**4g** saturated fat), **41mg** cholesterol, **0.6g** salt.

Turkey and bean chilli with avocado salsa

serves 8

PREPARATION TIME: 35 MINUTES

COOKING TIME: 1 HOUR AND 10 MINUTES

Beans, with their useful sugar-lowering soluble fibre content, should be on your menu weekly, and this full-flavoured chilli is a great way to enjoy them. We've lightened up the typical chilli by using turkey instead of beef and given it a Magic boost with an avocado salsa that's full of good fat. Offer a selection of garnishes, such as chopped spring onions, lime wedges, Tabasco sauce, Greek yoghurt and grated reduced-fat cheese, so your family and friends can flavour their chilli bowls to taste.

CHILLI

340g lean minced **turkey** breast (see Ingredient note, page 250)

4 tablespoons mild chilli powder

1 tablespoon ground cumin

1½ teaspoons dried oregano

2 teaspoons canola (rapeseed) oil

1 large **onion**, chopped

4 **garlic** cloves, finely chopped

200g jar jalapeño chillies, drained

2 x 400g cans chopped **tomatoes** (undrained)

400ml chicken stock made without salt

1½ x 400g cans black **beans**, drained and rinsed

1½ x 400g cans red kidney **beans**, drained and rinsed

AVOCADO SALSA

2 medium Hass **avocados**, diced

1 large plum **tomato**, deseeded and diced

4 tablespoons finely diced white or red **onion**

1 small fresh jalapeño or green chilli, deseeded and finely chopped

2 tablespoons chopped fresh coriander

2 tablespoons **lime** juice

¼ teaspoon salt, or to taste

1 **To make the chilli:** combine the turkey, chilli powder, cumin and oregano in a large non-stick frying pan. Cook over a medium-high heat, breaking up the meat and mixing in the spice, for 4–5 minutes or until lightly browned. Remove from the heat and set aside.

2 **Heat the oil** in a flameproof casserole or large saucepan over a medium heat. Add the onion and cook, stirring often, for 3–5 minutes or until softened. Add the garlic and jalapeño chillies and cook, stirring, for 1–2 minutes or until fragrant. Add the tomatoes, stock and browned spiced turkey. Bring to a simmer. Reduce the heat to low, cover the pot and simmer, stirring occasionally, for 45 minutes.

3 **Stir in the black beans** and kidney beans. Bring back to a simmer, cover again and simmer gently for 15–20 minutes or until the sauce is rich and thick.

4 **Meanwhile, make the avocado salsa:** combine the avocado, tomato, onion, fresh jalapeño (or green chilli), coriander, lime juice and salt in a medium bowl. Toss gently to mix.

5 **To serve, ladle the chilli into bowls** and spoon 2 tablespoons of salsa on to each serving. (The chilli will keep, covered, in the refrigerator for up to 2 days or in the freezer in an airtight container for up to 3 months. Make the salsa just before serving.)

PER SERVING: **250**kcal, **19g** protein, **24g** carbohydrate, **9g** fibre, **9g** total fat (**2g** saturated fat,) **24mg** cholesterol, **1.2g** salt.

Honey-mustard turkey burgers

serves 4

PREPARATION TIME: 20 MINUTES

COOKING TIME: 10–12 MINUTES

Next time you're longing for a burger, try this lean turkey version. A little reduced-fat mayonnaise helps keep the burgers moist, while mustard and honey perk up the flavour.

4 tablespoons coarse-grain mustard

2 tablespoons clear honey

1½ teaspoons Worcestershire sauce

450g lean minced **turkey** breast

1 tablespoon reduced-fat mayonnaise

1 **garlic** clove, finely chopped

½ teaspoon salt, or to taste

¼ teaspoon freshly ground black pepper

4 soft **wholemeal rolls** or baps, split open

1 **Stir the mustard,** honey and Worcestershire sauce together in a medium bowl. Reserve 2 tablespoons of this mixture to use as a basting glaze. Add the minced turkey, mayonnaise, garlic, salt and pepper to the mustard mixture remaining in the bowl. Mix with a potato masher. Divide into four portions and shape each one into a 1cm thick burger.

2 **Preheat the grill** to medium-high. Lightly oil the grill rack by rubbing with a piece of oil-soaked kitchen paper.

3 **Grill the burgers** for 4 minutes. Turn them over and brush the cooked sides with the reserved glaze. Cook for another 4 minutes. Turn the burgers over again and brush with the rest of the glaze. Grill for a further 2–4 minutes or until they are cooked through.

4 **Just before the burgers** are done, place the rolls or baps, cut side up, under the grill and toast for 30–60 seconds. Place a burger in each roll and add garnishes to taste (*see* below).

PER SERVING (without garnishes): **300**kcal,
34g protein, **33g** carbohydrate, **3g** fibre,
5g total fat (**0.8g** saturated fat), **65mg** cholesterol,
2g salt.

*Optional garnishes: **crisp lettuce leaves, sliced tomatoes, thinly sliced red or sweet white onions, tomato ketchup, reduced-fat mayonnaise, mustard.***

Turkey and bean chilli with avocado salsa
turkey • onion • garlic • tomatoes • beans • avocado • lime

Turkey meatballs in tomato sauce

serves
8

PREPARATION TIME: 40 MINUTES

COOKING TIME: 40–50 MINUTES

Made with lean minced turkey breast, these tender meatballs provide protein without the baggage of saturated fat. The Magic cinnamon seasoning in the meatballs adds a delightful accent to the tomato sauce. Spaghetti with meatballs is always a crowd-pleaser, and the recipe here will make enough to serve a hungry crowd. If you are cooking for one or two, make the whole batch of meatballs and sauce and freeze it in portion-size containers. Serve over wholemeal spaghetti, allowing 60g uncooked pasta per person, or use in sandwiches.

SAUCE

2 teaspoons **olive oil**

4 **garlic** cloves, cut into thin slivers

1/2 teaspoon dried oregano

Good pinch of crushed dried chillies

3 x 400g cans chopped **tomatoes** (undrained)

425ml **tomato** passata

MEATBALLS

450g lean minced **turkey** breast (see Ingredient note, page 250)

2 slices **wholemeal bread**, made into crumbs (see Tip)

1 medium **onion**, finely chopped

1 medium **egg**, lightly beaten

35g Parmesan **cheese**, freshly grated

3/4 teaspoon salt, or to taste

1/2 teaspoon ground **cinnamon**

1/4 teaspoon freshly ground black pepper

2 teaspoons **olive oil**

2 tablespoons chopped fresh parsley

1 **To make the sauce:** heat the oil in a large saucepan over a medium-low heat. Add the garlic, oregano and chillies and cook, stirring, for 1–2 minutes or until softened but not browned. Add the canned tomatoes and mash with a potato masher. Add the passata and stir well, then bring to a simmer over a medium-high heat. Reduce the heat to medium-low, cover and leave to simmer while you prepare the meatballs.

2 **To make the meatballs:** mix the minced turkey, breadcrumbs, onion, egg, cheese, salt, cinnamon and pepper together in a large bowl. Form into 1cm diameter meatballs.

3 **Heat 1 teaspoon** of the oil in a large non-stick frying pan over a medium-high heat. Add half of the meatballs and cook, turning occasionally, until browned on all sides. Transfer to a plate. Repeat with the remaining 1 teaspoon oil and meatballs.

4 **Add the browned meatballs** to the tomato sauce and simmer, covered, for 20 minutes. Uncover and simmer, stirring occasionally, for a further 20–40 minutes or until the meatballs are cooked through and the sauce has thickened slightly. Sprinkle with the parsley when serving. The meatballs and sauce can be kept, covered, in the refrigerator for up to 2 days or in the freezer in an airtight container for up to 3 months (thaw in the refrigerator). Reheat on the stovetop or in the microwave.

PER SERVING: **165**kcal, **19g** protein, **12g** carbohydrate, **2g** fibre, **4.5g** total fat, **1.5g** saturated fat, **66mg** cholesterol, **0.8g** salt.

Tip: **To make fresh breadcrumbs,** *tear slices of bread into small pieces and place in a food processor or blender. Pulse until broken down into fine crumbs.*

Fish and seafood

Plaice florentine

serves
4
PREPARATION TIME: 30 MINUTES
COOKING/BAKING TIME: 40–45 MINUTES

The term 'florentine' simply means with spinach, and this vegetable is the perfect partner for a delicate white fish such as plaice. The cheese sauce in this recipe not only enhances the fish and spinach, it also provides calcium, vitamin D and extra protein.

1 teaspoon grated lemon zest
400ml semi-skimmed **milk**
3 tablespoons plain flour
50g Parmesan **cheese**, freshly grated
¼ teaspoon salt, or to taste
Freshly ground black pepper to taste
Pinch of cayenne pepper
500g frozen **spinach**
4 x 115g **plaice** fillets (or **lemon sole** or
    orange roughy fillets)
2 teaspoons **lemon** juice
3 tablespoons fine fresh breadcrumbs
1 teaspoon **olive oil**

1 **Preheat the oven** to 220°C/gas 7. Coat a 20 x 30cm ovenproof dish (or similar 2 litre capacity dish) with cooking spray. Sprinkle the lemon zest over the bottom of the dish.

2 **Whisk 4 tablespoons** of the cold milk with the flour in a small bowl until smooth. Heat the remaining milk in a heavy saucepan over a medium heat until steaming. Add the flour mixture and cook, whisking constantly, for 2–3 minutes or until the sauce bubbles and thickens. Remove from the heat. Stir in 25g of the Parmesan, the salt, pepper and cayenne.

3 **While making the sauce,** cook the spinach according to the instructions on the pack. Drain and refresh under cold running water. When cool enough to handle, squeeze handfuls of spinach to press out all excess moisture.

4 **Spread the spinach** over the bottom of the ovenproof dish. Arrange the fish fillets, slightly overlapping, over the spinach. Sprinkle with the lemon juice. Spoon the cheese sauce evenly over the fish. Sprinkle the remaining Parmesan over the sauce. Mix the breadcrumbs and oil in a small bowl and sprinkle over the top.

5 **Place the dish in the oven** and bake for 30–35 minutes or until bubbling and the fish flakes when poked with a small sharp knife.

PER SERVING: **284**kcal, **31g** protein, **22g** carbohydrate, **3g** fibre, **8.8g** total fat (**4g** saturated fat), **67mg** cholesterol, **1.5g** salt.

Seared fish steaks with tomato and olive sauce

serves 4

PREPARATION TIME: 25 MINUTES
MARINATING TIME: 10–20 MINUTES
COOKING/BAKING TIME: 10–12 MINUTES

Firm fish like halibut and swordfish benefit from this easy two-step technique of first browning the steaks on one side and then finishing cooking in the oven (cooking the fish entirely in the frying pan could make the outside tough and requires more fat). The spicy tomato sauce sets off the succulent fish steaks beautifully.

1 tablespoon **lime** juice
4 teaspoons **olive oil**
Good pinch of salt, or to taste
Freshly ground black pepper to taste
4 x 125g **halibut** steaks, each 2.5cm thick (or 4 x 170g **swordfish** steaks of the same thickness)
$\frac{1}{2}$ medium **onion**, chopped
1 **garlic** clove, finely chopped
$\frac{1}{2}$ teaspoon ground cumin
$\frac{1}{4}$ teaspoon crushed dried chillies
400g can chopped **tomatoes** (undrained)
85ml water
1 tablespoon chopped green **olives**
2 teaspoons drained capers, rinsed
Lime wedges

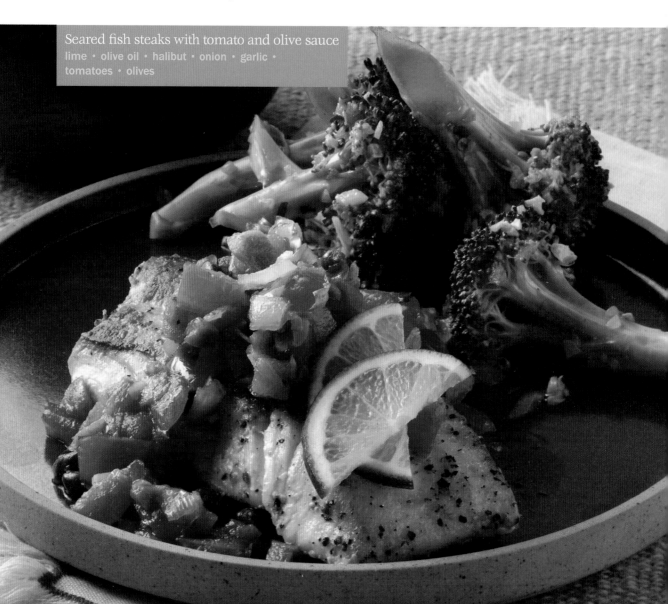

Seared fish steaks with tomato and olive sauce
lime · olive oil · halibut · onion · garlic · tomatoes · olives

1 **Preheat the oven** to 220°C/gas 7. Coat a baking tray with cooking spray.

2 **Mix the lime juice,** 1 teaspoon oil, the salt and pepper in a shallow glass dish. Add the fish steaks and turn to coat. Cover and leave to marinate in the refrigerator for 10–20 minutes.

3 **Meanwhile, heat 2 teaspoons oil** in a medium saucepan over a medium heat. Add the onion and cook, stirring often, for 3–4 minutes or until softened. Add the garlic, cumin and chillies. Cook, stirring, for 30 seconds. Add the tomatoes and water. Bring to a simmer. Cook over a medium heat, stirring occasionally, for about 10 minutes or until thickened.

4 **While the sauce is simmering,** cook the fish. Heat the remaining 1 teaspoon oil in a large non-stick frying pan over a medium-high heat. Add the fish and cook for 2–3 minutes or until browned on the underside. Transfer the fish to the baking tray, browned side up, and place in the oven. Bake for 8–10 minutes or until the fish is opaque in the centre.

5 **Stir the olives and capers** into the tomato sauce. Season with black pepper. To serve, top each fish steak with tomato and olive sauce and serve with lime wedges.

PER SERVING: **182**kcal, **28g** protein,
4g carbohydrate, **1g** fibre, **6g** total fat
(**1g** saturated fat), **44mg** cholesterol, **0.8g** salt.

*Tip: **The tomato and olive sauce** (Steps 3 and 5) is also delicious served over grilled or griddled chicken fillets.*

Mustard-glazed salmon with lentils

serves 4

PREPARATION TIME: **10 MINUTES**
COOKING TIME: **12–15 MINUTES**

It doesn't get much easier than this: canned lentil soup (well-drained so it has the consistency of braised lentils) topped with baked salmon. This delightful pairing of two Magic foods makes a French bistro classic.

3 x 400g cans **lentil** soup
450g **salmon** fillet, cut into 4 portions
Freshly ground black pepper to taste
3 tablespoons coarse-grain or Dijon mustard
2 teaspoons **olive oil**
1 bunch **spring onions**, chopped
½ teaspoon dried thyme
1 tablespoon **lemon** juice
Lemon wedges

1 **Preheat the oven** to 230°C/gas 8. Line a small roasting tin with foil and coat it with cooking spray.

2 **Pour the lentil soup** into a sieve set over a bowl. Set aside to drain for several minutes.

3 **Place the salmon fillets,** skin side down, in the roasting tin. Season with pepper and spread over the mustard. Bake the salmon for 12–15 minutes or until opaque in the centre.

4 **Meanwhile, heat the oil** in a medium saucepan over a medium heat. Add the spring onions and cook, stirring, for 1–2 minutes or until softened. Add the drained lentil soup and thyme and heat through. Stir in the lemon juice. Spoon the lentils on to four plates and top each with a salmon fillet. Garnish with lemon wedges.

PER SERVING: **300**kcal, **30g** protein,
13g carbohydrate, **4g** fibre, **14g** total fat
(**2g** saturated fat), **56mg** cholesterol, **2.9g** salt.

*Tip: **To cook salmon in the microwave**, place in a microwave-safe dish, cover with greaseproof paper and microwave on high for 5–7 minutes.*

Salmon with lemon and dill sauce

serves **4** PREPARATION TIME: **20 MINUTES**

BAKING TIME: **15–20 MINUTES**

Salmon is your best source of omega-3 fatty acids, which can actually *improve* insulin sensitivity, benefiting your blood sugar. Here's a foolproof way to prepare this fish that produces exceptionally moist and succulent results. The creamy sauce, a lighter, much easier version of Hollandaise, is brightened with herbs and lemon.

SALMON

450g centre-cut **salmon** fillet (about 3cm thick), cut into 4 portions
2 tablespoons dry white wine or water
2 tablespoons finely chopped **shallots**
¼ teaspoon salt, or to taste
Freshly ground black pepper to taste
Lemon wedges

SAUCE

4 tablespoons reduced-fat mayonnaise
4 tablespoons semi-skimmed **milk**
2 tablespoons chopped fresh dill
1 teaspoon grated lemon zest
1 tablespoon **lemon** juice
2 teaspoons Dijon mustard

1 **Preheat the oven** to 220°C/gas 7. Coat a shallow ovenproof dish with cooking spray. Place the salmon pieces, skin side down, in the dish. Sprinkle with the wine (or water), then with the shallots, and season with salt and pepper. Cover with foil. Bake for 15–20 minutes or until the salmon is opaque in the centre.

2 **Meanwhile, make the sauce:** place the mayonnaise in a small saucepan. Gradually whisk in the milk. Set the saucepan over a medium-low heat and cook, whisking constantly, for about 2 minutes or until the mixture is smooth and heated through but not bubbling. Remove from the heat and stir in the dill, lemon zest and juice, mustard and pepper. Keep warm.

3 **Divide the pieces of salmon** among four warmed plates. Pour the liquid remaining in the ovenproof dish into the sauce and stir to mix. Spoon the sauce over the salmon and serve with lemon wedges.

PER SERVING: **260**kcal, **24g** protein, **3g** carbohydrate, **0g** fibre, **17g** total fat (**3g** saturated fat), **60mg** cholesterol, **0.9g** salt.

Warm salmon salad with olive toasts

serves **4** PREPARATION TIME: **25 MINUTES**

COOKING TIME: **5 MINUTES**

Chunks of pink salmon contrast beautifully with leafy baby greens in this satisfying but light main-course salad, perfect for a warm summer evening. The olive oil dressing is sharpened with fresh lemon juice, which gives the salad an appealing kick and also dampens your blood sugar response to the meal. Crisp toasts topped with black olive spread garnish the salad. This is an excellent opportunity to enjoy the rye or pumpernickel bread that is recommended for Magic eating.

140g mixed baby salad leaves, rinsed and dried
2 tablespoons plus 2 teaspoons extra virgin **olive oil**
5 tablespoons **lemon** juice
½ teaspoon Dijon mustard
1 **garlic** clove, finely chopped
2 good pinches of salt
Freshly ground black pepper to taste
4 slices **rye** or **pumpernickel bread**
450g **salmon** fillet, skin removed, cut into 3cm chunks
1 small red **onion**, finely chopped
4 teaspoons drained capers, rinsed
2 tablespoons tapenade (black **olive** spread) or finely chopped Kalamata olives

1 **Place the mixed salad leaves** in a large bowl. Combine 2 tablespoons of the oil, 1 tablespoon lemon juice, the mustard, garlic, a good pinch of salt and pepper in a small bowl or screw-top jar. Whisk or shake to blend. Set the leaves and dressing aside. Toast the bread slices.

2 **Season the salmon** with the remaining salt and some pepper. Heat the remaining 2 teaspoons oil in a large non-stick frying pan over a medium-high heat. Add the salmon and cook, turning several times, for 3–4 minutes or until browned. Add the remaining lemon juice, the onion and capers. Cook, shaking the pan, for a further 30–60 seconds or until salmon is opaque in the centre.

3 **Drizzle the lemon dressing** over the salad leaves and toss to coat, then divide among four plates. Top with the salmon, onion, capers and pan juices. Cut each slice of toast in half and spread with the tapenade (or chopped olives). Garnish each salad with two olive toasts.

PER SERVING: **340**kcal, **26g** protein, **14g** carbohydrate, **2g** fibre, **21g** total fat (**3g** saturated fat), **56mg** cholesterol, **1.6g** salt.

VARIATION

Warm tuna salad with olive toasts

In Step 2, substitute fresh tuna for the salmon.

Prawn and scallop stew

serves 4

PREPARATION TIME: **25 MINUTES**
COOKING TIME: **15 MINUTES**

If you think seafood cookery is all about deep-frying, think again. This simple but elegant stew demonstrates how poaching keeps seafood moist and provides a flavourful base for the sauce. Cooking fish in wine is a classic method preferred by chefs, but it is also a good idea for home cooks because the acids in the wine have blood sugar–control benefits. Although butter is at the top of The Magic Foods Pyramid, just a little goes a long way here for a delicious finish.

2 teaspoons **olive oil**
1 large **leek**, white and pale green parts only, sliced
125ml dry white wine
180ml chicken stock made without salt
250g raw king or tiger **prawns**, peeled and deveined
250g **scallops**, halved horizontally
20g butter, cut into small pieces
2 teaspoons grated lemon zest
Good pinch of salt, or to taste
Freshly ground black pepper to taste
Pinch of cayenne pepper
2 tablespoons coarsely chopped fresh tarragon or snipped fresh chives

1 **Heat the oil** in a deep sauté pan over a medium-low heat. Add the leek and cook for 4–6 minutes or until tender but not browned. (Add 1 tablespoon water, if necessary, to prevent the leek catching.) Add the wine and stock and bring to a simmer. Add the prawns and scallops, cover and simmer over a medium-low heat for 4–5 minutes or until the prawns are pink and the scallops are opaque in the centre.

2 **Transfer the prawns** and scallops to a warm bowl using a slotted spoon. Cover and keep warm. Increase the heat under the pan and boil the cooking liquid for 2–3 minutes to reduce it and intensify the flavour. Remove from the heat. Add the butter, whisking until it is melted and incorporated into the sauce. Whisk in the lemon zest, salt, black pepper and cayenne. Spoon the sauce over the prawns and scallops and garnish with the tarragon (or chives).

PER SERVING: **183**kcal, **26g** protein, **3.5g** carbohydrate, **1.1g** fibre, **7g** total fat (**3g** saturated fat), **161mg** cholesterol, **0.9g** salt.

Prawn and orzo casserole

serves 6

PREPARATION TIME: 20 MINUTES
BAKING TIME: 20–25 MINUTES

This easy recipe for heart-healthy prawns is prepared Greek-style, with tomatoes, tangy feta cheese and rice-shaped orzo pasta cooked just until al dente. Convenient canned artichoke hearts are a surprisingly good source of fibre – another excellent reason to keep them in your storecupboard.

2 teaspoons **olive oil**
2 **garlic** cloves, finely chopped
½ teaspoon dried oregano
Pinch of crushed dried chillies
400g can chopped **tomatoes** (undrained)
400ml chicken stock made without salt
170g orzo **pasta** (see Ingredient note)
400g can artichoke hearts in water, drained,
    rinsed and quartered
1 teaspoon grated lemon zest
Freshly ground black pepper to taste
450g peeled, cooked king or tiger **prawns**
    (see Tip)
2 tablespoons chopped fresh parsley
85g feta **cheese**, crumbled

1 Preheat the oven to 220°C/gas 7. Coat a 20 x 30cm ovenproof dish (or a similar dish with a 2 litre capacity) with cooking spray.

2 Heat the oil in a large saucepan over a medium heat. Add the garlic, oregano and chillies and cook, stirring, for 30–60 seconds or until fragrant but not brown. Add the tomatoes and mash in with a potato masher. Add the stock and bring to a simmer. Stir in the orzo, artichoke hearts, lemon zest and pepper. Transfer to the ovenproof dish and cover tightly with foil.

3 Place in the oven and bake for 15 minutes. Stir the ingredients in the casserole, then stir in the prawns. Sprinkle with the parsley and then the feta. Bake, uncovered, for a further 5–10 minutes or until the orzo is al dente and the feta is starting to melt. Serve hot.

PER SERVING: **231**kcal, **23g** protein, **27g** carbohydrate, **2.7g** fibre, **4.9g** total fat (**2.2g** saturated fat), **156mg** cholesterol, **2g** salt.

*Tip: **To cook raw prawns,** place them in a large saucepan of lightly salted boiling water and simmer for 2–3 minutes or until the prawns turn pink, then drain. You can also use frozen cooked prawns. Thaw before using.*

*Ingredient note: **Wholemeal orzo** will provide extra fibre and wholegrain goodness. It's not yet widely available in shops, but can be ordered online at websites such as amazon.com. If you can't find orzo (regular or wholemeal), you can use other very small pasta shapes.*

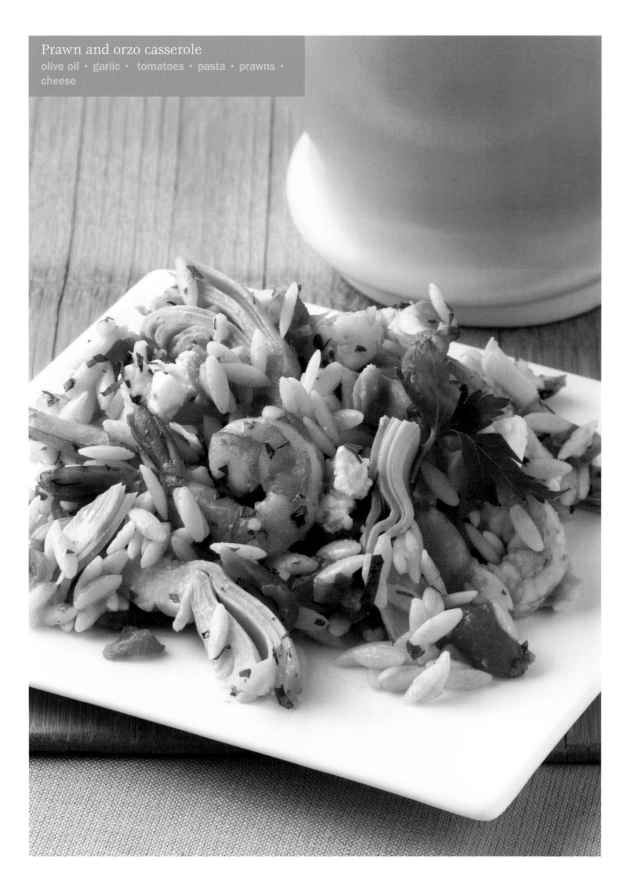

Prawn and orzo casserole
olive oil • garlic • tomatoes • pasta • prawns • cheese

Pasta and pizza

Penne with tomato and aubergine sauce

serves 6

PREPARATION TIME: 20 MINUTES

COOKING TIME: 25 MINUTES

Wholemeal pasta has come a long way in recent years, with supermarkets now stocking a wide variety of shapes. The nutty taste of wholemeal pasta pairs well with assertive flavours like those found in this tomato sauce, which has a rich, meaty taste thanks to the Magic aubergine, an excellent meat substitute.

4 teaspoons **olive oil**
1 large (250g) **aubergine**, cut into 2cm cubes
1 medium **onion**, chopped
4 **garlic** cloves, finely chopped
Good pinch of crushed dried chillies
2 x 400g cans chopped **tomatoes** (undrained)
3 tablespoons chopped fresh parsley or basil
Good pinch of salt, or to taste
Freshly ground black pepper to taste
340g **wholemeal penne pasta**, or other shapes
    such as rigatoni (see Tip)
75g feta **cheese**, crumbled
50g pine **nuts**, toasted (see Tip)

1 **Bring a large pan** of lightly salted water to the boil for cooking the pasta.

2 **Heat 2 teaspoons** of the olive oil in a large non-stick frying pan over a medium-high heat. Add the aubergine and cook, turning from time to time, for 5–7 minutes or until browned and tender. Transfer to a plate.

3 **Reduce the heat** to medium and add the remaining 2 teaspoons oil to the frying pan. Add the onion and cook, stirring often, for 2–3 minutes or until softened. Add the garlic and crushed chillies and cook, stirring, for about 30 seconds or until fragrant. Add the tomatoes and mash in with a potato masher.

4 **Bring to a simmer,** then add the aubergine and stir to mix. Simmer over a medium-low heat, stirring occasionally, for 15–20 minutes or until the sauce is rich and thick. (Add a little water if the sauce reduces too quickly.) Stir in 2 tablespoons of the parsley (or basil). Season with salt and pepper.

5 **Meanwhile, cook the pasta** in the pan of boiling water for 8–10 minutes, or according to packet instructions, until al dente. Drain and add to the sauce in the frying pan. Toss to coat well. Spoon the pasta on to warmed plates and sprinkle each serving with feta, pine nuts and the rest of the parsley (or basil).

PER SERVING: 337kcal, 12g protein,
    50g carbohydrate, 3.9g fibre, 11.5g total fat,
    (2.5g saturated fat), 9mg cholesterol, 0.8g salt.

Tips
■ *Toast the pine nuts in a small, dry frying pan over a medium-low heat, stirring constantly, for 1–3 minutes or until golden and fragrant.*
■ *Test the pasta often towards the end of cooking, so you will be sure to catch it when it has just become al dente (tender but still firm to the bite). When pasta is overcooked, not only does it lose its appeal, it has a higher GL.*

tomatoes their lycopene may have special power against diabetes

aubergine adding bulky veg like aubergine to pasta lowers the GL of the dish

pine nuts their 'good' fats help slow the digestion of your meal

cheese feta provides calcium, which may help boost your sensitivity to insulin

onions indispensable onions may lower high blood sugar

pasta wholemeal has three times the fibre per serving

Penne with tomato and aubergine sauce

garlic it helps keep blood clots and cholesterol in check

olive oil this liquid gold helps 'spike-proof' your meals

Penne with asparagus, ricotta and lemon

serves 4

PREPARATION TIME: 15 MINUTES

COOKING TIME: 8–10 MINUTES

Bulking up a pasta dish with vegetables can be as easy as tossing the veg into the boiling water to cook with the pasta – in most cases, add the vegetables halfway through the pasta cooking time. This super-simple pasta dish, highlighting asparagus, lemon and herbs and finished with a ricotta sauce, is perfect for a light spring supper.

120g ricotta **cheese**
50g Parmesan **cheese**, freshly grated
2 tablespoons chopped fresh parsley
2 teaspoons grated lemon zest
2 teaspoons **lemon** juice
$1/2$ teaspoon salt, or to taste
Freshly ground black pepper to taste
250g **wholemeal penne pasta**
450g asparagus, ends snapped off and spears cut into 4cm lengths

1 **Bring a large pan** of lightly salted water to the boil for cooking the penne.

2 **Combine the ricotta,** half the Parmesan, the parsley, lemon zest and juice, salt and pepper in a small bowl and stir until smooth.

3 **Add the penne** to the boiling water and cook for 4 minutes (or half the cooking time given on the packet). Add the asparagus, stir and cook for a further 4–6 minutes or until the penne is al dente and the asparagus is tender. Drain the pasta and asparagus, reserving 5 tablespoons of the cooking liquid, and place in a large bowl.

4 **Add the reserved** cooking liquid to the ricotta mixture and whisk until smooth. Toss the pasta with the ricotta sauce, sprinkle over the remaining Parmesan and serve.

PER SERVING: **326**kcal, **19g** protein, **44g** carbohydrate, **7g** fibre, **9g** total fat, **5g** saturated fat, **27mg** cholesterol, **1g** salt.

VARIATION

Penne with spinach, ricotta and lemon

Omit the asparagus, and in Step 3 cook the penne for 8–12 minutes or until al dente. Meanwhile, cook 300g frozen spinach according to the instructions on the pack. In Step 4, toss the penne with the ricotta sauce and spinach.

Macaroni cheese with spinach

serves 6

PREPARATION TIME: 15 MINUTES

COOKING/BAKING TIME: 45–55 MINUTES

A crusty macaroni cheese is pure comfort food – and it can be a Magic food as well. We've improved the dish with your blood sugar in mind by using wholemeal pasta, a lightened cheese sauce, a surprise layer of spinach and a topping of wheat germ. You can assemble the recipe to halfway through Step 5 in advance, then cover and keep in the refrigerator for up to 2 days before baking or freeze for up to 3 months (thaw in the refrigerator before baking).

400ml semi-skimmed **milk**
3 tablespoons plain flour
170g mature Cheddar **cheese**, grated
240g low-fat cottage **cheese**
Good pinch of grated nutmeg
$1/2$ teaspoon salt, or to taste
Freshly ground black pepper to taste
300g frozen **spinach**
250g **wholemeal macaroni**
4 tablespoons toasted **wheat germ**

1 **Preheat the oven** to 200°C/gas 6. Coat a 20cm square baking dish (2 litre capacity) with cooking spray. Bring a large pan of lightly salted water to the boil for cooking the macaroni.

2 **Whisk 4 tablespoons** of the cold milk with the flour in a small bowl until smooth. Heat the remaining milk in a heavy medium saucepan over a medium heat until steaming. Add the flour mixture and cook, whisking constantly, for 2–3 minutes or until the sauce boils and thickens. Remove from the heat. Add the Cheddar cheese, stirring until melted. Stir in the cottage cheese, nutmeg, salt and pepper.

3 **Cook the spinach** according to the instructions on the pack. Drain, refresh under cold water and press out excess moisture.

4 **Cook the macaroni,** stirring often, in the boiling water for 4–5 minutes or until not quite tender. (The macaroni will continue to cook during baking.) Drain, rinse with cold running water and drain again. Mix together the macaroni and cheese sauce in a large bowl.

5 **Spread half the macaroni cheese** in the baking dish. Spoon the spinach on top and cover with the remaining macaroni mix. Sprinkle with the wheat germ. Bake for 35–45 minutes or until bubbling and golden. Serve hot.

PER SERVING: **365**kcal, **23g** protein, **40g** carbohydrate, **5g** fibre, **12.8g** total fat (**7.5g** saturated fat), **33mg** cholesterol, **1.5g** salt.

VARIATION
Tex-Mex macaroni cheese

In Step 2, omit the nutmeg, and add 125g (or to taste) jalapeño chillies from a jar, drained, 15g chopped fresh coriander and a pinch of cayenne to the cheese sauce. In Step 3, omit the spinach. Instead, sauté 225g frozen mixed peppers in 1 teaspoon olive oil for 3–4 minutes or until tender. In Step 5, spread the peppers over the bottom layer of macaroni cheese.

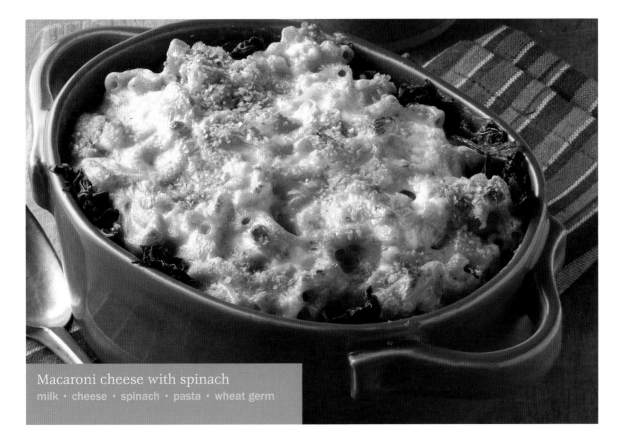

Macaroni cheese with spinach
milk · cheese · spinach · pasta · wheat germ

Wholemeal pasta with sausage, beans and greens

serves 6

PREPARATION TIME: 25 MINUTES

COOKING TIME: 20–25 MINUTES

A small amount of lean sausage goes a long way in imparting a full flavour to this quick pasta sauce. We've boosted the fibre content with cannellini beans and the vegetables with vibrant Swiss chard, which cooks conveniently in the pasta water.

125g spicy turkey or other low-fat sausage, skin removed

1 teaspoon **olive oil**

1 small **onion**, chopped

3 **garlic** cloves, finely chopped

400g can chopped **tomatoes** (undrained)

250ml tomato passata

400g can cannellini **beans**, drained and rinsed

4 tablespoons water

Freshly ground black pepper to taste

340g **wholemeal pasta** shapes (fusilli, penne or rigatoni)

450g **Swiss chard**, stalks trimmed off (see Tip), leaves washed and torn into bite-size pieces

6 tablespoons freshly grated Parmesan **cheese**

1 **Bring a large pan** of lightly salted water to the boil for cooking the pasta. Meanwhile, cook the sausage meat in a large non-stick frying pan over a medium heat, breaking up the sausage with a wooden spoon, for 3–5 minutes or until browned. Transfer the sausage to a plate lined with kitchen paper to drain.

2 **Add the olive oil** to the pan. Add the onion and cook, stirring often, for 1–2 minutes or until softened. Add the garlic and cook, stirring, for 10–20 seconds. Add the tomatoes and mash in with a wooden spoon or potato masher. Add the passata, beans, water and browned sausage meat. Bring to a simmer. Cook, uncovered, at a lively simmer over a medium-low heat, stirring from time to time, for 10–15 minutes or until the sauce is rich and thickened. Season with pepper.

3 **Meanwhile, add the pasta** to the boiling water and cook for 5 minutes (or half the cooking time given on the packet). Add the Swiss chard leaves and stir to immerse. Cook for a further 3–5 minutes or until the pasta is al dente and the chard has wilted. Drain well, then transfer to a large warmed bowl and toss with the tomato sauce. Sprinkle 1 tablespoon of Parmesan over each serving.

PER SERVING: **385**kcal, **23g** protein, **40g** carbohydrate, **5g** fibre, **12.8g** total fat (**7.5g** saturated fat), **33mg** cholesterol, **1.5g** salt.

Ingredient note: ***The celery-like stalks*** *of Swiss chard have a pleasant, mild taste. To serve them as a vegetable, cut into bite-size pieces and steam or boil for 6–8 minutes or until tender.*

Tip: ***If you have any leftovers,*** *transform them into a pasta gratin. Spread in a shallow baking dish coated with cooking spray. Moisten with a little water and top with grated Parmesan and breadcrumbs. Bake in a preheated 220 °C/ gas 7 oven for 25–30 minutes or until the top is golden and crusty.*

Quick spinach and sausage lasagne

serves 6

PREPARATION TIME: 30 MINUTES

COOKING/BAKING TIME: 1 HOUR

You can't beat lasagne for make-ahead convenience when entertaining. We've given the version here a healthier spin by lightening up the meat and cheese layers and bulking up the spinach layer. You can assemble the recipe in advance to the end of Step 4, then cover and keep in the refrigerator for up to 2 days or freeze for up to 3 months (thaw completely in the refrigerator before baking).

125g spicy turkey or other low-fat sausage, skin removed
750ml ready-made **tomato** pasta sauce, (eg napoletana)
1 teaspoon dried oregano
1/4 teaspoon crushed dried chillies
500g frozen chopped **spinach**
1 medium **egg**
425g ricotta **cheese**
50g Parmesan **cheese**, freshly grated
Good pinch of grated nutmeg
Freshly ground black pepper to taste
12 sheets no-cook lasagne (see Tip)
150g half-fat mozzarella **cheese**, grated

1 **Preheat the oven** to 200°C/gas 6. Coat a 23 x 33cm ovenproof dish with cooking spray.

2 **Cook the sausage** in a small non-stick frying pan over a medium heat, breaking it up with a wooden spoon, for 2–4 minutes or until browned. Drain the sausage on kitchen paper, then transfer to a medium bowl. Stir in the pasta sauce, oregano and chillies.

3 **Cook the spinach** according to the instructions on the pack. Drain and refresh under cold running water, then press out excess moisture. Whisk together the egg and ricotta in a medium bowl until smooth. Add the spinach, half of the Parmesan, the nutmeg and black pepper. Mix well.

4 **Place three of the lasagne sheets** in a deep dish or bowl and cover with warm water. Leave to soak while you assemble the lasagne. Spread about 180ml of the sausage sauce in the ovenproof dish. Arrange three of the remaining unsoaked lasagne sheets crossways over the sauce. Spread about one-third of the spinach mixture over the noodles. Spoon 125ml sauce over the spinach mixture and sprinkle with one-quarter of the mozzarella. Add another layer of unsoaked noodles, then spinach mixture, sauce and mozzarella as before. Repeat the layers one more time (there will be some mozzarella left over). Lift the soaked lasagne sheets from the water, shake off excess and arrange over the top. Spread the remaining sausage sauce evenly over the final layer of pasta.

5 **Cover the lasagne dish** with foil and bake for 35 minutes. Remove the foil. Sprinkle with the remaining Parmesan and mozzarella, then bake, uncovered, for a further 15 minutes or until the lasagne is golden brown and bubbling. Leave to stand for 5 minutes before serving.

PER SERVING: **426**kcal, **29g** protein, **40g** carbohydrate, **3g** fibre, **18g** total fat (**8g** saturated fat), **83mg** cholesterol, **2.3g** salt.

*Tip: **No-cook lasagne sheets** eliminate the step of boiling them before assembling the dish. However, even when the top layer of pasta is thoroughly covered with sauce, it never seems to get completely tender during baking. Soaking the sheets for the top layer in warm water first will solve this problem.*

Quick wholemeal pizza dough

1 pizza

PREPARATION TIME: **10 MINUTES**
RISING TIME: **10–20 MINUTES**

A food processor mixes and kneads this 'better-blood-sugar' pizza dough in just minutes. You can also make it in a bread machine – have the water at room temperature and place the ingredients in your bread machine in the order recommended by the manufacturer. This makes 340g dough, which is enough for a 30cm pizza.

85g **wholemeal flour**
85g white bread flour
2 teaspoons dried easy-blend yeast
   (see Ingredient note)
3/4 teaspoon salt
1/4 teaspoon caster sugar
125–150ml hot water (50–55°C)
2 teaspoons **olive oil**

1 **Combine the wholemeal flour,** bread flour, yeast, salt and sugar in a food processor. Pulse to mix. Combine the hot water and oil in a measuring jug. With the motor running, gradually pour the hot liquid through the hole in the lid and process until a ball of dough is formed. Process for 1 minute to knead. The dough should be quite soft. If it seems dry, add 1–2 tablespoons warm water. If it is too sticky, add 1–2 tablespoons more flour.

2 **Transfer the dough** to a lightly floured surface. Spray a sheet of cling film with cooking spray and place it, sprayed side down, over the dough. Leave the dough to rest for 10–20 minutes before rolling out.

Ingredient note: **Easy-blend yeast** *can be mixed directly with dry ingredients, so is quicker and easier to use than regular dried yeast.*

Mushroom and herb pizza

serves 4

PREPARATION TIME: **30 MINUTES**
COOKING/BAKING TIME: **20 MINUTES**

Yes, pizza can be part of your Magic Foods eating plan, especially when you make your own with a thin wholegrain crust, topped with lots of vegetables and a moderate amount of cheese. Using our Quick wholemeal pizza dough (left), you can bake your own wholesome pizza in about the same time it takes for a pizza to be delivered to your door. We offer three toppings, one with meaty-tasting mushrooms, one with broccoli and olives, and a third with mushrooms and prawns.

340g Quick wholemeal pizza dough, or ready-made
   pizza dough (preferably wholemeal)
Polenta for dusting
1 tablespoon **olive oil**
250g baby cremini or chestnut mushrooms, stalk
   ends trimmed, wiped clean and sliced
2 **garlic** cloves, finely chopped
2 tablespoons chopped fresh parsley
Pinch of salt
Freshly ground black pepper to taste
150ml ready-made **tomato** pasta sauce
   (eg napoletana) or pizza topping
2 tablespoons chopped fresh marjoram or oregano
Good pinch of crushed dried chillies
125g half-fat mozzarella **cheese**
1 small red **onion**, thinly sliced into shreds
25g Parmesan **cheese**, freshly grated

See method overleaf.

Mushroom and herb pizza
wholemeal flour · olive oil · garlic · cheese ·
onion · tomato

1 **Prepare the** Quick wholemeal pizza dough, if using, then leave it to rest.

2 **Place a baking stone,** or an inverted heavy baking tray, on the lowest rack of the oven. Preheat the oven to its highest setting. Coat a 32cm pizza tin (or another heavy baking tray) with cooking spray and dust with polenta.

3 **Heat 2 teaspoons** of the olive oil in a large non-stick frying pan over a medium-high heat. Add the mushrooms and cook, stirring them from time to time, for 3–4 minutes or until tender and lightly browned. Add the garlic and cook, stirring, for a further 30 seconds. Remove the pan from the heat and stir in the parsley, salt and pepper. Allow to cool slightly.

4 **Mix together the tomato pasta sauce,** marjoram (or oregano) and crushed chillies in a small bowl.

5 **On a lightly floured surface,** roll out the dough to a 33cm round. Transfer to the pizza tin (or baking tray). Turn the edge of the round under to make a slightly raised edge and brush the remaining 1 teaspoon oil over the edge. Spread the pasta sauce evenly over the pizza base, leaving the raised edge clear. Sprinkle the mozzarella over the sauce, then scatter the mushrooms over the mozzarella followed by the onion. Sprinkle with the Parmesan cheese.

6 **Place the pizza tin** on the heated baking stone (or baking tray) in the oven and bake for 10–14 minutes or until the pizza base is crisp and golden. Serve hot.

PER SERVING: **300**kcal, **15g** protein,
37g carbohydrate, **4g** fibre, **11g** total fat
(**2g** saturated fat), **26mg** cholesterol, **1.5g** salt.

VARIATIONS

Wholemeal pizza with broccoli and olives

In Step 3, omit the mushrooms and instead steam 225g broccoli florets, cut into 2cm pieces, for 2–3 minutes or until tender but still firm. In Step 4, mix the tomato pasta sauce with 1 teaspoon dried oregano and a good pinch of crushed dried chillies. In Step 5, after spreading the tomato pasta sauce over the pizza base and sprinkling with the mozzarella, scatter the broccoli over the top followed by 85g diced red onion and 35g coarsely chopped Kalamata olives. Spritz the top lightly with olive oil cooking spray. Bake the pizza as directed in Step 6.

Wholemeal pizza with prawns and mushrooms

In Step 3, mix the cooked mushrooms with the parsley and 150g peeled cooked prawns. Drain and chop a 50g can of anchovies, and add to the mushroom mix with 1 tablespoon capers. Season with pepper (the anchovies are salty). In Step 5, after spreading the tomato pasta sauce over the pizza base and sprinkling with the mozzarella, scatter the mushroom and prawn mixture over the top followed by 250g cherry tomatoes, halved. Spritz the top lightly with olive oil cooking spray. Bake the pizza as directed in Step 6.

Meatless main dishes

Spring vegetable stir-fry with tofu

serves 4

PREPARATION TIME: **25 MINUTES**
MARINATING TIME: **10 MINUTES**
COOKING TIME: **10 MINUTES**

This colourful stir-fry celebrates spring with seasonal asparagus and sweet onions. It is a protein-rich vegetarian dish, thanks to the tofu. And with its zesty sauce, it will appeal even to resolute meat-lovers. You can vary the recipe by using mangetout instead of asparagus and red pepper rather than carrots. Substitute sliced chicken breast fillet for the tofu, if you like – just be sure that it is cooked through when you brown it in Step 2.

400–450g firm **tofu**, drained
125ml orange juice
2 tablespoons reduced-salt soy sauce
1 tablespoon oyster sauce
1 tablespoon medium sherry or rice wine
1½ teaspoons Thai chilli sauce or other hot
    chilli sauce
1 teaspoon caster sugar
1½ teaspoons cornflour
1 tablespoon vegetable oil
1 tablespoon grated fresh root ginger
2 teaspoons grated orange zest
3 **garlic** cloves, finely chopped
1 small sweet or red **onion**, thinly sliced
450g asparagus, stalk ends snapped off and
    spears cut into 2.5cm lengths
125g baby **carrots**, quartered lengthways
4 tablespoons water

1 **Pat the tofu dry** and cut into 2cm pieces. Whisk the orange juice, soy sauce, oyster sauce, sherry (or wine), chilli sauce and sugar together in a medium bowl. Add the tofu and toss gently to coat. Leave to marinate for about 10 minutes, turning from time to time, while you prepare the vegetables.

2 **When you are ready** to cook, drain the tofu, reserving the marinade. Add the cornflour to the reserved marinade and whisk until smooth. Reserve for the sauce. Heat 2 teaspoons of the oil in a wok or non-stick frying pan over a high heat. Add the tofu and cook, turning from time to time, for 3–5 minutes or until browned and crusty. Transfer to a plate.

3 **Add the remaining** 1 teaspoon oil to the wok. Add the ginger, orange zest and garlic. Stir-fry for 10–20 seconds or until fragrant. Add the onion and stir-fry for 1 minute. Add the asparagus and carrots and stir-fry for 30 seconds. Add the water, cover the wok and cook for about 2 minutes or just until vegetables are tender. They should still be firm.

4 **Push the vegetables** to the sides of the wok. Stir the reserved sauce and pour it into the centre of the wok. Cook, stirring the sauce, for 1 minute or until it becomes glossy and thickens. Stir the vegetables into the sauce. Return the tofu to the wok and stir to coat. Serve immediately.

PER SERVING: **200**kcal, **15g** protein,
    16g carbohydrate, **3g** fibre, **9g** total fat
    (**1g** saturated fat), **0mg** cholesterol, **1.3g** salt.

Dhal with spinach

serves 6

PREPARATION TIME: 20 MINUTES
COOKING TIME: 45–50 MINUTES

Dhal (or dal) is one of those confusing terms that refer to both a preparation and an ingredient. As an ingredient, dhal encompasses a wide variety of dried pulses, including lentils and split peas, all of which are valuable sources of soluble fibre and vegetable protein. The preparation is a dish like this one, made with seasoned stewed pulses. We've squeezed three Magic seasonings – fenugreek, turmeric and garlic – into this spicy dish.

DHAL

200g yellow **split peas** or chana dhal (see Ingredient note), picked over and rinsed
750ml water
1/2 teaspoon **turmeric**
1 tablespoon canola (rapeseed) oil
1 teaspoon cumin **seeds**
1 medium **onion**, chopped
1 tablespoon grated fresh root ginger or 1/2 teaspoon ground ginger
3 **garlic** cloves, finely chopped
1 teaspoon ground **fenugreek** (optional)
1/4 teaspoon cayenne pepper
400g can chopped **tomatoes** (undrained)
300g frozen chopped **spinach**
1/2 teaspoon salt, or to taste

RAITA

225g low-fat plain **yoghurt**
4 teaspoons **lime** juice
1 teaspoon ground cumin
Good pinch of salt, or to taste

1 **To make the dahl:** combine the split peas (or chana dhal), water and turmeric in a large saucepan. Bring to a simmer. Partly cover, reduce the heat and cook for 40–45 minutes or until the split peas are tender.

2 **Meanwhile, heat the oil** in a large non-stick frying pan over a medium heat. Add the cumin seeds and cook, stirring, for 10–20 seconds or until fragrant. Add the onion and cook, stirring often, for 2–3 minutes or until softened. Add the ginger, garlic, fenugreek, if using, and cayenne. Stir and cook for a further 20–30 seconds. Add the tomatoes, stir well and cook for 5–10 minutes longer or until most of the liquid has evaporated and the mixture is rich and thick.

3 **Cook the chopped spinach** according to the instructions on the pack. Drain well, pressing out excess moisture.

4 **When the split peas** are tender, stir them (and any remaining cooking liquid) into the tomato mixture with the spinach. Cook for 2–3 minutes to blend the flavours. Season with salt.

5 **To make the raita:** mix all the ingredients in a small bowl. Serve the dhal with the raita. Any leftover dhal can be kept, covered, in the refrigerator for up to 2 days. Reheat gently in a saucepan, or in the microwave, adding a little additional water, if necessary.

PER SERVING: **176**kcal, **11g** protein,
26g carbohydrate, **4g** fibre, **3.5g** total fat
(**0.7g** saturated fat), **0mg** cholesterol, **0.8g** salt.

Ingredient note: **Chana dhal**, *which are a small, brown relation of the chickpea, are usually sold split, when they look like yellow split peas. You'll find them in most supermarkets and in Indian food shops.*

Barley risotto with asparagus and lemon

serves 4

PREPARATION TIME: 20 MINUTES
COOKING TIME: 35 MINUTES

A creamy risotto is traditionally made with a special short-grain rice, which falls in the top (undesirable) tier of the Magic Foods Carb Pyramid (*see page 43*). We've created this blood-sugar-friendly version, which swaps nutty-tasting, wholesome pearl barley for the white rice. The result is equally delicious.

320ml vegetable stock made without salt
180ml water
450g asparagus, stalk ends snapped off and
　　spears cut into 2.5cm pieces
1 tablespoon **olive oil**
50g **spring onions**, chopped
200g pearl **barley**
50g Parmesan **cheese**, freshly grated
4 tablespoons chopped fresh parsley or
　　snipped fresh chives
2 teaspoons grated lemon zest
1 tablespoon **lemon** juice
Pinch of salt
Freshly ground black pepper to taste

1 **Combine the stock** and water in a medium saucepan and bring to a simmer over a medium heat. Drop in the asparagus and cook for 2–4 minutes or until just tender. Transfer the asparagus to a plate using a slotted spoon and set aside. Reduce the heat to low and keep the stock at a bare simmer.

2 **Heat the oil** in a wide, heavy pan over a medium heat. Add the spring onions and cook, stirring, for about 1 minute or until they are softened. Add the barley and cook, stirring, for 30 seconds. Add a large ladleful of the hot stock and cook, stirring, for 1–1½ minutes or until most of the liquid has been absorbed.

3 **Continue to simmer** for about 30 minutes, adding the stock a small ladleful at a time and waiting until most of each batch has been absorbed before adding the next, until the barley grains are tender and the risotto has a creamy consistency. Stir frequently during cooking.

4 **Add the reserved asparagus** and stir for about 1 minute or until heated through. Remove the risotto from the heat. Stir in the Parmesan, parsley (or chives), lemon zest and juice, salt and pepper. Serve hot.

PER SERVING: **170**kcal, **9g** protein,
　　17g carbohydrate, **2g** fibre, **7.5g** total fat,
　　(**3g** saturated fat), **12mg** cholesterol, **0.5g** salt.

Lentil and bean chilli

serves 8 PREPARATION TIME: **20 MINUTES**
COOKING TIME: **50 MINUTES**

Nothing takes the chill out of a winter evening like a bowl of steaming, spicy chilli. The combination of lentils and beans here produces a vegetarian version that is rich in soluble fibre and protein, both strong allies in the battle against blood sugar spikes. Garnish the chilli with diced avocado, grated Cheddar, chopped coriander and spring onions, and Greek yoghurt.

2 teaspoons **olive oil**
1 medium **onion**, chopped
3 medium **carrots**, diced
3 **garlic** cloves, finely chopped
5 teaspoons mild chilli powder
4 teaspoons ground cumin
1 teaspoon dried oregano
1 litre vegetable stock made without salt
150g brown **lentils**, picked over and rinsed
2 x 400g cans chopped **tomatoes** (undrained)
2 x 400g cans red kidney **beans**, drained and rinsed
Freshly ground black pepper to taste

1 **Heat the oil** in a large saucepan over a medium heat. Add the onion and carrots and cook, stirring often, for 3–5 minutes or until softened. Add the garlic, chilli powder, cumin and oregano. Cook, stirring, for 30–60 seconds. Add the stock and lentils. Bring to a simmer, then reduce the heat to medium-low, cover the pan and simmer for 25 minutes.

2 **Add the tomatoes,** beans and pepper. Bring back to a simmer. Cook, covered, for a further 15–20 minutes or until the lentils are tender. Serve hot. Any leftovers can be kept, covered, in the refrigerator for up to 2 days. Reheat gently in a saucepan or in the microwave.

PER SERVING: **180**kcal, **12g** protein,
　　30g carbohydrate, **8.4g** fibre, **1.8g** total fat,
　　(**0.3g** saturated fat), **0mg** cholesterol, **0.9g** salt.

Black bean and sweet potato burritos

serves 8

PREPARATION TIME: 25 MINUTES

COOKING TIME: 20 MINUTES

Sweet potatoes and fibre-rich beans are a Magic marriage in this flavour-packed vegetarian main dish. If you are cooking for just one or two, make up the sweet potato and bean filling (to the end of Step 3) and keep, covered, in the refrigerator for up to 2 days. For a quick meal, just heat leftover filling and individual wraps in the microwave (*see* Tip).

2 teaspoons canola (rapeseed) oil

1 medium **onion**, chopped

2 **garlic** cloves, finely chopped

4 teaspoons ground cumin

$\frac{1}{2}$ teaspoon dried oregano

Good pinch of crushed chillies

180ml vegetable stock made without salt

1 medium **sweet potato**, peeled and diced

400g can chopped tomatoes (undrained)

425g can black **beans**, drained and rinsed

120g frozen sweetcorn

1 tablespoon fresh **lime** juice

4 tablespoons chopped fresh coriander

Good pinch of freshly ground black pepper

8 wholemeal wraps or flour tortillas (20cm in diameter)

120g Monterey Jack or mild Cheddar **cheese**, grated

125g Greek yoghurt

1 **Preheat the oven** to 160°C/gas 3.

2 **Heat the oil** in a large non-stick frying pan over a medium heat. Add the onion and cook, stirring often, for 2–3 minutes or until softened. Add the garlic, cumin, oregano and chillies. Cook, stirring, for 10–20 seconds or until fragrant. Add the stock and sweet potato. Bring to a simmer, then cover and cook for 5 minutes.

3 **Add the tomatoes,** beans and sweetcorn. Bring back to a simmer. Cook, covered, for a further 5–10 minutes or until the sweet potato is tender. Transfer about one-quarter of the vegetable mixture to a bowl and mash with a potato masher. Stir back into the unmashed vegetable mixture in the pan. Stir in the lime juice, coriander and pepper.

4 **Meanwhile, enclose** the wraps (or tortillas) in a foil parcel and heat in the oven for 10–15 minutes.

5 **To assemble,** lay out each wrap flat and spoon about one-eighth of the sweet potato filling down the centre. Sprinkle with about 2 tablespoons of the cheese. Fold in the top and bottom of the wrap, then fold one side over the filling and continue folding to wrap up the burrito. Serve with Greek yoghurt for dipping.

PER SERVING: **345**kcal, **14g** protein, **56g** carbohydrate, **5.7g** fibre, **8g** total fat (**4g** saturated fat), **15mg** cholesterol, **1.2g** salt.

*Tip: **To heat individual wraps** or flour tortillas in the microwave, place one wrap between two sheets of kitchen paper and microwave on high for 10–12 seconds.*

Side dishes

Bulghur wheat with ginger and orange

serves 4

PREPARATION TIME: 15 MINUTES
COOKING TIME: 25 MINUTES

Instead of cooking rice or potatoes (both high-GL foods) to accompany a chicken, beef or pork main dish, reach for the bag of bulghur wheat instead. Bulghur cooks in about the same time as white rice but offers the blood sugar benefits of a wholegrain rich in soluble fibre.

2 **oranges**, scrubbed
2 teaspoons canola (rapeseed) oil
2 tablespoons very finely chopped fresh
    root ginger
2 **garlic** cloves, finely chopped
155g **bulghur**, rinsed
2 teaspoons soft brown sugar
$1/4$ teaspoon salt, or to taste
70g **spring onions**, chopped
1 tablespoon reduced-salt soy sauce
40g slivered or flaked **almonds**, toasted (see Tip)

1 **Grate 1 tablespoon** of zest from the oranges and set aside. Squeeze the juice from the oranges and add enough water to make 375ml.

2 **Heat the oil** in a large, heavy saucepan over a medium-high heat. Add the ginger and garlic and cook, stirring, for about 30 seconds or until fragrant. Add the bulghur wheat and stir to coat with the flavoured oil. Add the orange juice, sugar and salt. Bring to a simmer, then reduce the heat to low, cover and simmer for 15–20 minutes or until the bulghur is tender and most of the liquid has been absorbed.

3 **Add the spring onions,** soy sauce and orange zest to the bulghur. Mix gently and fluff with a fork. Sprinkle with the almonds. Serve hot. Any leftovers can be kept, covered, in the refrigerator for up to 2 days. Reheat in the microwave.

PER SERVING: **255**kcal, **7g** protein, **41g** carbohydrate, **2.3g** fibre, **8g** total fat (**0.7g** saturated fat), **0mg** cholesterol, **0.7g** salt.

Tip: **Toast almonds** *in a small, dry frying pan over a medium-low heat, stirring constantly, for 2–3 minutes or until light golden and smelling nutty. Transfer to a plate and leave to cool.*

VARIATION

Bulghur wheat with carrot juice and sesame seeds

Substitute 375ml carrot juice for the orange juice and water mixture, and toasted sesame seeds for the almonds.

Mushroom and barley pilaf

serves 6

PREPARATION TIME: **15 MINUTES**

COOKING TIME: **30 MINUTES**

Taking its inspiration from barley and mushroom soup, this easy pilaf is an ideal side dish to accompany beef, pork or chicken. Finishing off the pilaf with a splash of vinegar heightens the flavours while dampening the blood-sugar effects of your whole meal.

4 teaspoons **olive oil**

1 medium **onion**, chopped

200g pearl **barley**

500ml chicken stock made without salt

250g mushrooms, stalk ends trimmed, caps wiped clean and sliced

1 medium red pepper, deseeded and diced

1 **garlic** clove, finely chopped

4 tablespoons chopped fresh dill

1 tablespoon balsamic **vinegar** or **lemon** juice

Freshly ground black pepper to taste

1 Heat 2 teaspoons of the olive oil in a large saucepan over a medium heat. Add the onion and cook, stirring often, for 2–3 minutes or until softened. Add the barley and cook, stirring, for 1 minute. Add the stock and bring to a simmer. Reduce the heat to low, then cover and simmer for about 30 minutes or until the barley is tender and the liquid has been absorbed.

2 Meanwhile, heat the remaining oil in a large non-stick frying pan over a medium-high heat. Add the mushrooms, red pepper and garlic and cook, stirring often, for 3–5 minutes or until tender. Add to the barley with the dill, vinegar and pepper. Stir gently to mix, then serve hot. The pilaf can be kept, covered, in the refrigerator for up to 2 days. Reheat in the microwave.

PER SERVING: **160**kcal, **4g** protein, **32g** carbohydrate, **1.1g** fibre, **3g** total fat, (**0.5g** saturated fat), **0mg** cholesterol, salt (trace).

Brown rice pilaf with lemon and toasted flaxseeds

serves 6

PREPARATION TIME: **10 MINUTES**

COOKING TIME: **45–55 MINUTES**

Nutty flaxseeds give a simple rice pilaf a boost of soluble fibre to help lower blood sugar. If you don't have time to cook brown rice, you can substitute white rice (reduce the quantity of water to 4 tablespoons and cook the pilaf for about 20 minutes). With its fresh lemon and parsley accent, this pilaf makes an excellent accompaniment to fish or chicken. Or use vegetable stock and serve the pilaf with a hearty vegetable stew or mixed vegetable kebabs.

2 teaspoons **olive oil**

1 medium **onion**, chopped

185g long-grain brown rice

400ml chicken or vegetable stock made without salt

180ml water

40g whole **flaxseeds**

2 teaspoons grated lemon zest

1 tablespoon **lemon** juice

4 tablespoons chopped fresh parsley

Freshly ground black pepper to taste

1 Heat the olive oil in a large, heavy saucepan over a medium heat. Add the onion and cook, stirring often, for 2–3 minutes or until softened. Add the rice and stir for 30 seconds. Pour in the stock and water and bring to a simmer. Reduce the heat to low, cover the pan and simmer for 45–55 minutes or until the rice is tender and the liquid has been absorbed.

2 Meanwhile, toast the flaxseeds in a small, dry frying pan over a medium-low heat, stirring constantly, for 2–3 minutes or until fragrant and starting to pop. Transfer to a small bowl and leave to cool. When cold, place the flaxseeds in a spice grinder or blender and pulse several times until broken down but not ground to a meal.

3 **When rice is ready,** add the flaxseeds, lemon zest and juice, parsley and pepper. Fluff and mix gently with a fork, then serve hot. Leftovers can be kept, covered, in the refrigerator for up to 2 days. Reheat in the microwave.

PER SERVING: 160kcal, **4g** protein,

26g carbohydrate, **2g** fibre, **4.5g** total fat,

(**0.5g** saturated fat), **0mg** cholesterol, salt (trace).

VARIATION

Brown rice pilaf with flaxseeds, lime and coriander

Substitute 1 teaspoon grated lime zest for the 2 teaspoons lemon zest; lime juice for the lemon juice; and chopped fresh coriander for the parsley.

Wheat berry salad with dried apricots and mint

serves 6

PREPARATION TIME: 25 MINUTES
COOKING TIME: 1½–1¾ HOURS

You may have to plan ahead when cooking wheat berries (which are also called whole wheat grain), but you'll be rewarded with a great-tasting wholegrain salad that's truly blood sugar–friendly. Here the chewy, nutty berries are complemented by a spiced citrus vinaigrette, dried fruits and nuts, and this makes a great side dish with lamb or poultry. Look for dried wheat berries in healthfood and wholefood shops, or order them from online sources.

145g dried **wheat berries**, rinsed (see Tip)
60g dried apricots, diced
4 tablespoons extra virgin **olive oil**
3 tablespoons orange juice
2 tablespoons **lemon** juice
½ teaspoon clear honey
½ teaspoon ground **cinnamon**
1 **garlic** clove, finely chopped
½ teaspoon salt, or to taste
Freshly ground black pepper to taste
50g **spring onions**, chopped
15g fresh mint, chopped
40g slivered or flaked **almonds**, or chopped
    pistachio nuts, toasted (see Tip, page 275)

1 **Place the wheat berries** in a large saucepan and cover generously with water. Bring to a simmer over a medium-high heat. Reduce the heat to medium-low, partly cover and cook for 1½–1¾ hours or until the wheat berries are tender. (Add more water, if necessary.) Drain and rinse with cold running water.

2 **Meanwhile,** place the apricots in a small bowl. Cover with boiling water and leave to soak for 5–10 minutes. Drain.

3 **Combine the oil,** orange juice, lemon juice, honey, cinnamon, garlic, salt and pepper in a medium bowl or a screw-top jar. Whisk or shake to blend.

4 **Combine the cooked** wheat berries, soaked dried apricots, spring onions and mint in a large bowl. Add the dressing and toss to coat well. Just before serving, sprinkle with the nuts. The salad can be kept, covered, in the refrigerator for up to 2 days.

PER SERVING: **215**kcal, **4g** protein,

25g carbohydrate, **1.3g** fibre, **12g** total fat,

(**1.5g** saturated fat), **0mg** cholesterol, **0.3g** salt.

Tip: ***If you soak the wheat berries*** *for at least 8 hours or overnight in a large bowl of water, you can reduce the cooking time to about 1 hour (discard the soaking water and cook the wheat berries in fresh water).*

Sweet potato mash with fresh ginger and orange

serves 6

PREPARATION TIME: 20 MINUTES

COOKING TIME: 12–15 MINUTES

Like chips, mashed potatoes are usually blood sugar nightmares – but not if they're made from sweet potatoes, one of our favourite Magic foods. In this dish, fresh citrus and ginger provide delicious accents. Boiling the orange juice to reduce it enhances its natural sweetness, while just a touch of butter provides exceptional enrichment with a minimum of saturated fat. This mash is special enough for a celebration meal, but it is also easy enough for a simple weeknight supper. Serve it with roast or grilled chicken, turkey or pork tenderloin.

700g **sweet potatoes**, peeled and cut
into 4–5cm chunks
300ml fresh orange juice (from about 4 oranges)
1 tablespoon grated fresh root ginger
1 **garlic** clove, finely chopped
Small knob of unsalted butter (about 10g)
¼ teaspoon salt, or to taste
Freshly ground black pepper to taste

1 **Place the sweet potatoes** in a large saucepan, add enough water to cover and bring to the boil. Reduce the heat to medium, cover and simmer for 10–12 minutes or until the sweet potatoes are tender.

2 **Meanwhile, combine** the orange juice, fresh ginger and garlic in a small saucepan and bring to the boil. Reduce the heat to medium and simmer for 5–8 minutes or until the juice is reduced to about 180ml. Remove the pan from the heat. Add the butter and stir until melted. Keep warm.

3 **When the sweet potatoes** are done, drain them well and return to the saucepan. Mash with a potato masher, or beat with a hand-held electric mixer, until smooth.

4 **Gradually add** the reduced orange juice mixture, stirring with a wooden spoon or beating at low speed with the electric mixer. Season with the salt and pepper. Serve hot. Any leftovers can be kept, covered, in the refrigerator for up to 2 days. Reheat in the microwave.

PER SERVING: **130**kcal, **2g** protein,
29g carbohydrate, **3g** fibre, **1.7g** total fat
(**1g** saturated fat), **3mg** cholesterol, **0.3g** salt.

Quinoa with chillies and coriander

serves 6

PREPARATION TIME: 15 MINUTES

COOKING TIME: 30 MINUTES

Quinoa, a delicately flavoured wholegrain that originated in South America, is higher in protein than any other grain. You can find it in healthfood and whole food shops and in many large supermarkets. The good news for busy cooks is that it takes no longer to cook than white rice. Accented with South American flavours, this versatile side dish is good with seafood, poultry or pork.

175g **quinoa**
2 teaspoons canola (rapeseed) oil
1 medium **onion**, chopped
1 fresh green chilli, deseeded and finely chopped
2 **garlic** cloves, finely chopped
400ml chicken or vegetable stock made without salt
45g fresh coriander, coarsely chopped
50g **spring onions**, chopped
35g **pumpkin seeds**, toasted (see Tip)
2 tablespoons **lime** juice
¼ teaspoon salt, or to taste

1 **Put the quinoa** in a large, dry frying pan over a medium heat and toast, stirring often, for 3–5 minutes or until it crackles and becomes aromatic. Transfer to a fine sieve and rinse thoroughly with cold running water. Shake the sieve to drain the quinoa.

2 **Heat the oil** in a large saucepan over a medium heat. Add the onion and cook, stirring often, for 2–3 minutes or until softened. Add the green chilli and garlic and cook, stirring, for 30 seconds.

3 **Add the stock** and quinoa and stir well, then bring to a simmer. Reduce the heat to low, cover the pan and cook for 20–25 minutes or until the quinoa is tender and most of the liquid has been absorbed.

4 **Add the coriander,** spring onions, pumpkin seeds, lime juice and salt to the quinoa. Mix gently and fluff with a fork. Serve hot.

PER SERVING: **140**kcal, **6g** protein, **19g** carbohydrate, **0.7g** fibre, **5g** total fat, (**0.7g** saturated fat), **0mg** cholesterol, **0.3g** salt.

Tip: **Toast the pumpkin seeds** *in a small, dry frying pan over a low heat for 3–5 minutes.*

Quinoa with chillies and coriander
quinoa • onion • garlic • spring onions • pumpkin seeds • lime

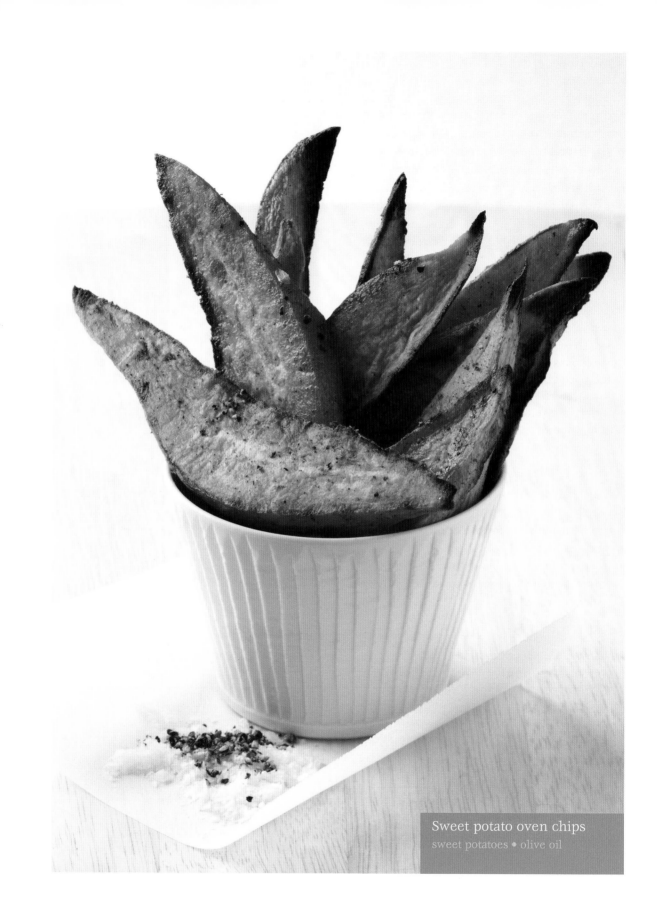

Sweet potato oven chips
sweet potatoes • olive oil

Jerusalem artichoke drop scones

serves 4

PREPARATION TIME: 20 MINUTES
COOKING/BAKING TIME: 25 MINUTES

Believe it or not, you can enjoy delicious savoury 'potato' drop scones without the potatoes – by using Jerusalem artichokes instead. These low-GL tubers are slightly sweet and have plenty of potato-like starch, which makes them perfect for these drop scones.

450g **Jerusalem artichokes**
1 medium **onion**, halved
1 medium **egg**
3 tablespoons plain flour
$\frac{1}{2}$ teaspoon salt, or to taste
Freshly ground black pepper to taste
4 teaspoons vegetable oil
125g low-fat plain **yoghurt**

1 **Preheat the oven** to 220°C/gas 7. Coat a large baking tray with cooking spray.

2 **Peel the artichokes,** then grate with the onion in a food processor fitted with the grating disc, or on a box grater.

3 **Whisk the egg** in a large bowl. Add the grated artichoke mixture, flour, salt and pepper, and mix well with a fork.

4 **Brush 2 teaspoons** of the oil over a large non-stick griddle or frying pan, then set it over a medium-high heat. Allowing a heaping tablespoon of the artichoke mixture per scone, drop four scones on to the griddle, spacing evenly. Flatten each scone with the back of a fish slice. Cook for $1\frac{1}{2}$–$2\frac{1}{2}$ minutes on each side or until golden. Transfer the scones to the prepared baking tray. Repeat with the remaining artichoke mixture and oil to make two more batches of scones (12 in all) using 1 teaspoon oil for each batch.

5 **Place the baking tray** in the oven and bake for about 10 minutes or until the scones are crisp and heated through. Serve topped with yoghurt. One serving is three drop scones.

PER SERVING: **160**kcal, **6.5g** protein, **25g** carbohydrate, **4.5g** fibre, **5g** total fat (**1g** saturated fat), **60mg** cholesterol, **0.6g** salt.

Tip: **Once peeled and grated,** *Jerusalem artichokes will discolour quickly, so make the batter and cook the drop scones straightaway.*

Ingredient note: **Jerusalem artichokes** *are knobby in shape. Choose smooth, unblemished tubers that are firm, not soft.*

Sweet potato oven chips

serves 4

PREPARATION TIME: 10 MINUTES
COOKING TIME: 25–30 MINUTES

Chips are one of the top 10 worst foods for blood sugar. But these chips, made in the oven with sweet potatoes, have a dramatically lower GL and more nutrients. They're so tasty you might even prefer them to regular chips.

2 **sweet potatoes** (340–450g total weight), peeled
2 teaspoons **olive oil**
$\frac{1}{2}$ teaspoon paprika
$\frac{1}{4}$ teaspoon salt, or to taste
Good pinch of freshly ground black pepper

1 **Preheat the oven** to 230°C/gas 8. Coat a baking tray or a large roasting tin with cooking spray.

2 **Cut the sweet potatoes** in half crossways, then lengthways into 1cm wide wedges. Place on the baking tray. Toss with the oil, paprika, salt and pepper.

3 **Bake the sweet potatoes** chips, turning them over several times, for 25–30 minutes or until golden brown and tender.

PER SERVING: **87** kcal, **1g** protein, **18g** carbohydrate, **2g** fibre, **1.8g** total fat (**0.3g** saturated fat), **0mg** cholesterol, **0.3g** salt.

Crushed curried butternut squash

Ingredient note: Freshly ground fenugreek will give the most wonderful flavour, so try to buy fenugreek seeds and grind them yourself in a spice mill or an electric coffee grinder reserved for spices.

serves 4

PREPARATION TIME: **10 MINUTES**

COOKING TIME: **30–35 MINUTES**

A departure from the many butternut squash preparations with sweet spicing, this recipe has an exotic flavour thanks to a simple seasoning of fenugreek seeds and turmeric, two Magic spices. Fenugreek seeds have a distinctive aroma reminiscent of curry.

1 tablespoon vegetable oil
2 medium **onions**, chopped
2 teaspoons ground **fenugreek** seeds (see Ingredient note)
½ teaspoon **turmeric**
Pinch of cayenne pepper
550g peeled, seeded butternut squash, cut into 4cm cubes
250ml water
½ teaspoon salt, or to taste
2 teaspoons **lemon** juice

1 **Heat the oil** in a heavy saucepan over a medium heat. Add the onions and cook, stirring often, for 2–3 minutes or until softened but not browned. Add the fenugreek seeds, turmeric and cayenne and stir for a few seconds until fragrant.

2 **Add the squash,** water and salt and stir to mix. Bring back to a simmer, then cover the pan and cook over a medium-low heat for 25–30 minutes or until the squash is very tender. (Add a little additional water, if necessary.)

3 **Crush the squash** coarsely with a fork or potato masher, then stir in the lemon juice. Serve hot. Any leftovers can be kept, covered, in the refrigerator for up to 2 days. Reheat in the microwave.

PER SERVING: **92**kcal, **2g** protein, **15g** carbohydrate, **2.9g** fibre, **3g** total fat (**0.5g** saturated fat), **0mg** cholesterol, **0.5g** salt.

Cauliflower and spinach gratin

serves 6

PREPARATION TIME: **20 MINUTES**

COOKING/BAKING TIME: **50 MINUTES**

This crisp-topped gratin will be sure to win over even fussy eaters who claim they don't like vegetables. It's great when you have friends over for supper because it can be prepared in advance and baked just before serving (prepare to the end of Step 5, then cover and keep in the refrigerator for up to 2 days). For convenience, frozen vegetables can be used instead of fresh: substitute 450g frozen cauliflower florets and 300g frozen spinach, and cook them according to the instructions on the packs.

3 tablespoons plain dried breadcrumbs
1 teaspoon **olive oil**
¼ teaspoon paprika
1 medium **cauliflower** (about 1.25kg), cored and cut into 4cm florets
400g fresh **spinach**, coarse stalks trimmed off and leaves thoroughly washed (or buy ready-washed spinach)
400ml semi-skimmed **milk**
3 tablespoons plain flour
160g mature Cheddar **cheese**, grated
1½ teaspoons dry mustard
½ teaspoon salt, or to taste
Freshly ground black pepper to taste

1 **Preheat the oven** to 220°C/gas 7. Coat a 30 x 20cm gratin dish or other shallow ovenproof dish (about 2.5 litre capacity) with cooking spray. Set aside.

2 **Mix the breadcrumbs** with the oil and paprika in a small bowl.

3 **Drop the cauliflower florets** into a large saucepan of lightly salted boiling water and cook for about 6 minutes or until tender. Stir in the spinach and cook for a further 1 minute or until the spinach has wilted. Drain the cauliflower and spinach in a colander and refresh under cold running water to stop further cooking. Drain the vegetables thoroughly, shaking the colander, and spread out in the gratin dish.

4 **Whisk 4 tablespoons** of the cold milk with the flour in a small bowl until smooth. Heat the remaining milk in a heavy medium saucepan over a medium heat until steaming. Remove from the heat and whisk in the flour mixture.

5 **Return to the heat** and cook, whisking constantly, for 2–3 minutes or until the sauce bubbles and thickens. Remove from the heat. Stir in the cheese, mustard, salt and pepper until smoothly blended. Pour the sauce over the vegetables, spreading evenly. Sprinkle with the breadcrumb mixture.

6 **Place the dish in the oven** and bake for 30–35 minutes or until the gratin is golden and bubbling. Serve hot.

PER SERVING: **277**kcal, **20g** protein, **20g** carbohydrate, **5.5g** fibre, **13g** total fat (**7g** saturated fat), **30mg** cholesterol, **1.3g** salt.

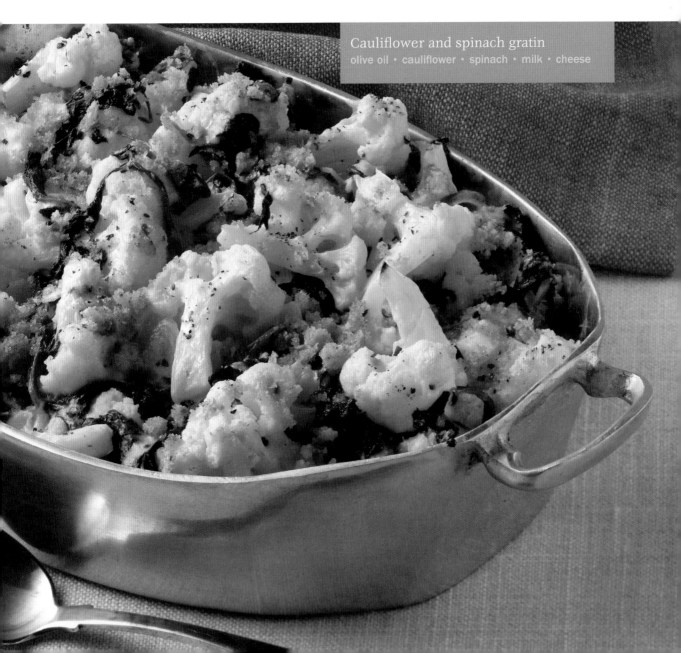

Cauliflower and spinach gratin
olive oil · cauliflower · spinach · milk · cheese

Spiced cauliflower with peas

serves **6** PREPARATION TIME: **25 MINUTES**
COOKING TIME: **15 MINUTES**

This Indian-style dish of braised vegetables gets its golden hue from the spice turmeric, which boasts anti-inflammatory properties and is believed to have positive affects on blood sugar. The aromatic spice mixture transforms plain old cauliflower and peas into a star-attraction side dish to accompany chicken or a dhal (stewed lentils). Since the complex flavours of the spice blend develop as the dish sits, it will benefit from being made ahead.

1 tablespoon canola (rapeseed) oil
1 teaspoon cumin seeds
2 medium **onions**, thinly sliced
2 green chillies, deseeded and finely chopped
4 **garlic** cloves, finely chopped
1 tablespoon grated fresh root ginger
1 tablespoon ground coriander
1 teaspoon ground cumin
½ teaspoon **turmeric**
250ml water
1 medium **cauliflower**, cut into florets
¾ teaspoon salt, or to taste
1 large plum **tomato**, diced
145g frozen **peas**, rinsed under cold water
    to thaw
20g fresh coriander, chopped
Lime wedges

1 **Heat the oil** in a large, heavy saucepan over a medium-high heat. Add the cumin seeds and cook, stirring, for 10–20 seconds or until they sizzle. Add the onions, chillies, garlic and ginger. Cook, stirring often, for 2–3 minutes or until the onions are softened. Add the ground coriander, cumin and turmeric and stir for 10–20 seconds or until fragrant. Pour in the water, then add the cauliflower and salt. Stir well to mix. Cover and cook for about 8 minutes or until the cauliflower is almost tender.

2 **Stir in the tomato and peas.** Cover again and cook for a further 2–3 minutes or until the cauliflower is tender and the peas are heated through. Sprinkle with the fresh coriander and serve hot, with lime wedges. Any leftovers can be kept, covered, in the refrigerator for up to 2 days. Reheat in the microwave.

PER SERVING: **140**kcal, **7g** protein, **10g** carbohydrate, **3g** fibre, **8g** total fat (**3g** saturated fat), **13mg** cholesterol, **0.9g** salt.

Sautéed Brussels sprouts with red pepper and caraway seeds

serves **4** PREPARATION TIME: **15 MINUTES**
COOKING TIME: **12 MINUTES**

Brussels sprouts are a traditional part of the Christmas feast, but usually ignored the rest of the year. That's a shame, because this hardy vegetable is loaded with Magic benefits. Sautéed with colourful red pepper, sprouts make a superb side dish to accompany lean meat or poultry for a simple midweek supper.

300g **Brussels sprouts**, trimmed and cored
2 teaspoons canola (rapeseed) oil
1 medium **onion**, sliced
1 medium red pepper, deseeded and cut
    into 5cm long slivers
1½ teaspoons caraway **seeds**
125ml vegetable or chicken stock made
    without salt
3 tablespoons cider **vinegar**
¼ teaspoon salt, or to taste
Freshly ground black pepper to taste

1 **Quarter the Brussels sprouts** with a sharp knife, or shred them in a food processor fitted with the slicing disc.

2 **Heat the oil** in a large non-stick frying pan over a medium-high heat. Add the onion and red pepper and cook, stirring frequently, for 3–4 minutes or until softened. Add the caraway seeds and cook, stirring, for 30 seconds.

3 **Add the Brussels sprouts** and sauté them, stirring, for 2 minutes. Pour in the stock. Cover the pan and cook for a further 2–3 minutes or until the sprouts are tender but still have a bit of bite. Stir in the cider vinegar, salt and pepper and serve hot.

PER SERVING: **66**kcal, **3.3g** protein, **7.5g** carbohydrate, **4g** fibre, **2.7g** total fat (**0.5g** saturated fat), **0mg** cholesterol, **0.3g** salt.

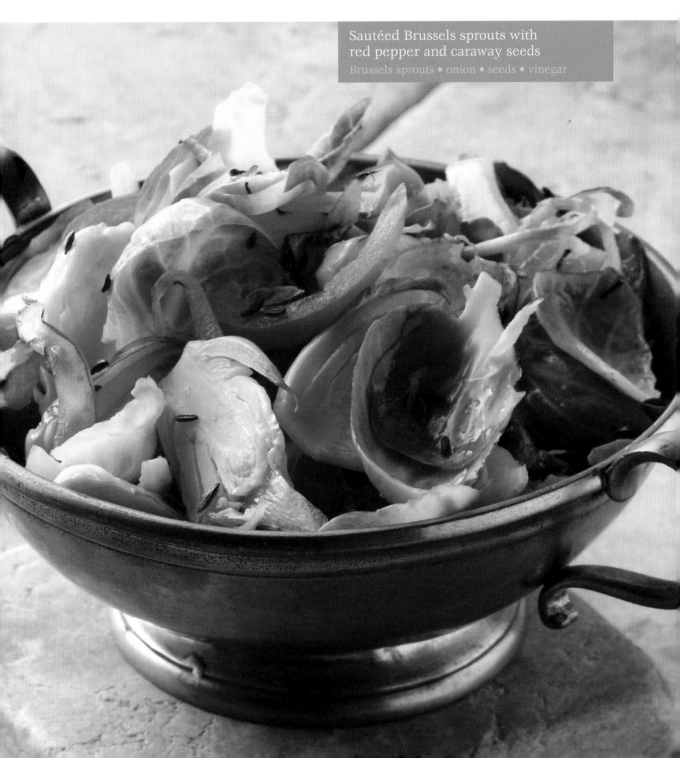

Sautéed Brussels sprouts with red pepper and caraway seeds
Brussels sprouts • onion • seeds • vinegar

Spinach with pine nuts and currants

serves 4

PREPARATION TIME: 10 MINUTES

COOKING TIME: 10 MINUTES

Even if you haven't had time to buy fresh vegetables, you can include a side dish of Magic spinach in your weekly menu plan, because frozen spinach works perfectly in this adaptation of a traditional Spanish recipe. Use the frozen chopped spinach that is packed loose, rather than spinach frozen in a block, as it is easier to sauté.

50g currants or coarsely chopped raisins
2 teaspoons extra virgin **olive oil**
35g pine **nuts**
1 medium **onion**, finely chopped
1 **garlic** clove, finely chopped
500g frozen chopped **spinach**
1 tablespoon balsamic **vinegar**
$^{1}/_{2}$ teaspoon salt, or to taste
Freshly ground black pepper to taste

1 **Place the currants** (or raisins) in a small bowl and pour in enough boiling water to cover. Leave to plump up for 5–10 minutes. Drain, reserving the soaking liquid.

2 **Heat the oil** in a large non-stick frying pan over a medium-low heat. Add the pine nuts and cook, stirring, for 1–2 minutes or until light golden brown. Transfer the pine nuts to a small bowl and set aside.

3 **Add the onion** and garlic to the pan. Cook, stirring, for 2–3 minutes or until softened and light golden. Add the frozen spinach and 2 tablespoons of the reserved soaking liquid. Increase the heat to medium-high and cook, stirring, for 3–5 minutes or until the spinach is completely thawed and piping hot. Stir in the currants and pine nuts. Season with the vinegar, salt and pepper, and serve.

PER SERVING: **152**kcal, **5g** protein,
13g carbohydrate, **3.4g** fibre, **8.6g** total fat
(**0.7g** saturated fat), **0mg** cholesterol, **0.9g** salt.

Moroccan spiced carrots

serves 4

PREPARATION TIME: 10 MINUTES

COOKING TIME: 8 MINUTES

It is hard to believe that humble carrots can be transformed into such a rich-tasting yet low-calorie dish. The secret is the Moroccan spice blend, which includes a subtle hint of Magic cinnamon. And, of course, we've used olive oil instead of butter.

700g **carrots**, peeled and cut into 6 x 1cm sticks
1 tablespoon extra virgin **olive oil**
1 **garlic** clove, finely chopped
$^{3}/_{4}$ teaspoon paprika
$^{1}/_{2}$ teaspoon ground cumin
Good pinch of ground **cinnamon**
Pinch of cayenne pepper
3 tablespoons **lemon** juice
2 tablespoons chopped fresh parsley or coriander
$^{1}/_{4}$ teaspoon salt, or to taste

1 **Steam the carrots** for 4–6 minutes or until they are just tender but still have a bite. Remove from the heat and keep warm.

2 **Heat the oil** in a large non-stick frying pan over a medium-low heat. Add the garlic, paprika, cumin, cinnamon and cayenne. Cook, stirring, for 1–2 minutes or until fragrant. Add the carrots, lemon juice, parsley (or coriander) and salt and stir to coat the carrots with the spice mixture. Serve hot.

PER SERVING: **86**kcal, **1g** protein,
14g carbohydrate, **4g** fibre, **3.5g** total fat
(**0.5g** saturated fat), **0mg** cholesterol, **0.4g** salt.

Sautéed spinach with ginger and soy sauce

serves 2

PREPARATION TIME: 10 MINUTES
COOKING TIME: 5–8 MINUTES

You cannot have enough recipes for simple spinach side dishes in your repertoire. This one has an oriental flair and uses aromatic sesame oil, which is low in saturated fat.

300g fresh **spinach**, large stalks trimmed off
    and leaves thoroughly washed
1 tablespoon reduced-salt soy sauce
2 teaspoons rice **vinegar**
1 teaspoon toasted sesame oil
¼ teaspoon soft brown sugar
2 teaspoons canola (rapeseed) oil
1 **garlic** clove, finely chopped
1½ teaspoons finely chopped fresh root ginger
Pinch of crushed dried chillies
1 tablespoon sesame **seeds**, toasted (see Tip,
    page 227)

1 **Sauté the spinach** (with just the water clinging to the leaves after washing) in a large, wide pan over a medium-high heat for 3–5 minutes or until wilted. Drain, rinse with cold water and press out excess moisture.

2 **Mix the soy sauce,** vinegar, sesame oil and sugar together in a small bowl. Heat the oil in a large non-stick frying pan over a medium-high heat. Add the garlic, ginger and chillies, and stir-fry for about 10 seconds or until fragrant but not browned. Add the spinach and cook, stirring often, for 2–3 minutes or until heated through. Stir in the soy sauce mixture and toss to coat well. Sprinkle with the sesame seeds and serve.

PER SERVING: **129**kcal, **6g** protein,
    5g carbohydrate, **4g** fibre, **10g** total fat
    (**1.5g** saturated fat), **0mg** cholesterol, **1.32g** salt.

Broccoli with lemon vinaigrette

serves 4

PREPARATION TIME: 10 MINUTES
COOKING TIME: 5–8 MINUTES

Heaping your plate with a generous portion of broccoli is an excellent strategy for Magic eating, as long as you don't drown it in butter or cheese sauce. Instead use a flavourful olive oil and lemon dressing to moisten steamed broccoli. For convenience, you can substitute 450g frozen broccoli florets for fresh (cook according to the instructions on the pack).

1 teaspoon grated **lemon** zest
2 tablespoons **lemon** juice
1 tablespoon extra virgin **olive oil**
2 **garlic** cloves, finely chopped
¼ teaspoon salt, or to taste
Good pinch of crushed dried chillies
Freshly ground black pepper to taste
700g **broccoli**

1 **Whisk together the lemon zest** and juice, oil, garlic, salt, chillies and pepper in a large bowl. Set aside.

2 **Separate the broccoli florets** and cut into 2.5cm pieces. Trim about 7.5cm from the stalks. Peel the remaining portions of stalk, then cut into 1cm thick slices. Rinse all the broccoli. Place in a steamer basket over boiling water, cover and steam for 5–8 minutes or until tender but still with a bit of a bite.

3 **Add the hot broccoli** to the bowl with the lemon dressing and toss to coat well. Serve immediately (if left, the lemon juice will cause the broccoli to discolour).

PER SERVING: **82**kcal, **8g** protein,
    3g carbohydrate, **4.5g** fibre, **4g** total fat
    (**0.7g** saturated fat), **0mg** cholesterol, **0.3g** salt.

Desserts

Blueberry and melon compote with green tea and lime

serves 8

PREPARATION TIME: 10 MINUTES
COOKING TIME: 0 MINUTES

Blueberries and orange-fleshed melon are a natural pairing of Magic foods. Here a tart lime flavouring and light green tea syrup give a distinctive and thoroughly refreshing finish to this low-calorie dessert, which could also be served as a breakfast compote.

2 green **tea** bags
150ml boiling water
2 tablespoons sugar
1 teaspoon grated lime zest
2 tablespoons **lime** juice
1 orange-fleshed **melon** (canteloupe or Charentais), peeled and cut into 4cm cubes
300g **blueberries**, rinsed and dried

1 **Place the tea bags** in the boiling water and leave to steep for 3–4 minutes. Remove the tea bags. Add the sugar to the tea and stir until dissolved. Stir in the lime zest and juice. Leave to cool to room temperature.

2 **Combine the melon** and blueberries in a large bowl. Pour the green tea mixture over the fruit and toss to coat well. The compote can be kept, covered, in the refrigerator for up to 2 days.

PER SERVING: **51**kcal, **0.8g** protein,
7.5g carbohydrate, **0.8g** fibre, **0g** total fat
(**0g** saturated fat), **0mg** cholesterol, salt (trace).

Pink grapefruit brûlée

serves 2

PREPARATION TIME: 5 MINUTES
COOKING TIME: 5–7 MINUTES

Chilled fresh grapefruit is always a refreshing breakfast treat, but when it is caramelised with a cinnamon-scented honey drizzle and warmed, it becomes a simple yet satisfying winter dessert.

1 pink **grapefruit**
2 teaspoons clear honey
Pinch of ground **cinnamon**

1 **Preheat the grill.** Line a small baking tray with foil (the caramelised drippings can be hard to remove). Cut the grapefruit in half horizontally. Use a paring knife or grapefruit knife to separate the flesh from the rind and membrane. Drizzle 1 teaspoon honey over each grapefruit half and spread evenly, then sprinkle with the cinnamon.

2 **Set the grapefruit** halves on the foil-lined baking tray and grill for 5–7 minutes or until the grapefruit skin is lightly browned in places and the grapefruit is warmed through.

PER SERVING: **38**kcal, **0.7g** protein,
9g carbohydrate, **1g** fibre, **0g** total fat
(**0g** saturated fat), **0mg** cholesterol, salt (trace).

Nectarine, plum and mixed berry soup

serves 8

PREPARATION TIME: **20 MINUTES**

COOKING TIME: **0 MINUTES**

Don't let the title mislead you – this 'soup' is actually a cool, refreshing dessert. Made with some of our favourite Magic berries and stone fruits, it bursts with flavour but contains surprisingly few calories and no fat.

4 tablespoons orange juice
1 tablespoon **lemon** juice
3 tablespoons caster sugar
2 medium **nectarines**, stoned and cut
    into 2.5 x 1cm pieces
3 medium **plums**, stoned and cut
    into 2.5 x 1cm pieces
150g **blueberries**, rinsed
150g **blackberries**, rinsed
2 ice cubes, crushed (see Tip)
125g fat-free vanilla **yoghurt**
Mint sprigs to garnish

1 **Combine the orange juice,** lemon juice and sugar in a large bowl. Stir to dissolve the sugar. Gently stir in the nectarines, plums, blueberries and blackberries. Transfer 180ml of the fruit and juices to a blender. Add the ice cubes and blend until smooth. Scrape the purée into the bowl containing the remaining fruit and stir gently to combine. Chill for at least 1 hour.

2 **To serve, stir the 'soup',** then ladle into dessert bowls and garnish each serving with a dollop of yoghurt and a mint sprig.

PER SERVING: **70**kcal, **2.5g** protein,
    12g carbohydrate, **1.4g** fibre, **0g** total fat
    (**0g** saturated fat), **0mg** cholesterol, salt (trace).

*Tip: **To crush ice cubes,** place them in a sturdy plastic bag, close tightly and smash with a rolling pin or the base of a heavy saucepan.*

Instant strawberry frozen yoghurt

serves 6

PREPARATION TIME: **5 MINUTES**

COOKING TIME: **0 MINUTES**

Home-made desserts are rarely as fast and easy as this one. Even if you haven't got an ice cream maker, you can still enjoy frozen yoghurt that tastes better – and is better for you – than anything ready-made you can buy. Start with unsweetened frozen fruit and use your food processor to whirl in yoghurt for a low-calorie frozen treat in just minutes.

450g unsweetened frozen **strawberries**
100g caster sugar
125g plain fat-free **yoghurt**
1 tablespoon lemon juice

1 **Place the strawberries** and sugar in a food processor and pulse until coarsely chopped. Mix the yoghurt and lemon juice in a measuring jug. With the motor running, gradually pour the yoghurt mixture through hole in the lid. Process until smooth and creamy, stopping once or twice to scrape down the side of bowl.

2 **Serve the frozen yoghurt** directly from the food processor or place it in the freezer for 30 minutes to harden before serving.

PER SERVING: **100**kcal, **1.7g** protein,
    23g carbohydrate, **0.8g** fibre, **0g** total fat,
    (**0g** saturated fat), **0mg** cholesterol, salt (trace).

VARIATIONS
Instant berry or peach frozen yoghurt

Substitute unsweetened frozen raspberries, blueberries or peaches for the strawberries.

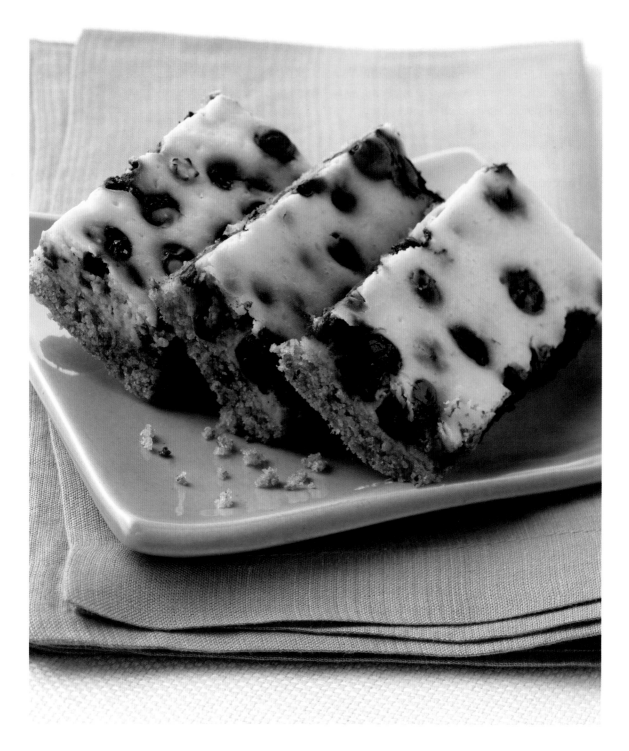

Lemony blueberry cheesecake bars

24 bars

PREPARATION TIME: 25 MINUTES
COOKING TIME: 55–60 MINUTES

If you love cheesecake – and who doesn't? – you will certainly enjoy these wholesome little bars. We've used naturally sweet blueberries to stretch the creamy filling and also replaced the traditional shortbread base (made with white flour and a copious amount of butter) with a wholemeal flour mixture, which contains more fibre and a fraction of the saturated fat.

BASE

175g **wholemeal flour**
$1/4$ teaspoon baking powder
$1/4$ teaspoon bicarbonate of soda
$1/4$ teaspoon salt
30g unsalted butter, softened
2 tablespoons canola (rapeseed) oil
100g caster sugar
1 medium **egg**, lightly beaten
1 teaspoon pure vanilla extract

FILLING

340g low-fat soft **cheese**
100g caster sugar
1 tablespoon cornflour
2 medium **eggs**, lightly beaten
4 teaspoons grated lemon zest
$1^1/2$ teaspoons pure vanilla extract
450g fresh, or partially thawed frozen,
    blueberries

1 **Preheat the oven** to 180°C/gas 4. Coat a 23 x 33cm baking tin or ovenproof dish with cooking spray. Set aside.

2 **To make the base:** whisk together the flour, baking powder, bicarbonate of soda and salt in a medium bowl. Beat the butter, oil and sugar with an electric mixer in a mixing bowl until smooth. Add the egg and vanilla extract and beat until smooth. Add the flour mixture and fold in with a rubber spatula just until the dry ingredients are moistened. Transfer the dough to the prepared tin or dish. Use a piece of cling film to press it into an even layer.

3 **Bake for about 20 minutes** or until the biscuit base is puffed and starting to brown around the edges.

4 **To make the filling:** beat the soft cheese with the caster sugar and cornflour using an electric mixer, or mix in a food processor, until smooth and creamy. Add the eggs, lemon zest and vanilla extract, and beat or process until smooth again. Spread out the blueberries over the biscuit base. Pour the filling mixture over the blueberries, spreading evenly.

5 **Bake for 35–40 minutes** or until the filling has set. Leave to cool completely in the tin or dish set on a wire rack, then cut into 24 bars using a sharp knife that has been coated with cooking spray. One serving is one bar. The bars can be kept, covered, in the refrigerator for up to 4 days or in the freezer for up to 1 month.

PER SERVING: **117**kcal, **2.7g** protein, **16g** carbohydrate, **0.5g** fibre, **4g** total fat (**2g** saturated fat), **52mg** cholesterol, **0.2g** salt.

Pumpkin custards

serves 6

PREPARATION TIME: 20 MINUTES

BAKING TIME: 50–55 MINUTES

These delicate custards have a generous amount of cinnamon, which not only makes them taste good, it also helps with blood sugar control.

2 medium **eggs**
2 medium **egg** whites (see Tip, page 211)
135g caster sugar
185g canned unseasoned pumpkin purée
1½ teaspoons ground **cinnamon**
½ teaspoon grated nutmeg
¼ teaspoon salt
1 teaspoon pure vanilla extract
375ml semi-skimmed **milk** (or **soya milk**)
3 heaped tablespoons whipped cream

1 **Preheat the oven** to 160°C/gas 3. Line a roasting tin with a folded tea towel (this will prevent the ramekins from sliding around). Put a kettle of water on to boil for the bain-marie.

2 **Whisk the eggs,** egg whites and sugar in a large bowl until smooth. Add the pumpkin purée, cinnamon, nutmeg, salt and vanilla extract. Whisk until blended. Gently whisk in the milk.

3 **Divide the mixture** among six 180ml ramekins or custard pots. Skim any foam from the surface of the custards. Set the ramekins on the towel in the roasting tin and pour enough boiling water into the tin to come halfway up the sides of the ramekins. Place the tin in the oven and bake for 50–55 minutes or until the custards are set.

4 **Transfer the ramekins** to a wire rack and leave to cool, then cover the custards and chill in the refrigerator for at least 1 hour. Just before serving, top each custard with a dollop of whipped cream.

PER SERVING: **183**kcal, **6g** protein, **27g** carbohydrate, **0.5g** fibre, **6.5g** total fat (**3g** saturated fat), **91mg** cholesterol, **0.4g** salt.

Orange and pomegranate compote

serves 4

PREPARATION TIME: 15 MINUTES

COOKING TIME: 0 MINUTES

The best strategy for making Magic desserts is to celebrate the fruits of the season. This simple but elegant compote will brighten a winter meal with two seasonal favourites – sweet oranges and pomegranates – and a splash of orange liqueur. Ruby-red pomegranate seeds, renowned for their antioxidant content and high in fibre, lend an exquisite, tart flavour and an appealing crunch.

2 tablespoons orange liqueur, such as Grand Marnier or Cointreau, or orange juice
1 tablespoon caster sugar
3 medium-large navel **oranges**
½ pomegranate

1 **Stir the orange liqueur** (or orange juice) and sugar together in a medium bowl. Peel the oranges, removing all the white pith. Quarter the oranges, then slice. Add the orange pieces to the bowl. Toss to coat with the orange liqueur.

2 **Scoop the seeds** from the pomegranate half into a small bowl, discarding all the membrane. Sprinkle the pomegranate seeds over the oranges. The compote can be kept, covered, in the refrigerator for up to 2 days.

PER SERVING: **93**kcal, **1.6g** protein, **18g** carbohydrate, **3g** fibre, **0g** total fat, (**0g** saturated fat), **0mg** cholesterol, salt (trace).

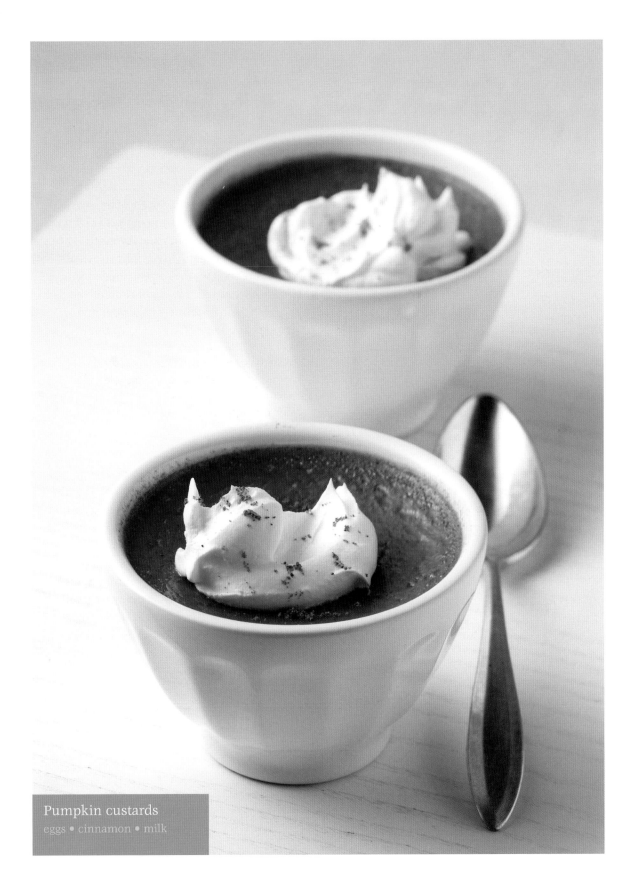

Pumpkin custards
eggs • cinnamon • milk

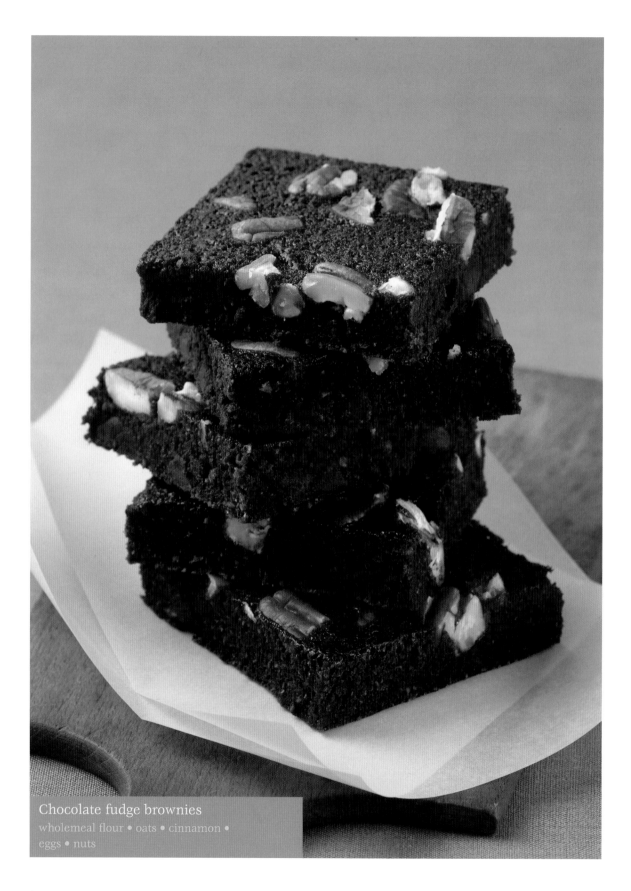

Chocolate fudge brownies
wholemeal flour • oats • cinnamon •
eggs • nuts

Chocolate fudge brownies

24 squares

PREPARATION TIME: 20 MINUTES

BAKING TIME: 20–25 MINUTES

Nearly everyone has a craving for a chewy chocolate treat from time to time. Here is a way to indulge yourself – with a wholegrain brownie that contains much less saturated fat than traditional recipes. We've lowered the GL by replacing some of the flour with oat bran and seasoning the brownies with cinnamon, a delicious complement to the chocolate.

85g plain dark chocolate (see Ingredient note, page 299)

80g **wholemeal flour**

80g **oat** bran

½ teaspoon ground **cinnamon**

¼ teaspoon salt

30g cocoa powder

4 medium **egg** whites (see Tip, page 211)

3 medium **eggs**

270g soft light brown sugar

180ml unsweetened apple purée (see Ingredient note)

4 tablespoons canola (rapeseed) oil

1 teaspoon pure vanilla extract

100g plain dark chocolate chips

40g chopped **pecan nuts** or **walnuts**

1 **Preheat the oven** to 180°C/gas 4. Coat a 23 x 33cm baking tin or ovenproof dish with cooking spray.

2 **Melt the chocolate** in a heatproof bowl set over a pan of barely simmering water, or in the microwave. Stir until smooth.

3 **Combine the flour,** oat bran, cinnamon and salt in a medium bowl. Sift in the cocoa powder. Whisk to blend the dry ingredients.

4 **Beat the egg whites** with the whole eggs and sugar in a large mixing bowl, using an electric mixer or a whisk, until smooth. Add the apple purée, oil and vanilla extract and beat until blended. Mix in the melted chocolate.

5 **Add the flour mixture** and beat into the egg mixture at low speed, or whisk together gently, just until all the dry ingredients are moistened. Stir in the chocolate chips. Scrape the mixture into the prepared baking tin or ovenproof dish, spreading evenly. Sprinkle with the chopped nuts.

6 **Bake the brownies** for 20–25 minutes or until the top springs back when touched lightly. Leave to cool completely in the tin set on a wire rack, then cut into 24 squares. One serving is one 5cm square.

PER SERVING: **163**kcal, **4g** protein, **24g** carbohydrate, **2.5g** fibre, **7g** total fat (**2g** saturated fat), **30mg** cholesterol, **0.1g** salt (trace).

*Ingredient note: **Fruit purées,** such as apple and prune, can be used very successfully as a fat replacement in baking. Ready-made apple sauce is normally sweetened with sugar, so make your own apple purée from sweet dessert apples. Another alternative is to use apple purée prepared for babies, as this will be sweetened with fruit concentrate.*

Maple-walnut baked apples

serves 4

PREPARATION TIME: 15 MINUTES

BAKING TIME: 30–40 MINUTES

While a crisp apple is one of the tastiest, healthiest snacks, when cooked, apples can also be the starting point for an easy low-calorie dessert. Our sophisticated yet simple baked apples feature walnuts for a dose of protein and 'good' fat and maple syrup, rather than brown sugar, to sweeten.

125g maple syrup
3 tablespoons apple juice
Small knob of unsalted butter (about 10g)
2 large Bramley **apples**
2 tablespoons chopped **walnuts**
250ml reduced-fat vanilla ice cream or vanilla frozen yoghurt

1 **Preheat the oven** to 200°C/gas 6. Coat a 20cm square ovenproof dish with cooking spray. Set aside.

2 **Combine the maple syrup,** apple juice and butter in a small saucepan. Bring to a simmer, stirring. Remove from the heat.

3 **Wash and dry the apples,** then cut in half lengthways (leave the skin on) and remove the cores. Place the apple halves, cut side up, in the ovenproof dish. Pour the maple syrup mixture over the apples. Cover with foil.

4 **Bake for 20 minutes,** then baste the apples with the maple syrup mixture in the dish. Sprinkle with the walnuts. Return to the oven and bake, uncovered, for 10–20 minutes or until the apples are tender and glazed, basting once or twice. Let cool slightly, then place an apple half in each bowl. Drizzle over the syrup and add a scoop of vanilla ice cream (or frozen yoghurt).

PER SERVING: **214**kcal, **2.5g** protein, **39g** carbohydrate, **1.6g** fibre, **6g** total fat (**1g** saturated fat), **5mg** cholesterol, salt (trace).

Orange-glazed baked plums

serves 4

PREPARATION TIME: 15 MINUTES

BAKING TIME: 30–40 MINUTES

Baking brings out the natural sweetness in fruits and is a delicious way to prepare fibre-rich stone fruits. Here, an orange-scented syrup provides a delicate balance to tart plums.

1 teaspoon grated orange zest or grated fresh root ginger
Juice of 1 orange
3 tablespoons soft brown sugar
Small knob of unsalted butter (about 10g)
4 medium **plums** (450–600g total weight), halved and stoned
2 tablespoons slivered or flaked **almonds**
125g fat-free vanilla **yoghurt**

1 **Preheat the oven** to 200°C/gas 6. Coat a 20cm square ovenproof dish with cooking spray. Set aside.

2 **Combine the orange zest** (or ginger), orange juice and brown sugar in a small saucepan. Bring to a simmer, stirring to dissolve the sugar. Remove from the heat. Add the butter and stir until melted.

3 **Place the plum halves,** cut side up, in the ovenproof dish. Pour over the orange juice mixture and cover with foil. Bake for 20–25 minutes or until the plums are almost tender.

4 **Baste the plums** with the orange syrup and sprinkle over the almonds. Bake, uncovered, for a further 10–15 minutes or until tender and glazed, basting once or twice. Serve the plums warm or chilled, with the syrup drizzled over and topped with a dollop of yoghurt.

PER SERVING: **170**kcal, **4g** protein, **25g** carbohydrate, **2.5g** fibre, **7g** total fat (**2g** saturated fat), **6mg** cholesterol, **0.1g** salt.

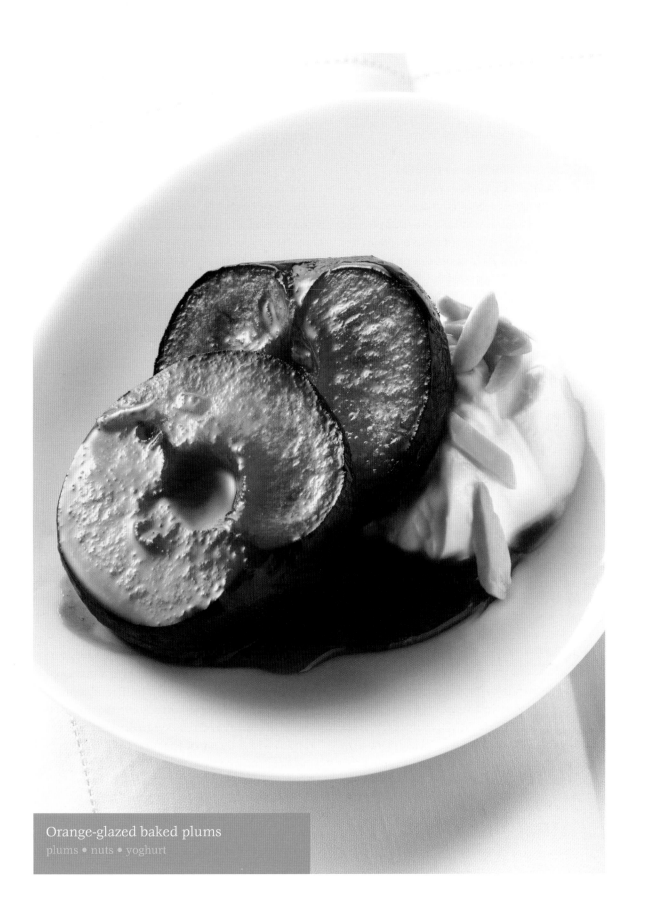

Orange-glazed baked plums
plums • nuts • yoghurt

Chocolate and raspberry cheesecake

serves 12

PREPARATION TIME: 40 MINUTES

BAKING TIME: 60–70 MINUTES

This fabulously rich-tasting cheesecake plays on the delicious contrast of tart raspberries and dark chocolate to make a truly impressive dessert. No one will ever guess that it is relatively low in calories and saturated fat. The secret ingredient is silken tofu, which bakes into a velvety filling, and the protein it provides helps to offset the carbohydrates in the dessert.

CRUST

125g plain chocolate biscuits (see
    Ingredient note)

40g **walnut halves**

4 teaspoons soft light brown sugar

Good pinch of ground **cinnamon**

3 tablespoons canola (rapeseed) oil

FILLING

125g plain dark chocolate (see Ingredient note)

350g silken **tofu**

250g low-fat soft **cheese**

150g soft light brown sugar

100g caster sugar

60g cocoa powder

2 tablespoons cornflour

2 teaspoons pure vanilla extract

3 medium **eggs**, lightly beaten

180g **raspberries**

GARNISH

250g **raspberries**

30g chocolate shavings (see Tip)

Icing sugar for dusting

Raspberry Coulis (see opposite page)

1 **Preheat the oven** to 160°C/gas 3. Coat a 23cm springform cake tin with cooking spray. Wrap a double thickness of foil around the outside of the tin, to ensure that no water from the bain-marie seeps into the cheesecake while it is baking.

2 **To make the crust:** combine the biscuits, walnuts, brown sugar and cinnamon in a food processor. Pulse until fine crumbs form. Add the oil and pulse just until the crumbs are moistened and starting to clump together. Transfer to the cake tin and use the bottom of a glass to press the crumb mixture evenly over the bottom of the tin and 1cm up the sides. Bake the crust for 10–15 minutes or until firm to the touch. Set aside to cool. (Wash and dry the food processor bowl.)

3 **To make the filling:** melt the chocolate in a heatproof bowl set over a pan of barely simmering water, or in the microwave. Stir the chocolate until smooth. Set aside.

4 **Place the tofu** in the food processor and process until smooth, stopping to scrape down the sides of the bowl once or twice. Add the soft cheese, brown sugar, caster sugar, cocoa powder, melted chocolate, cornflour and vanilla extract. Process until well blended. Add the eggs and pulse just until they are mixed in.

5 **Put a kettle of water on** to boil for the bain-marie. Rinse the raspberries and pat thoroughly dry, then scatter them evenly over the baked crust. Scrape the chocolate filling mixture into the tin and spread evenly. Place the tin in a shallow roasting tin and pour enough boiling water into the roasting tin to come 1cm up the sides of the cake tin.

6 **Bake the cheesecake** for 50–55 minutes or until set around the edges but the centre still wobbles slightly when the tin is tapped. Turn off the oven and prop the oven door open with a wooden spoon. Leave the cheesecake to cool in the oven for 1 hour.

7 **Remove the foil wrapping** and place the cake tin on a wire rack to cool completely. Cover with cling film and chill for at least 4 hours (or keep in the refrigerator for up to 4 days).

8 **To prepare the garnish:** rinse the raspberries and pat thoroughly dry. Run a small, sharp knife between the cheesecake and the side of the tin to loosen, then unclip and remove the tin side. Set the cheesecake on a serving platter and arrange the raspberries on top. Sprinkle with chocolate shavings and dust with icing sugar. Serve with the raspberry coulis.

PER SERVING: **408**kcal, **10g** protein,
   53g carbohydrate, **3g** fibre, **18g** total fat
   (**7.5g** saturated fat), **61mg** cholesterol, **0.2g** salt.

Tip: **To make chocolate shavings,** *warm a chunk or piece of dark plain chocolate on low power in the microwave for a few seconds, just until pliable but not melted. Use a vegetable peeler to shave off curls.*

Ingredient notes:

■ **Look for plain chocolate biscuits,** *not chocolate-covered biscuits, without any filling. Chocolate cantucci or chocolate amaretti would both be suitable.*
■ **For the best chocolate flavour** *in this cheesecake, use a plain dark chocolate with a high cocoa content – 70 per cent minimum. Those chocolates with a higher cocoa content are also richer in antioxidants.*

Raspberry coulis

serves 12

PREPARATION TIME: **5 MINUTES**
COOKING TIME: **0 MINUTES**

This elegant sauce is made simply by puréeing raspberries (frozen berries work well and are very convenient) and then sweetening the purée slightly. In addition to serving it with the cheesecake, use it to dress up a compote of fresh strawberries or mixed berries, or as a topping for reduced-fat vanilla ice cream or frozen yoghurt. If serving with a sweetened dessert, remember that the coulis contains sugar too, and keep an eye on the serving size.

300g frozen unsweetened **raspberries**, thawed
40g icing sugar, sifted
1 tablespoon orange juice

Put the raspberries, sugar and orange juice in a food processor. Process until puréed. Press the purée through a fine nylon sieve set over a medium bowl using a large spoon or rubber spatula. Discard the pips left in the sieve. Chill the coulis before serving. One serving is about 2 tablespoons.

PER SERVING: **20**kcal, **0.5g** protein,
   5g carbohydrate, **0.6g** fibre, **0g** total fat
   (**0g** saturated fat), **0mg** cholesterol, (salt) trace.

VARIATION
Fresh berry coulis

Substitute 350g fresh raspberries, or 175g each fresh raspberries and strawberries, for the frozen raspberries. If using strawberries, you can reduce the amount of icing sugar to 2 tablespoons, or to taste. Use either orange juice or lemon juice.

Cherry clafoutis

serves 8

PREPARATION TIME: 25 MINUTES
BAKING TIME: 35–40 MINUTES

Cherries are one of our favourite low-GL foods, and it's hard to think of a more delicious way to enjoy them than in a clafoutis. In this rustic French pudding the fruit is baked in a thick, sweet pancake batter. The pudding is simple to make and ever so comforting. If you're using fresh cherries, a cherry stoner will speed up the preparation. Or use frozen cherries, which are already stoned.

125g caster sugar
75g plain flour
2 medium **eggs**
2 medium **egg** whites (see Tip, page 211)
250ml semi-skimmed **milk**
15g unsalted butter, melted
1 teaspoon pure vanilla extract
450g fresh **cherries**, stoned, or partially thawed frozen cherries
Icing sugar for dusting

1 **Preheat the oven** to 200°C/gas 6. Coat a 23–24cm round ovenproof dish or baking tin with cooking spray. Sprinkle with 1 tablespoon of the caster sugar and tilt to coat evenly.

2 **Place 100g** of the remaining caster sugar, the flour, eggs, egg whites, milk, butter and vanilla extract in a food processor or blender. Process to make a smooth batter.

3 **Spread out the cherries** in the ovenproof dish or tin. Pour the batter over the cherries and sprinkle with the remaining 1 tablespoon sugar. Bake the clafoutis for 35–40 minutes or until light brown and slightly puffed. Leave to cool slightly (the clafoutis will sink as it cools), then dust with icing sugar and serve warm. (Leftovers are also delicious chilled.)

PER SERVING: **181**kcal, **5g** protein, **34g** carbohydrate, **0.8g** fibre, **4g** total fat (**2g** saturated fat), **55mg** cholesterol, **0.15g** salt.

VARIATION
Pear and berry clafoutis

In Step 2, add 2 teaspoons grated lemon zest to the batter. In Step 3, substitute 2 firm dessert pears, peeled and sliced, and 120g fresh raspberries, or partially thawed frozen raspberries, for the cherries.

Mixed berry and almond gratin

serves 6

PREPARATION TIME: 30 MINUTES
BAKING TIME: 30–40 MINUTES

In this special dessert, fruit is baked in a rich-tasting almond cream. Tofu may seem a surprising ingredient, but it works well here as a healthy substitute for butter.

40g slivered or flaked **almonds**
70g caster sugar
1 tablespoon plain flour
Pinch of salt
1 medium **egg**
1 medium **egg** white
125g silken **tofu**
15g unsalted butter, softened
¼ teaspoon almond essence
375g mixed fresh **berries** (eg raspberries, blackberries and blueberries) or frozen and partially thawed berries
Icing sugar for dusting

1 **Preheat the oven** to 190°C/gas 5. Coat a 24cm round ovenproof dish or baking tin with cooking spray.

2 **Spread the almonds** in a small baking tray. Toast in the oven for 4–6 minutes or until light golden and fragrant. Cool.

3 **Combine the almonds,** caster sugar, flour and salt in a food processor. Process until the almonds are ground. Add the egg, egg white, tofu, butter and almond essence. Process until smooth.

4 Spread out the berries in the ovenproof dish or tin and cover evenly with the tofu mixture. Bake the gratin for 30–40 minutes or until light golden and firm to the touch. Leave to cool slightly, then dust with icing sugar. Serve warm or at room temperature.

PER SERVING: **193**kcal, **6g** protein, **25g** carbohydrate, **1g** fibre, **8g** total fat (**2g** saturated fat), **45mg** cholesterol, **0.2g** salt.

VARIATIONS

Cherry and almond gratin

In Step 4, substitute 450g fresh cherries, stoned, or frozen and partially thawed cherries, for the mixed berries.

Pear and dried cranberry gratin

In Step 4, substitute 3 firm dessert pears, peeled and sliced, and 70g plumped dried cranberries (microwave with 2 tablespoons water on high for 1 minute) for the cherries.

Cranberry and apple crumble

serves 8

PREPARATION TIME: **20 MINUTES**
BAKING TIME: **40–55 MINUTES**

With its emphasis on wholegrains and fruit, this could be the ideal Magic pudding. We've replaced the white flour in the typical recipe with wholemeal to make a 100 per cent wholegrain topping, and substituted fruit juice concentrate and oil for much of the butter. This is an extremely versatile concept – there are crumble recipes overleaf for every season. Top each serving with a dollop of fat-free vanilla yoghurt.

4–5 dessert **apples**, peeled and sliced
100g fresh or frozen **cranberries**
70g granulated sugar
100g **wholemeal flour**
40g rolled **oats**
100g soft light brown sugar
2 teaspoons ground **cinnamon**
Pinch of salt
15g unsalted butter, cut into small pieces
1 tablespoon canola (rapeseed) oil
3 tablespoons apple juice concentrate
1 tablespoon chopped **walnuts**

1 Preheat the oven to 190°C/gas 5. Coat a 20cm square ovenproof dish (2 litre capacity) with cooking spray.

2 Combine the apples, cranberries and granulated sugar in the ovenproof dish. Toss to mix. Cover with foil and bake for 20 minutes (25 minutes, if using some frozen fruit).

3 Meanwhile, mix the flour, oats, brown sugar, cinnamon and salt with a fork in a medium bowl. Add the butter and rub in with your fingertips until the mixture resembles coarse crumbs. Add the oil, then add the apple juice concentrate. Stir and toss until the dry ingredients are moistened.

4 When the fruit has baked for 20 minutes, sprinkle the crumble topping evenly over the top. Scatter on the walnuts. Bake, uncovered, for 20–30 minutes or until the fruit is bubbling and tender and the topping is lightly browned. Leave to cool for at least 10 minutes before serving warm or at room temperature.

PER SERVING: **218**kcal, **3g** protein, **43g** carbohydrate, **3g** fibre, **5g** total fat (**1g** saturated fat), **4mg** cholesterol, **0.1g** salt.

Rhubarb and blackberry crumble

PER SERVING: **225**kcal, **4g** protein, **45g** carbohydrate, **3.5g** fibre, **5g** total fat (**1g** saturated fat), **4mg** cholesterol, salt (trace).

serves 8

PREPARATION TIME: 20 MINUTES

BAKING TIME: 40–55 MINUTES

If you enjoy the tart taste of rhubarb, you'll adore this sweet and tangy early summer pudding with its cinnamon-spiced topping.

700g rhubarb, cut into 1cm pieces
145g fresh or partially thawed frozen **blackberries**
100g granulated sugar
1 tablespoon cornflour
100g **wholemeal flour**
40g rolled **oats**
100g soft light brown sugar
1 teaspoon ground **cinnamon**
Pinch of salt
15g unsalted butter, cut into small pieces
1 tablespoon canola (rapeseed) oil
3 tablespoons apple juice concentrate
1 tablespoon chopped **almonds**

1 **Preheat the oven** to 190°C/gas 5. Coat a 20cm square ovenproof dish (2 litre capacity) with cooking spray.

2 **Combine the rhubarb,** blackberries, granulated sugar and cornflour in the ovenproof dish. Toss to mix. Cover with foil and bake for 20 minutes.

3 **Meanwhile, mix the flour,** oats, brown sugar, cinnamon and salt with a fork in a medium bowl. Add the butter and rub in with your fingertips until the mixture resembles coarse crumbs. Add the oil and then add the apple juice concentrate. Stir and toss until the dry ingredients are moistened.

4 **When the fruit has baked** for 20 minutes, sprinkle the crumble mixture evenly over the top. Scatter over the almonds. Bake, uncovered, for 20–30 minutes or until the fruit is bubbling and tender and the topping is lightly browned. Leave to cool for at least 10 minutes before serving warm or at room temperature.

VARIATIONS

Peach and raspberry crumble

In Step 2, combine 1kg peaches, peeled and sliced, 120g raspberries, 2 tablespoons granulated sugar, 1 tablespoon cornflour and 1 tablespoon lemon juice in the ovenproof dish and toss to mix.

Cherry and raspberry crumble

In Step 2, combine 700g cherries, stoned, 120g raspberries, 70g granulated sugar, 1 tablespoon cornflour and 1 tablespoon lemon juice in the ovenproof dish and toss to mix.

Plum and walnut crumble

In Step 2, combine 1kg plums, sliced, 70g granulated sugar, 2 teaspoons grated orange zest and 1 tablespoon orange juice in the ovenproof dish. Toss to mix.
In Step 4, substitute walnuts for the almonds.

7-day meal plans

Incorporating a few Magic foods into your diet is as easy as can be. But you may be wondering what a whole day of Magic eating looks like. Also, how do you know if you're eating too many carbohydrates – or not enough? And how do you know if you're eating too much food?

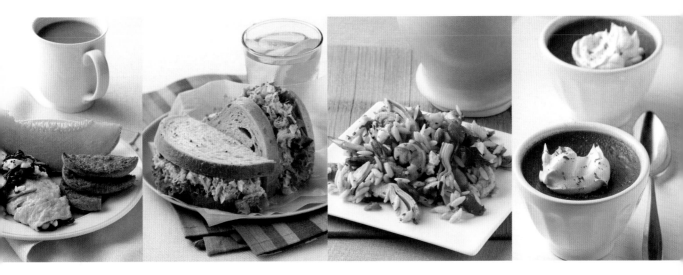

To help you put the *Magic Foods* approach to work on your plate, we have designed week-long meal plans based on three different calorie goals. Each meal, snack and dessert incorporates the 'Seven secrets of Magic eating', and each day features at least a dozen different Magic foods.

You'll see for yourself not only how much food you should be eating but also what a good breakdown of carbohydrates, protein and fat looks like; what constitutes three daily servings of whole grains; and what five or more daily servings of fruits and vegetables look like.

If you're not sure which calorie goal is right for you or you think you need to lose weight, consult your doctor or dietician and he or she will help you to decide. Remember that controlling portion sizes and calories is key to controlling your blood sugar. Broadly speaking, the 1400kcal target is appropriate for most smaller women or women trying to lose weight, the 1800kcal target is appropriate for most larger women and average-size men and for larger men who want to lose weight; and the 2200kcal target appropriate for larger or highly active men.

These are rough targets for you to aim for. You'll notice that some day plans are slightly over and some slightly under the suggested target but the small calorie difference will not affect your dietary goals.

Whichever plan you decide to try, we don't necessarily expect you to follow the menu choices to the letter (although if you want to, all the better). But do try one or two days to see what the *Magic Foods* approach is like – and how good it makes you feel.

1400 kcal meal plan

	monday	tuesday	wednesday
breakfast	1 pot (200g) low-fat yoghurt plus 2 tbsp sugar-free muesli 1 orange Coffee or tea	1 serving **Porridge with apple and flaxseeds** *page 192* Coffee or tea	30g Fruit 'n Fibre cereal with 80g strawberries & 150ml semi-skimmed milk Coffee or tea
lunch	1 serving **Turkey and bean chilli with avocado salsa** *page 252* 1 pear Sugar-free drink or water	Turkey sandwich with: 2 slices wholemeal bread 2 tsp unsaturated margarine 100g cooked turkey Plenty of salad 1 banana Sugar-free drink or water	1 serving **Grilled chicken salad with orange** *page 214* 1 slice pumpernickel bread Sugar-free drink or water
snacks	1 serving **Oriental peanut dip** *page 206* with 50g carrot sticks	1 serving **White bean spread with Italian flavours** *page 208* 4 **Wholemeal pitta crisps** *page 210*	1 serving **Mediterranean split pea spread** *page 208* 4 **Wholemeal pitta crisps** *page 210*
evening meal	1 serving **Chicken sauté with apples** *page 246* 1 serving **Mushroom and barley pilaf** *page 276* 80g French beans Sugar-free drink or water	1 serving **Greek pasta and beef casserole** *page 240* 1 serving **Broccoli with lemon vinaigrette** *page 287* Sugar-free drink or water	1 serving **Mustard-glazed salmon with lentils** *page 257* 1 serving **Brown rice pilaf with lemon and toasted flaxseeds** *page 276* 6 asparagus spears Sugar-free drink or water
dessert	1 portion (150g) fresh fruit salad	1 slice of fresh pineapple	1 serving **Pumpkin custard** *page 292*
nutritional information	Kcal: 1,367 Protein: 77g Carbohydrate: 197g Fat: 32g Fibre: 28g Percentage of calories from carbs: 57; protein: 22; fat: 21	Kcal: 1,412 Protein: 90g Carbohydrate: 165g Fat: 45g Fibre: 20g Percentage of calories from carbs: 47; protein: 25; fat: 28	Kcal: 1,345 Protein: 90g Carbohydrate: 150g Fat: 42g Fibre: 25g Percentage of calories from carbs: 45; protein: 27; fat: 28

thursday	friday	saturday	sunday
30g sugar-free muesli with 200ml semi-skimmed milk & 80g blueberries 125ml orange juice	30g sugar-free muesli with 200ml Greek yoghurt (0% fat) & 80g raspberries Coffee or tea	2 **Multigrain griddle cakes** *page 192* with syrup and berries 200ml semi-skimmed milk	1 **Spinach and goat's cheese omelette** *page 194* 2 slices (160g) melon Coffee or tea
1 **Tuna and carrot sandwich on rye** *page 229* 2 tbsp **Spiced almonds** *page 205* 1 peach Sugar-free drink or water	Wholemeal pitta stuffed with small can drained tuna in water, 2 tbsp canned sweetcorn 2 tbsp light mayo 1 apple Sugar-free drink or water	1 serving **Curried red lentil soup** *page 230* 2 tbsp (50g) hummus plus vegetable crudités Sugar-free drink or water	1 serving **Wholemeal noodles with peanut sauce and chicken** *page 220* 2 slices (100g) fresh pineapple Sugar-free drink or water
1 **Oat and peanut butter bar** *page 211*	Low-fat fruit yoghurt	1 pot Greek yoghurt (0% fat) with 80g blueberries	small banana plus 2 oatcakes
1 serving **Rump steak with balsamic sauce** *page 237* 100g (cooked weight) brown rice 1 mixed salad with 50g canned chickpeas and 1 tbsp olive oil and balsamic vinegar dressing Sugar-free drink or water	1 serving **Prawn and orzo casserole** *page 260* 80g French beans Mixed salad with 1 tbsp olive oil and balsamic vinegar dressing Mineral water	1 serving **Slow-cooker beef and red wine stew** *page 238* 1 slice **Wholemeal flaxseed bread** *page 196* Mixed salad with 1 tbsp olive oil and balsamic vinegar dressing Sugar-free drink or water	1 serving **Spring vegetable stir-fry with tofu** *page 271* 100g (cooked weight) brown rice Sugar-free drink or water
1 pear	1 serving (150g) fresh fruit salad	1 serving **Orange and pomegranate compote** *page 292*	1 serving **Instant strawberry frozen yoghurt** *page 289*
Kcal: 1,350 Protein: 80g Carbohydrate: 180g Fat: 42g Fibre: 26g Percentage of calories from carbs: 50; protein: 23; fat: 28	Kcal: 1,399 Protein: 84g Carbohydrate: 172g Fat: 42g Fibre: 26g Percentage of calories from carbs: 49; protein: 24; fat: 27	Kcal: 1,399 Protein: 85g Carbohydrate: 170g Fat: 45g Fibre: 27g Percentage of calories from carbs: 47; protein: 24; fat: 29	Kcal: 1,361 Protein: 80g Carbohydrate: 160g Fat: 42g Fibre: 25g Percentage of calories from carbs: 47; protein: 24; fat: 28

1800
kcal meal plan

	monday	tuesday	wednesday
breakfast	1 pot (200g) low-fat yoghurt plus 3 tbsp sugar-free muesli 1 orange 180ml unsweetened fruit juice Coffee or tea	1 serving **Porridge with apple and flaxseeds** *page 192* plus 15g toasted almonds Coffee or tea	40g Fruit 'n Fibre with 80g strawberries and 200ml skimmed milk Coffee or tea
lunch	1 serving **Turkey and bean chilli with avocado salsa** *page 252* 1 slice **Wholemeal flaxseed bread** *page 196* with 1 tsp unsaturated margarine 1 pot (200g) Greek yoghurt (0% fat) plus 80g raspberries Sugar-free drink or water	Turkey sandwich with 2 slices wholemeal bread 2 tsp unsaturated margarine 100g cooked turkey and plenty of salad 1 banana plus 1 pot (200g) low-fat fruit yoghurt Sugar-free drink or water	1 serving **Grilled chicken salad with orange** *page 214* 2 slices pumpernickel bread 1 peach Sugar-free drink or water
snacks	1 serving **Oriental peanut dip** *page 206* plus 50g carrot sticks 1 pear	1 **Blueberry and oat muffin** *page 198*	1 serving **Mediterranean split pea spread** *page 208* 4 **Wholemeal pitta crisps** *page 210*
evening meal	1 serving **Chicken sauté with apples** *page 246* 1 serving **Mushroom and barley pilaf** *page 276* 125g French beans Sugar-free drink or water	1 serving **Greek pasta and beef casserole** *page 240* 1 serving **Broccoli with lemon vinaigrette** *page 287* Sugar-free drink or water	1 serving **Mustard-glazed salmon with lentils** *page 257* 1 serving **Brown rice pilaf with lemon and toasted flaxseeds** *page 276* 6 asparagus spears Sugar-free drink or water
dessert	1 serving (150g) fresh fruit salad		1 serving **Pumpkin custard** *page 292*
nutritional information	Kcal: 1,767kcal Protein: 103g Carbohydrate: 258g Fat: 35g Fibre: 37g Percentage of calories from carbs: 58; protein: 23; fat: 18	Kcal: 1,840 Protein: 118g Carbohydrate: 211 g Fat: 58g Fibre: 23g Percentage of calories from carbs: 46; protein: 26; fat: 28	Kcal: 1,820 Protein: 120g Carbohydrate: 190g Fat: 64g Fibre: 38g Percentage of calories from carbs: 42; protein: 26; fat: 32

thursday	friday	saturday	sunday
40g sugar-free muesli plus 80g blueberries and 200ml semi-skimmed milk 180ml unsweetened fruit juice Coffee or tea	1 grapefruit 1 **Apple bran muffin** *page 198* 180ml unsweetened fruit juice Coffee or tea	2 **Multigrain griddle cakes** *page 192* with syrup and berries 180ml unsweetened fruit juice 200ml skimmed milk	1 **Spinach and goat's cheese omelette** *page 194* 1 slice **Wholemeal flaxseed bread** *page 196* 2 slices (160g) melon Coffee or tea
1 **Tuna and carrot sandwich on rye** *page 229* 4 **Wholemeal pitta crisps** *page 210* 2 tbsp **Spiced almonds** *page 205* 1 portion (150g) fresh fruit salad Sugar-free drink or water	1 wholemeal pitta stuffed with 1 small can drained tuna in water 2 tbsp canned sweetcorn 2 tbsp light mayonnaise 1 pot (200g) Greek yoghurt (0% fat) plus 2 passion fruit Sugar-free drink or water	1 serving **Curried red lentil soup** *page 230* 2 tbsp (50g) reduced-fat hummus plus vegetable crudités and 4 **Wholemeal pitta crisps** *page 210* 1 peach Sugar-free drink or water	1 serving **Wholemeal noodles with peanut sauce and chicken** *page 220* 2 slices (100g) fresh pineapple Sugar-free drink or water
1 **Oat and peanut butter bar** *page 211* 2 oatcakes plus 1 tbsp reduced-fat hummus	1 pot (150g) low-fat fruit yoghurt 2 oatcakes each spread with 1 tsp reduced-fat hummus	1 pot (200g) Greek yoghurt (0% fat) plus 80g blueberries 1 **Lemony blueberry cheesecake bar** *page 291*	Small banana plus 2 oatcakes 2 tbsp **Spiced almonds** *page 205* **Peachy iced tea** *page 213*
1 serving **Rump steak with balsamic sauce** *page 237* 100g (cooked weight) brown rice Mixed salad with 50g canned chickpeas and 1 tbsp oil and balsamic vinegar dressing 1 pear Sugar-free drink or water	1 serving **Prawn and orzo casserole** *page 260* 80g French beans Mixed salad with 1 tablespoon olive oil and balsamic vinegar dressing Sugar-free drink or water	1 serving **Slow-cooker beef and red wine stew** *page 238* 1 slice **Wholemeal flaxseed bread** *page 196* with 1 tsp unsaturated margarine Mixed salad with 1 tbsp oil and balsamic vinegar dressing Sugar-free drink or water	1 serving **Spring vegetable stir-fry with tofu** *page 271* 100g (cooked weight) brown rice Sugar-free drink or water
		1 serving **Orange and pomegranate compote** *page 292*	1 serving **Instant strawberry frozen yoghurt** *page 289* plus 1 apple
Kcal: 1,800 Protein: 115g Carbohydrate: 210g Fat: 55g Fibre: 32g Percentage of calories from carbs: 47; protein: 26; fat: 27	Kcal: 1,363 Protein: 82g Carbohydrate: 165g Fat: 42g Fibre: 22g Percentage of calories from carbs: 48; protein: 24; fat: 28	Kcal: 1,730 Protein: 105g Carbohydrate: 215g Fat: 51g Fibre: 35g Percentage of calories from carbs: 50; protein: 24; fat: 26	Kcal: 1,771 Protein: 105g Carbohydrate: 215g Fat: 55g Fibre: 36g Percentage of calories from carbs: 48; protein: 24; fat: 28

	monday	tuesday	wednesday
breakfast	1 pot (200g) low-fat yoghurt plus 4 tbsp sugar-free muesli 180ml unsweetened fruit juice 1 orange Coffee or tea	1 serving **Porridge with apples and flaxseeds** *page 192* plus 15g toasted almonds 180ml unsweetened fruit juice 1 peach Coffee or tea	40g Fruit 'n Fibre cereal with 80g strawberries 15g flaked almonds and 200ml semi-skimmed milk 180ml unsweetened fruit juice Coffee or tea
lunch	1 serving **Turkey and bean chilli with avocado salsa** *page 252* 2 slices **Wholemeal flaxseed bread** *page 196* with 1 tbsp unsaturated margarine 1 pot (200g) Greek yoghurt (0% fat) plus 80g raspberries Sugar-free drink or water	Turkey sandwich with 2 slices wholemeal bread 2 tsp unsaturated margarine 100g cooked turkey and plenty of salad 1 pot (200g) low-fat fruit yoghurt plus 1 banana Sugar-free drink or water	1 serving **Grilled chicken salad with orange** *page 214* plus ½ avocado 2 slices pumpernickel bread Peach Sugar-free drink or water
snacks	1 serving **Oriental peanut dip** *page 206* plus 50g carrot sticks plus 4 **Wholemeal pitta crisps** *page 210* **Berry and flaxseed smoothie** *page 201*	1 **Blueberry and oat muffin** *page198* 2 oatcakes with low-fat soft cheese **Iced coffee frappé** *page 213*	1 pot (150g) low-fat vanilla yoghurt plus 1 kiwi fruit 1 small pitta bread with 50g reduced-fat hummus
evening meal	1 serving **Chicken sauté with apples** *page 246* 1 serving **Mushroom and barley pilaf** *page 276* 80g French beans Sugar-free drink or water	1 serving **Greek pasta and beef casserole** *page 240* 1 serving **Broccoli with lemon vinaigrette** *page 287* Sugar-free drink or water	1 serving **Mustard-glazed salmon with lentils** *page 257* 1 serving **Brown rice pilaf with lemon and toasted flaxseeds** *page 276* 6 asparagus spears Sugar-free drink or water
dessert	1 portion (150g) fresh fruit salad	1 serving **Maple-walnut baked apples** *page 296*	1 serving **Pumpkin custard** *page 292*
nutritional information	Kcal: 2,250 Protein: 123g Carbohydrate: 310g Fat: 59g Fibre: 45g Percentage of calories from carbs: 55; protein: 21; fat: 24	Kcal: 2,210 Protein: 129g Carbohydrate: 280g Fat: 63g Fibre: 35g Percentage of calories from carbs: 51; protein: 23; fat: 26	Kcal: 2,175 Protein: 120 g Carbohydrate: 280g Fat: 65g Fibre: 42g Percentage of calories from carbs: 51; protein: 22; fat: 27

thursday	friday	saturday	sunday

thursday	friday	saturday	sunday
40g sugar-free muesli with 80g blueberries and 200ml semi-skimmed milk 180ml unsweetened fruit juice Coffee or tea	1 grapefruit 1 **Apple bran muffin** *page 198* 180ml unsweetened fruit juice Coffee or tea	2 **Multigrain griddle cakes** *page 192* with syrup and berries 180ml unsweetened fruit juice 180ml semi-skimmed milk	1 **Spinach and goat's cheese omelette** *page 194* 1 slice **Wholemeal flaxseed bread** *page 196* 2 slices (160g) melon Coffee or tea
1 **Tuna and carrot sandwich on rye** *page 229* 4 **Wholemeal pitta crisps** *page 210* plus 4 tbsp tomato salsa 2 tbsp **Spiced almonds** *page 205* 1 pot (200g) Greek yoghurt (0% fat) with 1 kiwi fruit Sugar-free drink or water	Wholemeal pitta stuffed with 1 small can drained tuna in water 2 tbsp canned sweetcorn 2 tbsp light mayonnaise 1 pot (200g) Greek yoghurt (0% fat) with 1 banana Sugar-free drink or water	1 serving **Curried red lentil soup** *page 230* 4 **Wholemeal pitta crisps** *page 210* with 2 tbsp (50g) reduced-fat hummus and vegetable crudités 1 portion (150g) fresh fruit salad Sugar-free drink or water	1 serving **Wholemeal noodles with peanut sauce and chicken** *page 220* 2 slices (100g) fresh pineapple Sugar-free drink or water
1 **Oat and peanut butter bar** *page 211* 3 oatcakes plus 2 tbsp reduced-fat hummus	3 oatcakes spread with reduced-fat soft cheese 1 **Lemony blueberry cheesecake bar** *page 291*	1 pot (200g) Greek yoghurt with 80g blueberries 1 banana	1 small banana plus 2 oatcakes 2 tbsp **Spiced almonds** *page 205* **Peachy iced tea** *page 213*
1 serving **Rump steak with balsamic sauce** *page 237* 100g (cooked weight) brown rice Mixed salad plus 50g canned chickpeas and 1 tbsp olive oil and balsamic vinegar dressing Sugar-free drink or water	1 serving **Prawn and orzo casserole** *page 260* 80g French beans Mixed salad with 1 tbsp olive oil and balsamic vinegar dressing Sugar-free drink or water	1 serving **Slow-cooker beef and red wine stew** *page 238* 1 slice **Wholemeal flaxseed bread** *page 196* Mixed salad plus 1 small avocado and 1 tbsp olive oil and balsamic vinegar dressing Sugar-free drink or water	1 serving **Spring vegetable stir-fry with tofu** *page 271* 150g (cooked weight) brown rice Sugar-free drink or water
1 serving **Cherry clafoutis** *page 300*		1 serving **Orange and pomegranate compote** *page 292*	1 serving **Mixed berry and almond gratin** *page 300*
Kcal: 2,200 Protein: 122g Carbohydrate: 285g Fat: 63g Fibre: 41g Percentage of calories from carbs: 52; protein: 22; fat: 26	Kcal: 2,150 Protein: 123g Carbohydrate: 270g Fat: 65g Fibre: 39g Percentage of calories from carbs: 50; protein: 23; fat: 27	Kcal: 2,175 Protein: 120g Carbohydrate: 280g Fat: 62g Fibre: 37g Percentage of calories from carbs: 52; protein: 22; fat: 26	Kcal: 2,190 Protein: 125g Carbohydrate: 285g Fat: 62g Fibre: 40g Percentage of calories from carbs: 52; protein: 23; fat: 25

Index

Recipes are indicated in *italic*

Project Staff
Editor Rachel Warren Chadd
Assistant editor Celia Coyne
Art editor Conorde Clarke
Designers Nigel Soper and David Whelan
Proofreader Ron Pankhurst
Indexer Hilary Bird

Reader's Digest Books
Editorial director Julian Browne
Art director Anne-Marie Bulat
Managing editor Nina Hathway
Head of book development Sarah Bloxham
Picture resource manager Sarah Stewart-Richardson
Pre-press account manager Dean Russell
Product production manager Claudette Bramble
Senior production controller Katherine Bunn

Origination Colour Systems Limited, London
Printing and binding MOHN Media, Germany

Picture credits
© Reader's Digest/Elizabeth Watts
apart from the following:

Front & back cover background: iStockphoto.com
10 iStockphoto.com/Pavel Losevsky
12 CL iStockphoto.com
17 Photolibrary Group/Walter Hodges
23 ShutterStock, Inc/Iofoto
27 ShutterStock, Inc/Tomo Jesenicnik
29T iStockphoto.com/Eric Gevaert
31 iStockphoto.com/Graeme Gilmour
33 Getty Images Ltd/Superstudio
34 Photolibrary Group/Dennis Galante
38 Getty Images Ltd/Noel Hendrickson
41 ShutterStock, Inc/Galina Barskaya
42 ShutterStock, Inc/AG Photographer
45 iStockphoto.com/Olga Lyubkina
48 ShutterStock, Inc/Ronen Boidek
51 iStockphoto.com/Ivan Mateev
52 ShutterStock, Inc/Maja Schon
54 ShutterStock, Inc/Dan Peretz
59 Getty Images Ltd/Superstudio
71 ShutterStock, Inc/Graca Victoria
83-88, 91, 97,109,113,116 © Reader's Digest/
Ian Hofstetter
125 iStockphoto.com/Robyn Mackenzie
130,156 © Reader's Digest /Ian Hofstetter
166 iStockphoto.com
169, 178 TL TR & BR © Reader's Digest /Ian Hofstetter
179 CL ShutterStock, Inc/Harris Shiffman
179 CR© Reader's Digest

Magic Foods for Better Blood Sugar was published by The Reader's Digest Association Limited, London

First edition copyright © 2008
The Reader's Digest Association Limited
11 Westferry Circus, Canary Wharf
London E14 4HE

This book was adapted from *Magic Foods for Better Blood Sugar*, published by The Reader's Digest Association, Inc. USA
Copyright © 2007

We are committed both to the quality of our products and the service we provide to our customers.
We value your comments, so please do contact us on **08705 113366** or via our website at
www.readersdigest.co.uk
If you have any comments or suggestions about the content of our books, email us at
gbeditorial@readersdigest.co.uk

Concept Code US4951/IC
Book Code 400-346 UP0000-1
Oracle Code 250010106H.00.24
ISBN 978 0 276 44339 8